Eating Disorders
SOURCEBOOK

Third Edition

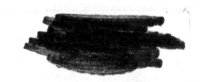

Health Reference Series

Third Edition

Eating Disorders
SOURCEBOOK

Basic Consumer Health Information about Anorexia Nervosa, Bulimia Nervosa, Binge Eating Disorder, and Other Eating Disorders and Related Concerns, Such As Compulsive Exercise, Female Athlete Triad, and Body Dysmorphic Disorder, Including Details about Risk Factors, Warning Signs, Adverse Health Effects, Methods of Prevention, Treatment Options, and the Recovery Process

Along with Suggestions for Maintaining a Healthy Weight, Improving Self-Esteem, and Promoting a Positive Body Image, a Glossary of Related Terms, and a Directory of Resources for More Information

Edited by
Sandra J. Judd

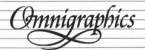

P.O. Box 31-1640, Detroit, MI 48231

Bibliographic Note

Because this page cannot legibly accommodate all the copyright notices, the Bibliographic Note portion of the Preface constitutes an extension of the copyright notice.

Edited by Sandra J. Judd

Health Reference Series

Karen Bellenir, *Managing Editor*
David A. Cooke, MD, FACP, *Medical Consultant*
Elizabeth Collins, *Research and Permissions Coordinator*
Cherry Edwards, *Permissions Assistant*
EdIndex, Services for Publishers, *Indexers*

* * *

Omnigraphics, Inc.

Matthew P. Barbour, *Senior Vice President*
Kevin M. Hayes, *Operations Manager*

* * *

Peter E. Ruffner, *Publisher*

Copyright © 2011 Omnigraphics, Inc.

ISBN 978-0-7808-1143-0

Library of Congress Cataloging-in-Publication Data

Eating disorders sourcebook : basic consumer health information about anorexia nervosa, bulimia nervosa, binge eating disorder, and other eating disorders and related concerns, such as compulsive exercise, female athlete triad, and body dysmorphic disorder, including details about risk factors, warning signs, adverse health effects, methods of prevention, treatment options, and the recovery process ... / edited by Sandra J. Judd. -- 3rd ed.
    p. cm. -- (Health reference series)
    Summary: "Provides basic consumer health information about risk factors, causes, and complications of eating disorders, along with facts about prevention, treatment, and recovery. Includes index, glossary of related terms, and other resources"-- Provided by publisher.
    Includes bibliographical references and index.
    ISBN 978-0-7808-1143-0 (hardcover : alk. paper) 1. Eating disorders. 2. Consumer education. I. Judd, Sandra J. II. Title. III. Series.

    RC552.E18E287 2011
    616.85'26--dc22

                                        2010053167

Table of Contents

Visit www.healthreferenceseries.com to view *A Contents Guide to the Health Reference Series*, a listing of more than 15,000 topics and the volumes in which they are covered.

Part II: Risk Factors for Eating Disorders

Part III: Causes of Eating Disorders

Part IV: Medical Complications of Eating Disorders

Part V: Recognizing and Treating Eating Disorders

Part VI: Preventing Eating Disorders and Achieving a Healthy Weight

Part VII: Additional Help and Information

Preface

About This Book

According to the Eating Disorders Coalition, the incidence of eating disorders has doubled since the 1960s, and these disorders are occurring increasingly in younger and older age groups and in diverse ethnic and sociocultural groups. The physical and psychological toll is high. Suicide, depression, and severe anxiety are common, and eating disorders can lead to major medical complications, including cardiac arrhythmia, cognitive impairment, osteoporosis, infertility, or even death. Furthermore, although eating disorders can be successfully treated—even to complete remission—estimates suggest that only one in ten people with an eating disorder receives treatment.

Eating Disorders Sourcebook, Third Edition provides basic consumer health information about anorexia nervosa, bulimia nervosa, binge eating disorder, and other eating disorders and related concerns, such as compulsive exercise, female athlete triad, the abuse of laxatives and diet pills, and body dysmorphic disorder. It explains the factors that put people at risk for developing eating disorders, and it discusses their adverse health affects and the methods used to prevent, diagnose, and treat them. Tips for determining a healthy weight and promoting self-esteem and a positive body image are also included, along with guidelines for safe weight loss and exercise, and a glossary of terms related to eating disorders, and a list of resources for further information.

How to Use This Book

This book is divided into parts and chapters. Parts focus on broad areas of interest. Chapters are devoted to single topics within a part.

Part I: What Are Eating Disorders? defines eating disorders and explains how they differ from disordered and normal eating patterns. It describes the most common types of eating disorders and other related concerns, such as body dysmorphic disorder and compulsive exercising, that often accompany them.

Part II: Risk Factors for Eating Disorders describes the populations most at risk for eating disorders and offers suggestions to help prevent eating disorders in these groups. It also describes problems, such as anxiety disorders, depression, sexual abuse, and substance abuse, that may increase the risk of developing an eating disorder.

Part III: Causes of Eating Disorders explains what is known about the biological factors and genetic predispositions that may lead to the development of eating disorders. Environmental factors, such as bullying and boundary invasion, that can cause eating disorders are also described, as well as the effect of the media in distorting body image and encouraging these disorders.

Part IV: Medical Complications of Eating Disorders provides information about the adverse—and sometimes fatal—physical health effects of eating disorders, including infertility, oral health problems, osteoporosis, and cardiovascular disorders.

Part V: Recognizing and Treating Eating Disorders describes the physiological and behavioral warning signs of an eating disorder and provides suggestions for confronting a person with an eating disorder. It explains the treatment process, from determining the level of care needed to choosing a therapist and treatment facility, and it details the different treatment options available, including medications, psychotherapeutic approaches, and nutritional support. Issues common to the recovery process are also discussed.

Part VI: Preventing Eating Disorders and Achieving a Healthy Weight offers guidelines for the prevention of eating disorders, including tips for promoting self-esteem and a positive body image. It explains how people can determine a medically optimal weight for themselves and offers suggestions for safe weight gain, loss, and maintenance. Nutrition guidelines and suggestions for exercising safely are also included.

Part VII: Additional Help and Information includes a glossary of terms related to eating disorders and a directory of resources for additional help and support.

Bibliographic Note

This volume contains documents and excerpts from the following U.S. government agencies and publications: Centers for Disease Control and Prevention; Department of Health and Human Services, Office on Women's Health; *Medline Plus Magazine*; National Institute of Diabetes and Digestive and Kidney Diseases; National Institute of Mental Health; National Institutes of Health; National Women's Health Information Center; President's Council on Physical Fitness and Sports; and the Substance Abuse and Mental Health Services Administration.

In addition, this volume contains copyrighted documents from the following organizations, individuals, and publications: About-Face; A.D.A.M., Inc.; Alliance for Eating Disorders Awareness; American Pregnancy Association; Anxiety Disorders Association of America; Beyond Blue; Center for Young Women's Health; Cleveland Center for Eating Disorders; Mary Anne Cohen; Cornell University Family Life Development Center; Diabetes Australia; Eating Disorder Hope; Eating Disorder Referral and Information Center; Eating Disorders Foundation of Victoria (Australia); Families Empowered and Supporting Treatment; Great Valley Publishing Company; Gurze Books; Harris Center for Education and Advocacy in Eating Disorders at Massachusetts General Hospital; Deborah J. Kuehnel; McGraw-Hill; McLean Hospital; Multi-Service Eating Disorder Association; NAMI: The Nation's Voice on Mental Illness; Abigail H. Natenshon; National Association of Anorexia Nervosa and Associated Disorders; National Center on Addiction and Substance Abuse at Columbia University; National Eating Disorders Association; Nemours Foundation; Ohio State University Body Image Health Task Force; Ohio State University Extension; Pauline Powers; PsychCentral; Ellyn Satter; Talk About Sleep; University of Arizona Cooperative Extension; University of California San Diego News Center; University of North Carolina Health Care System; University of Texas Health Science Center at Houston—*Health Leader*; University of Virginia—*UVa Today*; and the Washington State Department of Health, Office of Health Promotion.

Acknowledgements

Thanks go to the many organizations, agencies, and individuals who have contributed materials for this *Sourcebook* and to medical consultant Dr. David Cooke and prepress service provider WhimsyInk. Special thanks go to managing editor Karen Bellenir and permissions coordinator Liz Collins for their help and support.

About the Health Reference Series

The *Health Reference Series* is designed to provide basic medical information for patients, families, caregivers, and the general public. Each volume takes a particular topic and provides comprehensive coverage. This is especially important for people who may be dealing with a newly diagnosed disease or a chronic disorder in themselves or in a family member. People looking for preventive guidance, information about disease warning signs, medical statistics, and risk factors for health problems will also find answers to their questions in the *Health Reference Series*. The *Series*, however, is not intended to serve as a tool for diagnosing illness, in prescribing treatments, or as a substitute for the physician/patient relationship. All people concerned about medical symptoms or the possibility of disease are encouraged to seek professional care from an appropriate healthcare provider.

A Note about Spelling and Style

Health Reference Series editors use *Stedman's Medical Dictionary* as an authority for questions related to the spelling of medical terms and the *Chicago Manual of Style* for questions related to grammatical structures, punctuation, and other editorial concerns. Consistent adherence is not always possible, however, because the individual volumes within the *Series* include many documents from a wide variety of different producers and copyright holders, and the editor's primary goal is to present material from each source as accurately as is possible following the terms specified by each document's producer. This sometimes means that information in different chapters or sections may follow other guidelines and alternate spelling authorities. For example, occasionally a copyright holder may require that eponymous terms be shown in possessive forms (Crohn's disease vs. Crohn disease) or that British spelling norms be retained (leukaemia vs. leukemia).

Locating Information within the Health Reference Series

The *Health Reference Series* contains a wealth of information about a wide variety of medical topics. Ensuring easy access to all the fact sheets, research reports, in-depth discussions, and other material contained within the individual books of the series remains one of our highest priorities. As the *Series* continues to grow in size and scope, however, locating the precise information needed by a reader may become more challenging.

A Contents Guide to the Health Reference Series was developed to direct readers to the specific volumes that address their concerns. It presents an extensive list of diseases, treatments, and other topics of general interest compiled from the Tables of Contents and major index headings. To access *A Contents Guide to the Health Reference Series*, visit www.healthreferenceseries.com.

Medical Consultant

Medical consultation services are provided to the *Health Reference Series* editors by David A. Cooke, MD, FACP. Dr. Cooke is a graduate of Brandeis University, and he received his M.D. degree from the University of Michigan. He completed residency training at the University of Wisconsin Hospital and Clinics. He is board-certified in Internal Medicine. Dr. Cooke currently works as part of the University of Michigan Health System and practices in Ann Arbor, MI. In his free time, he enjoys writing, science fiction, and spending time with his family.

Our Advisory Board

We would like to thank the following board members for providing guidance to the development of this series:

Dr. Lynda Baker, Associate Professor of Library and Information Science, Wayne State University, Detroit, MI

Nancy Bulgarelli, William Beaumont Hospital Library, Royal Oak, MI

Karen Imarisio, Bloomfield Township Public Library, Bloomfield Township, MI

Karen Morgan, Mardigian Library, University of Michigan-Dearborn, Dearborn, MI

Rosemary Orlando, St. Clair Shores Public Library, St. Clair Shores, MI

Health Reference Series *Update Policy*

The inaugural book in the *Health Reference Series* was the first edition of *Cancer Sourcebook* published in 1989. Since then, the *Series* has been enthusiastically received by librarians and in the medical community. In order to maintain the standard of providing high-quality health information for the layperson the editorial staff at Omnigraphics felt it was necessary to implement a policy of updating volumes when warranted.

Medical researchers have been making tremendous strides, and it is the purpose of the *Health Reference Series* to stay current with the most recent advances. Each decision to update a volume is made on an individual basis. Some of the considerations include how much new information is available and the feedback we receive from people who use the books. If there is a topic you would like to see added to the update list, or an area of medical concern you feel has not been adequately addressed, please write to:

Editor
Health Reference Series
Omnigraphics, Inc.
P.O. Box 31-1640
Detroit, MI 48231
E-mail: editorial@omnigraphics.com

Part One

What Are Eating Disorders?

Chapter 1

Eating Disorders: A Statistical Overview

Facts and Findings

Facts

- More than five million Americans experience eating disorders.[3]
- Anorexia nervosa, bulimia nervosa, and binge-eating disorder are real, treatable illnesses that take on a life of their own.[22]
- About 90 percent of individuals with anorexia nervosa or bulimia nervosa[18] and about 60 percent of those with binge eating disorder[26] are female.
- A young woman with anorexia is twelve times more likely to die than other women her age without anorexia.[19]
- Thirteen percent of young women have substantially disordered eating behaviors.[24]
- Between 10 and 15 percent of those diagnosed with bulimia nervosa are men.[2]
- Thirty-seven percent of fourth-graders report that they have dieted to lose weight during the past year and 30 percent report that they are currently dieting.[6]

- About half of those with anorexia or bulimia have a full recovery, 30 percent have a partial recovery, and 20 percent have no substantial improvement.[20,27]

Findings

- A recent study of seventh- and tenth-graders revealed a decrease in body satisfaction and an increase in depression associated with viewing magazine images of idealized females.[12]

- In a study of almost five thousand adolescents, researchers found a significant association between weight-teasing and disordered eating behaviors among overweight and non-overweight girls and boys.[23]

- In a study of 220 women treated for bulimia with either cognitive behavioral therapy or interpersonal psychotherapy, early change in the frequency of purging was the best predictor of response to treatment.[13]

- Females who participate in elite competitive sports, such as figure-skating, gymnastics, dance, and crew, in which body shape and size are a factor in performance, are at higher risk for developing eating disorders than females who do not participate in such sports. Males who participate in these sports or in wrestling are also at increased risk.[29]

Frequently Asked Questions

How many people have eating disorders?

- Between 0.5 and 3.7 percent of females develop anorexia nervosa.[1]
- Between 1.1 and 4.2 percent of females develop bulimia nervosa.[1]
- Approximately 85 percent of eating disorders begin during adolescence.[3]

Do boys and men get eating disorders?

- One study showed that males comprised 10 to 15 percent of all subjects diagnosed with bulimia nervosa.[8]

- In research conducted on a large sample, 28 percent of ninth-grade males reported one or more of the following to lose or control weight: fasting or skipping meals, diet pills, vomiting, laxatives, or cigarette smoking.[9]

- Beginning in about the third grade, boys show significantly less desire to lose weight than girls, but express dissatisfaction with the upper rather than the lower body and use dieting to achieve specific external goals rather than to aspire to a cultural norm.[2]

- In a recent study, adolescent boys were most satisfied with their bodies when they were average weight and most dissatisfied with their bodies when they were either above or below average weight.[25]

- Research conducted on 10,583 adolescents indicated that gay/bisexual boys were more concerned with trying to look like men in the media and more likely to binge eat than heterosexual boys.[4]

What does research tell us about children with respect to eating behaviors or eating disorders?

- Expectations regarding thinness among females are evident as early as six and seven years old.[11]

- In a study of 252 fourth-graders, 37 percent reported that they had dieted to lose weight during the past year.[6]

- In another study, girls were tested for eating attitudes and dieting at ages five, seven, and nine. Girls who reported high body size and shape concerns across ages five to seven were more likely than girls without such concerns to restrict their food intake at age nine, and these associations were independent of what the girls actually weighed.[10]

- Girls who present with eating disorders before they have begun to menstruate may have a long history of poor weight gain and slowed growth prior to the onset of weight loss.[30]

Are there any statistics on adolescents with respect to eating behaviors or eating disorders?

In a national survey of 6,728 adolescents, 45 percent of the girls and 20 percent of the boys reported that they had, at some point, been on a diet. Thirteen percent of the girls and 7 percent of the boys reported disordered eating.[24]

What are the statistics regarding eating disorders and college students?

In a study of 1,899 college students, 4.5 percent of the women and 1.4 percent of the men reported previous treatment for an eating disorder. Four percent of the men and 10.9 percent of the women were considered at risk for eating disorders.[14]

What causes eating disorders?

- Although no one variable has been found to "cause" an eating disorder, research has discerned that certain personality characteristics, genetic disposition, environment, and biochemistry all play significant roles in the development of eating disorders.

- Body dissatisfaction (having a negative view of one's size or shape), weight concerns, and dieting are associated with the development of eating disorders.[15]

- Many people with eating disorders are perfectionistic and often excel at academics and sports. People with anorexia tend to avoid taking risks. People with bulimia often have difficulties dealing with stress and may binge and purge to try to cope with intense feelings.[18]

- Studies show that anorexia nervosa and bulimia nervosa run in families.[7,18,21,28,32]

- Studies are underway to identify the specific genes that may increase the risk of developing an eating disorder.[16,17,22]

- Increasing evidence points to alterations in central nervous system pathways as contributing to eating disorders. Many people with these illnesses have disturbances in brain serotonin, a neurotransmitter, which helps regulate appetite and mood.[18]

What are the best treatments for eating disorders?

- Eating disorders are most successfully treated when diagnosed early. The longer abnormal eating behaviors persist, the more difficult it is to overcome the disorder and its effects on the body.[22]

- Once the eating disorder is diagnosed, the clinician can assess whether hospitalization is necessary or if the person can be treated as an outpatient.[1,22]

- Conditions warranting hospitalization include the following:
  - Excessive and rapid weight loss
  - Serious metabolic disturbances
  - Clinical depression

- Risk of suicide
- Severe binge eating and purging
- Psychosis
- Many treatment plans are comprehensive due to the complex interaction of emotional and psychological problems in eating disorders.[1,22]
- Treatment often involves a combination of interventions including medical monitoring; individual, group, and family psychotherapy; nutritional counseling; cognitive therapy; behavioral therapy; and antidepressant medication.[1]
- Ongoing emotional support is necessary for the individual, as recovery is a long process and relapse is common.

What are the recovery rates for those with eating disorders?

Approximately half of those with anorexia or bulimia have a full recovery, approximately 30 percent have a partial recovery, and 20 percent have no substantial improvement in symptoms.[18,20,27]

Can eating disorders cause death?

The mortality rate associated with anorexia nervosa is twelve times higher than the mortality rate among young women in the general population.[19]

Are there any statistics about eating disorders and the effects of the media?

- A study of seventh- and tenth-graders revealed a decrease in body satisfaction and an increase in depression associated with viewing magazine images of idealized females.[12]
- Another study showed that two of the most common adolescent dieting methods—restricting calories and taking diet pills—were associated with the reading of women's beauty and fashion magazines.[31]
- Research on Fijian schoolgirls found that a dramatic increase in eating disorders symptoms was tied to the introduction of television to this area, despite a traditional culture that had previously protected girls from developing these disorders.[5]

References

1. American Psychiatric Association Work Group on Eating Disorders (2000). American Practice Guideline for the Treatment of Patients with Eating Disorders (revision). *American Journal of Psychiatry*; 157(1 Suppl):1–39.

2. Andersen AE, & Holman JE. (1997). Males with eating disorders: Challenges for treatment and research. *Psychopharmacology Bulletin*; 33(3):391–97.

3. Anonymous (2001). Position of the American Dietetic Association: Nutrition intervention in the treatment of anorexia nervosa, bulimia nervosa, and eating disorders not otherwise specified (EDNOS). *Journal of the American Dietetic Association*; 101(7): 810–19.

4. Austin SB, Ziyadeh N, Kahn JA, Camago CA Jr, Colditz GA, Field AE. (2004). Sexual orientation, weight concerns, and eating-disordered behaviors in adolescent girls and boys. *Journal American Academy Child Adolesc Psychiatry*; 43(9):1115–23.

5. Becker AE, Burwell RA, Gilman SE, Herzog DB, Hamburg P. (2002). Eating behaviours and attitudes following prolonged exposure to television among ethnic Fijian adolescent girls. *British Journal of Psychiatry*; 180:509–14.

6. Bronner Y, Welch C, Serpa M. (1999). Body size, body image perception and dieting behavior among urban fourth graders. *Journal of the American Dietetic Association*; 99(9, supplement).

7. Bulik CM, Sullivan PF, Wade TD, Kendler KS. (2000). Twin studies of eating disorders; a review. *International Journal of Eating Disorders*;27(1):1–20.

8. Carlat, DJ, & Carmago, CA. (1991). Review of bulimia nervosa in males. *American Journal of Psychiatry*; 148:831–43.

9. Croll J, Neumark-Sztainer D, Story M, Ireland M. (2002). Prevalence and risk and protective factors related to disordered eating behaviors among adolescents: relationship to gender and ethnicity. *J Adolescent Health*; 31(2):166–75.

10. Davison KK, Markey CN, Birch LL. (2003). A longitudinal examination of patterns in girls' weight concerns and body dissatisfaction from ages 5 to 9 years. *International Journal of Eating Disorders*; 33(3):320–32.

11. Dohnt HK, Tiggemann M. (2004). Development of perceived body size and dieting awareness in young girls. *Percept. Mot Skills*; 99 (3 Pt 1):790–92.

12. Durkin SJ, Paxton SJ. (2002). Predictors of vulnerability to reduced body image satisfaction and psychological wellbeing in response to exposure to idealized female images in adolescent girls.
Journal of Psychosomatic Research; 53 (5): 961–62.

13. Fairburn CG, Agras WS, Walsh BT, Wilson GT, Stice E. (2004).
Prediction of outcome in bulimia nervosa by early change in treatment. *American Journal of Psychiatry*; 161 (12): 2322–24.

14. Hoerr SL, Bokram R, Lugo B, Bivins T, Keast DR. (2002). Risk for
disordered eating relates to both gender and ethnicity for college students. *Journal of the American College of Nutrition*; 21(4):307–14.

15. Jacobi C, Hayward C, de Zwaan M, Kraemer H, Agras W. (2004).
Coming to terms with risk factors for eating disorders: application
of risk terminology and suggestions for a general taxonomy. *Psychological Bulletin*; 130(1):19–65.

16. Kaye WH, Devlin B, Barbarich N, Bulik CM, Thornton L, Bacanu
SA, Fichter MM, Halmi KA, Kaplan AS, Strober M, Woodside DB,
Bergen AW, Crow S, Mitchell J, Rotondo A, Mauri M, Cassano G,
Keel P, Plotnicov K, Pollice C, Klump KL, Lilenfeld LR, Ganjei JK,
Quadflieg N, Berrettini WH. (2004). Genetic analysis of bulimia
nervosa: methods and sample description. *Int J Eat Disord*;
35(4):556–70.

17. Kaye WH, Lilenfeld LR, Berrettini WH, Strober M, Devlin B,
Klump KL, Goldman D, Bulik CM, Halmi KA, Fichter MM, Kaplan A, Woodside DB, Treasure J, Plotnicov KH, Pollice C, Rao
R, McConaha CW. (2000). A search for susceptibility loci for
anorexia nervosa: methods and sample description. *Biol Psychiatry*; 47(9):794–803.

18. Keel PK. (2005). *Eating Disorders*. Upper Saddle River, N.J.: Pear-
son/Prentice Hall.

19. Keel PK, Dorer, DJ, Eddy, KT, Franko, DL, Charatan, DL, Herzog,
DB. (2003). Predictors of mortality in eating disorders. *Archives of
General Psychiatry*; 60(2):179–83.

20. Keel PK, Mitchell JE. (1997). Outcome in bulimia nervosa. *American Journal of Psychiatry*; 154(3):313–21.

21. Kendler KS, MacLean C, Neale M, Kessler R, Heath A, Eaves L.
(1991). The genetic epidemiology of bulimia nervosa. *American
Journal of Psychiatry*; 148(12):1627–37.

22. National Institute of Mental Health. (2001). *Eating disorders:
facts about eating disorders and the search for solutions*. NIH
Publication No. 94-3477. Rockville, MD.

23. Neumark-Sztainer D, Falkner M, Story M, Perry C, Hannan PJ and Mulert S. (2002). Weight-teasing among adolescents: correlations with weight status and disordered eating behaviors. *International Journal of Obesity*; 26 (1):123–31.

24. Neumark-Sztainer D, Hannan PJ. (2000). Weight-related behaviors among adolescent girls and boys: results from a national survey. *Arch Perdiatr Adolesc Med*; 154(6):569–77.

25. Presnell K, Bearman SK, Stice E. (2004). Risk factors for body dissatisfaction in adolescent boys and girls: a prospective study. *International Journal of Eating Disorders*; 36(4):389–401.

26. Spitzer, RL, Devlin, MJ, Walsh BT, & Hasin D, Wing R, Marcus M, et al. (1992). Binge eating disorder: a multisite field trial of the diagnostic criteria. *International Journal of Eating Disorders*; 11:191–203.

27. Steinhausen HC. (2002). The outcome of anorexia nervosa in the 20th century. *American Journal of Psychiatry*; 159(8):1284–93.

28. Strober M, Freeman R, Lampert C, Diamond J, Kaye W. (2000). Controlled family study of anorexia and bulimia nervosa: evidence of shared liability and transmission of partial syndromes. *American Journal of Psychiatry*; 157(3):393–401.

29. Sundgot-Borgen J, Torstveit MK. (2004). Prevalence of eating disorders in elite athletes is higher than in the general population. *Clinical Journal Sport Med*; 14(1):25–32.

30. Swenne I, Thurfjell B. (2003). Clinical onset and diagnosis of eating disorders in premenarcheal girls is preceded by inadequate weight gain and growth retardation. *Acta Paediatr*; 92(10):1133–37.

31. Thomsen SR, Weber MM, Brown LB. (2002). The relationship between reading beauty and fashion magazines and the use of pathogenic dieting methods among adolescent females. *Adolescence*; 37(145):1–18.

32. Walters EE, Kendler KS. (1995). Anorexia nervosa and anorexic-like syndromes in a population-based female twin sample. *American Journal of Psychiatry*; 152:64–71.

Chapter 2

Normal Eating, Disordered Eating, and Eating Disorders

Chapter Contents

Section 2.1

Do You Have a Healthy Relationship with Food?

"Do You Have a Healthy Relationship with Food?" © Rebecca Manley, MS, Multi-service Eating Disorder Association (MEDA), 1994. Reprinted with permission. For additional information, contact MEDA at 866-343-6332, or www.medainc.org. Reviewed by Dr. Cooke, M.D., FACP, September 2010.

1. I am preoccupied with the desire to be thinner.
2. I am terrified of gaining weight.
3. I feel that food controls my life.
4. My day revolves around the number on the scale and whether it went up or down.
5. I watch what other people eat and use that to determine what and how much I will eat.
6. Often, I eat when I am not hungry.
7. Often, I do not eat when I am hungry.
8. I feel guilty after eating.
9. Often, I purge after meals.
10. I have certain rituals around eating that other people tell me are not normal.
11. I react to stressful situations by using food.
12. Often, exercise and/or eating get in the way of my job, school, work, or other activities.
13. I often feel out of control around food.
14. My moods feel out of control and frequently change and are unstable.
15. If I were only thinner, my life would be better.

If you found yourself answering yes to these statements, there may be reason for concern.

Section 2.2

What Is Normal Eating?

Normal eating is going to the table hungry and eating until you are satisfied. It is being able to choose food you like and eat it and truly get enough of it—not just stop eating because you think you should. Normal eating is being able to give some thought to your food selection so you get nutritious food, but not being so wary and restrictive that you miss out on enjoyable food. Normal eating is giving yourself permission to eat sometimes because you are happy, sad, or bored, or just because it feels good. Normal eating is mostly three meals a day, or four or five, or it can be choosing to munch along the way. It is leaving some cookies on the plate because you know you can have some again tomorrow, or it is eating more now because they taste so wonderful. Normal eating is overeating at times, feeling stuffed and uncomfortable. And it can be undereating at times and wishing you had more. Normal eating is trusting your body to make up for your mistakes in eating. Normal eating takes up some of your time and attention, but keeps its place as only one important area of your life.

In short, normal eating is flexible. It varies in response to your hunger, your schedule, your proximity to food, and your feelings.

Section 2.3

Emotional Eating

"Emotional Eating" by Abigail H. Natenshon, MA, LCSW, GCFP. © 2010. Reprinted with permission. Abigail H. Natenshon has been a psychotherapist specializing in eating disorders for four decades. As the director of Eating Disorder Specialists of Illinois: A Clinic Without Walls, she has authored two books, *When Your Child Has an Eating Disorder: A Step-by-Step Workbook for Parents and Caregivers* and *Doing What Works: An Integrative System for the Treatment of Eating Disorders from Diagnosis to Recovery.* Natenshon, who is also a Guild Certified Feldenkrais Practitioner, hosts three informative websites, including www.empoweredparents.com, www.empoweredkidz.com, and www.treatingeatingdisorders.com.

Are you concerned that you may be eating too much or too little? Do you feel out of control of what you eat, when you eat, how you eat, and how much you eat? Do you wonder how to go about establishing a healthier eating lifestyle?

First, it would be helpful for you to become aware of the following:

- The quality of your relationship with food
- What prompts you to eat or not to eat
- Whether your emotions rule your eating
- Whether your eating rules your emotions
- Whether there is a compulsive, impulsive, or choiceless quality about your eating, or a sense of being powerless to make sought-after changes

Food and feelings are frequently bound together. When people use food and eating to produce or cover up certain feelings, they may be engaging in "emotional eating." Emotional eating often creates a "food fog" that distracts or anesthetizes feelings, disguising genuine needs, and in so doing, preventing effective problem resolving.

No one is emotionally neutral about eating all the time. On a blustery cold winter morning, it is normal to crave a warm and filling comfort food such as oatmeal; on Halloween, it is fun to get into the spirit of the holiday by overindulging on the treats in your sack. If overly nervous about a first day at work or taking an exam, it is not uncommon to lose one's appetite. Become aware, however, of whether you might be a person whose eating is primarily and consistently stimulated by your emotional states and needs. When eating or restricting food is primarily motivated by feelings other than by hunger or satiety, it can become disordered eating, which can lead to conditions such as obesity or clinical eating disorders in those with such genetic propensities.

Emotional states that might make a person vulnerable to the emotional use of food include depression, anxiety, boredom and loneliness, anger, and jealousy. If you have difficulty recognizing your emotional state at times, ask yourself, "What might be happening right now? Am I feeling mad, sad, glad, or scared?"

Are You an Emotional Eater?

- I always eat when I am happy.
- I always eat when I feel sad.
- I always eat when I feel anxious or nervous.
- I always eat when I feel angry.
- I always eat when I feel frustrated.
- I always eat when I am bored.
- I always eat when I don't want to do other things that I have been putting off, like homework.
- I always eat when I feel frightened.
- I don't eat when I feel frightened about becoming fat.
- I am afraid that I will not be popular if I gain any weight.
- I believe that I will be more popular if I weigh less.
- Dieting gives me a sense of purpose and of being in control.
- I feel good about skipping meals.
- I feel out of control in many areas of my life, beyond eating.
- I am not good at recognizing my feelings.
- When I am feeling bad, sometimes I "feel fat" even though I know that "fat" is not a feeling.

Fat has become a commonly used code word to camouflage real feelings. When a person adds "fat" to his or her list of feelings, emotional

15

eating may cross the line into disordered eating. If "fat" becomes a feeling, it is wise to look for deeper significance; you may be suffering from body image distortions or disturbances. Such disturbances can exacerbate emotional eating or food restriction (or both, intermittently), magnifying negative feelings, and leading to more serious forms of disordered eating or eating disorders.

What to Do If You Have a Problem

Once you learn to identify the emotions and circumstances that stimulate emotional eating, you will become better able to separate unwanted eating episodes from their triggers, and respond more appropriately to your feelings without having to turn to food. This provides greater options for solving problems at their source. Remember that there is no exact science to eating "right," and it is not unusual for us to harbor some idiosyncrasies or quirkiness about what and how we eat. What differentiates a benign quirk from a disordered eating pattern? The disordered pattern is invariably marked by rigidity and inflexibility, by an all-or-nothing, extreme, and compulsive quality.

It is important to find better ways to respond to feelings than to develop habits that are self-defeating. Here are ten things you might do:

1. Recognize your real feelings.

2. Keep a "feeling" journal. In this journal, make note of: what triggers your eating behaviors; what kinds of things you would you like to change about your eating; how easily you are able to make changes in your eating; and what helps you the most in attaining your eating goals.

3. Name your feelings. This gives you power. You can't resolve a problem without first defining it.

4. Discover which feelings and/or thoughts act as eating triggers for you.

5. By identifying your feelings, you can more precisely know and accomplish what you need and want.

6. Find a friend whom you can confide in or go to parents to talk out what might be concerning you.

7. Take a bike ride, shoot baskets, or take your dog for a walk instead of eating.

8. Keep in mind what healthy eating is really about. Healthy eating is regular, nutritious, varied, balanced, and fearless eating.

9. Never skip a meal.

10. If you find that it is not possible to resolve these issues on your own, don't hesitate to ask for assistance from people you trust, from your doctor, a nutritionist, or psychotherapist.

By eating enough of the right kinds of foods at least three times a day at every meal, you will regulate your hunger and will not be so prone to turn to food mindlessly. By eating healthfully and exercising regularly, you will also insure your physical fitness, learn to trust your body, and feel more in control of food as well as other aspects of your life, your self, and your happiness.

Section 2.4

Disordered Eating and Eating Disorders: What's the Difference?

Disordered eating refers to mild and transient changes in eating patterns that occur in relation to a stressful event, an illness, or even a desire to modify the diet for a variety of health and personal appearance reasons. The problem may be no more than a bad habit, a style of eating adapted from friends or family members, or an aspect of preparing for athletic competition.

While disordered eating can lead to weight loss or weight gain and to certain nutritional problems, it rarely requires in-depth professional attention. On the other hand, disordered eating can develop into an eating disorder. If disordered eating becomes sustained, distressing, or starts to interfere with everyday activities, then it may require professional evaluation.

Given Americans' interest in being fit and the widespread practice of dieting, it can sometimes be difficult to tell where disordered eating stops and an eating disorder begins. Indeed, many eating disorders get their start from a simple diet or inadvertent weight loss.

It is known that disordered eating or dieting can precipitate an eating disorder, and it is important to understand that when we talk of an eating disorder, we are talking about an illness. Eating disorders involve physiological changes associated with food restricting, binge eating, purging, and fluctuations in weight. They also involve a number of emotional and cognitive changes that affect the way a person perceives and experiences his or her body.

An eating disorder is not a diet, a sign of personal weakness, or a problem that will go away by itself. An eating disorder requires professional attention.

Table 2.1. Disordered Eating and Eating Disorders

	Disordered Eating	**Eating Disorders**
Essential Distinction	A reaction to life situations. A habit. Problematic behaviors.	An illness.
Psychological Symptoms	Infrequent thoughts and behaviors about body, foods, and eating that do not lead to health, social, school, and work problems.	Frequent and persistent thoughts and behaviors about body, foods, and eating that do lead to health, social, school, and work problems.
Associated Medical Problems	Transient weight changes or nutritional problems; rarely causes major medical complications.	Potential for major medical complications that lead to hospitalization or even death.
Treatment	Mental health services and nutritional counseling can be helpful but are not usually essential. Problem may go away without treatment, but disordered eating is a risk for an eating disorder.	Requires specific professional medical and mental health treatment.

Chapter 3

How Are Eating Disorders and Obesity Related?

Eating disorders and obesity are part of a range of weight-related problems. These problems include anorexia nervosa, bulimia nervosa, anorexic and bulimic behaviors, unhealthy dieting practices, binge eating disorder, and obesity. Adolescent girls may suffer from more than one disorder or may progress from one problem to another at varying degrees of severity. It is important to understand this range of weight-related problems in order to avoid causing one disorder, such as bulimia, while trying to prevent another, such as obesity.[1]

Body dissatisfaction and unhealthy dieting practices are linked to the development of eating disorders, obesity, and other problems. High numbers of adolescent girls are reporting that they are dissatisfied with their bodies and are trying to lose weight in unhealthy ways, including skipping meals, fasting, and using tobacco. A smaller number of girls are even resorting to more extreme methods such as self-induced vomiting, diet pills, and laxative use.[2]

These attitudes and behaviors place girls at a greater risk for eating disorders, obesity, poor nutrition, growth impairments, and emotional problems such as depression.[3] Research shows, for example, that overweight girls are more concerned about their weight, more dissatisfied with their bodies, and more likely to diet than their normal-weight peers.[4]

Excerpted from "Eating Disorders and Obesity: How Are They Related?" Body-Wise, Department of Health and Human Services Office on Women's Health. The full text of this document is available online at http://www.womenshealth.gov/BodyImage/bodyworks/CompanionPiece.pdf; accessed March 2010.

Binge eating is common among people with eating disorders and people who are obese. People with bulimia binge eat and then purge by vomiting, using laxatives, or other means. Binge eating that is not followed by purging may also be considered an eating disorder and can lead to weight gain. More than one-third of obese individuals in weight-loss treatment programs report difficulties with binge eating.[5] This type of eating behavior contributes to feelings of shame, loneliness, poor self-esteem, and depression.[6] Conversely, these kinds of feelings can cause binge eating problems.[7] A person may binge or overeat for emotional reasons, including stress, depression, and anxiety.[8]

Depression, anxiety, and other mood disorders are associated with both eating disorders and obesity. Adolescents who are depressed may be at an increased risk of becoming obese. One recent study found that depressed adolescents were two times more likely to become obese at the one year follow up than teens who did not suffer from depression.[9] In addition, many people with eating disorders suffer from clinical depression, anxiety, personality or substance abuse disorders, or in some cases obsessive compulsive disorder.[10] Therefore, a mental health professional may need to be involved in treating an adolescent who is obese or suffers from an eating disorder or other weight-related problem.

The environment may contribute to both eating disorders and obesity. The mass media, family, and peers may be sending children and adolescents mixed messages about food and weight that encourage disordered eating.[11] Today's society idealizes thinness and stigmatizes fatness, yet high-calorie foods are widely available and heavily advertised.[12] At the same time, levels of physical activity are at record lows as television and computers replace more active leisure activities, travel by automobile has replaced walking, and many communities lack space for walking and recreation.[13]

Health Risks of Eating Disorders and Obesity

Eating disorders may lead to the following health problems:

- Stunted growth
- Delayed menstruation
- Damage to vital organs such as the heart and brain
- Nutritional deficiencies, including starvation
- Cardiac arrest
- Emotional problems such as depression and anxiety

Obesity increases the risk for the following health problems:

- High blood pressure
- Stroke
- Cardiovascular disease
- Gallbladder disease
- Diabetes
- Respiratory problems
- Arthritis
- Cancer
- Emotional problems such as depression and anxiety

Notes

1. Neumark-Sztainer, D. "Obesity and Eating Disorder Prevention: An Integrated Approach?" *Adolescent Medicine*, Feb;14(1):159–73 (Review), 2003.

2. Neumark-Sztainer, D., Story, M., Hannan, P.J., et al. "Weight-Related Concerns and Behaviors Among Overweight and Non-Overweight Adolescents: Implications for Preventing Weight-Related Disorders." *Archives of Pediatrics and Adolescent Medicine*, Feb;156(2):171–78, 2002.

3. Neumark-Sztainer, D. "Obesity and Eating Disorder Prevention: An Integrated Approach?" 2003.

4. Burrows, A., Cooper, M. "Possible Risk Factors in the Development of Eating Disorders in Overweight Pre-Adolescent Girls." *International Journal of Obesity and Related Metabolic Disorders*, Sept;26(9):1268–73, 2002; Davison, K.K., Markey, C.N., Birch, L.L. "Etiology of Body Dissatisfaction and Weight Concerns Among 5-year-old Girls." *Appetite*, Oct;35(2):143–51, 2000; Vander Wal, J.S., Thelen, M.H. "Eating and Body Image Concerns Among Obese and Average-Weight Children." *Addictive Behavior*, Sep–Oct;25(5):775–78, 2000.

5. Yanovski, S.Z. "Binge Eating in Obese Persons." In Fairburn, C.G., Brownell, K.D. (eds), *Eating Disorders and Obesity*, 2nd ed. New York: Guilford Press, 403–7, 2002.

6. Waller, G. "The Psychology of Binge Eating." In Fairburn, C.G., Brownell, K.D. (eds) *Eating Disorders and Obesity*, 2nd ed. New York: Guilford Press, 98–102, 2002.

7. Fairburn, C., *Overcoming Binge Eating*. New York: The Guilford Press, 1995, 80–99.

8. Goodman, E, Whitaker, R. "A Prospective Study of the Role of Depression in the Development and Persistence of Adolescent Obesity." *Pediatrics*, 2002 Sep;110(3):497–504. Lumeng, J.C., Gannon, K., Cabral, H.J., Frank, D.A., Zuckerman, B. "Association between clinically meaningful behavior problems and overweight in children." *Pediatrics*. 2003 Nov;112(5):1138–45.

9. Goodman, E., Whitaker, R.C. "A Prospective Study of the Role of Depression in the Development and Persistence of Adolescent Obesity." *Pediatrics*. Sep;110(3):497–504, 2002.

10. National Mental Health Association. "Teen Eating Disorders." 1997.

11. Irving, L.M., Neumark-Sztainer, D. "Integrating the Prevention of Eating Disorders and Obesity: Feasible or Futile?" *Preventive Medicine*, 34:299–309, 2002. Stice, E. "Sociocultural Influences on Body Image and Eating Disturbance." In Fairburn, C.G., Brownell, K.D. (eds) Eating Disorders and Obesity, 2nd ed. New York: Guilford Press, 103–7, 2002.

12. Battle, E.K., Brownell, K.D. "Confronting a Rising Tide of Eating Disorders and Obesity: Treatment vs. Prevention and Policy." *Addictive Behavior*, 21:755-65 (Review), 1996.

13. French, S.A, Story, M., Jeffery, R. "Environmental Influences on Eating and Physical Activity." *Annual Review of Public Health*, 22:309–35 (Review), 2001.

Chapter 4

Understanding Eating Disorders

Chapter Contents

Section 4.1

Basic Facts about Eating Disorders

"Understanding Eating Disorders," *Medline Plus Magazine*,
National Institutes of Health, Spring 2008: volume 3, number 2.

Eating disorders, such as anorexia nervosa, bulimia nervosa, and binge eating, are among the most frustrating and difficult-to-treat conditions anyone can face. Research efforts at several National Institutes of Health (NIH) institutes are helping healthcare professionals and their patients better understand what can be done to deal with these conditions.

Eating disorders can affect girls and boys, women and men, people of all races and backgrounds. But because of the stigma or misperceptions, some people may not get the help they need. Mental health experts say it is important for people to understand what eating disorders are and what they are not. Eating disorders are not a silly desire to be thin, a figment of one's imagination, or a failing.

"The most important thing to recognize is that these are real disorders that require treatment," says Dr. Thomas Insel, the director of the National Institute of Mental Health (NIMH).

Eating disorders are serious, even life-threatening, medical illnesses that have biological and psychological causes. They are treatable. Recovery is possible.

"I tell my patients they are fighting an uphill battle against their biology. That does not mean it is not a fightable battle, because it is," says Cynthia Bulik, Ph.D., director of the eating disorders program at the University of North Carolina at Chapel Hill, which receives NIH funding for research.

What Are Eating Disorders?

Eating disorders are marked by extremes. People with an eating disorder may severely reduce the amount of food they eat, or eat an unusually large amount of food, or be extremely concerned about their weight or shape. They may start out simply eating smaller or larger portions than usual, but at some point the urge to eat more or less spirals out of control.

There are three main types of eating disorders: anorexia nervosa, bulimia nervosa, and binge-eating disorder. People with anorexia nervosa see themselves as overweight even though they are dangerously thin from starving themselves. People with bulimia nervosa eat unusually large amounts of food (binge eat) and then compensate by purging (vomiting, taking laxatives or diuretics), fasting, or excessive exercise. People with binge-eating disorder binge but do not purge, and they often become overweight or obese. Eating disorders may occur along with depression, substance abuse, or anxiety disorders, and can cause heart and kidney problems, even death. The disorders show up most frequently during the teenage years, but there are indications they may develop earlier or later in life.

Dr. Bulik and others in the field say they have seen an increase in adult women with eating disorders. At any given time, more than half the women in her program are older than thirty, which was not the case ten or twenty years ago, she adds. Dr. Bulik notes that environmental triggers, like the expectation to lose weight quickly after pregnancy, or to look young, can lead to extreme dieting or exercise.

"There are such extraordinary pressures on us not to let age show on our body," she says. "So, we are seeing more women caught up in extreme behaviors, and it's those behaviors that can trigger an eating disorder in a vulnerable individual."

There are clues as to what makes people likely to develop an eating disorder.

"There have been a number of studies showing that people who develop anorexia nervosa have certain traits in childhood that put them at risk, such as anxiety and perfectionism. If people do not have those traits, they are probably less likely to develop an eating disorder," says Walter Kaye, M.D. He directs the eating disorders program at the University of California, San Diego, and also receives NIH funding for his research.

Studies also show eating disorders run in families. But is it nature or nurture, inherited or learned behavior? Studies of twins suggest that genes play a role. To help further research into the genetics of eating disorders, Drs. Kaye, Bulik, and other researchers are collecting deoxyribonucleic acid (DNA) and blood samples from people in families where more than one person has anorexia nervosa. NIMH is supporting the research and will maintain a bank of the DNA and cell lines collected, so they can be used by researchers trying to identify variations in genes that affect the risk for anorexia and bulimia nervosa.

"By identifying these factors, we could see who is at risk, intervene early, and prevent people from coming into the emergency room," says Dr. Insel.

In addition to studying genes, researchers are using sophisticated imaging tools to see what is, or is not, happening in the brains of people with eating disorders.

"When it comes to hunger, it's hard for most people to stay on a diet. But, people with anorexia nervosa can diet every day and die from starvation. Why don't systems kick in that make them want to eat?" asks Dr. Kaye. By uncovering and understanding the differences in the brain circuitry and genes of people with eating disorders, researchers can work to develop new treatments.

Current treatment options may include mental health therapy, nutritional counseling, and medicines. One large-scale study suggests an online-intervention program may help some college-aged women who are at high risk of developing an eating disorder. The program includes online discussion groups moderated by psychologists, as well as reading and writing assignments.

Researchers are also studying the effectiveness of "family-based therapy" to treat children and teens with anorexia and bulimia. In family-based therapy, parents play an important and active role in a child's treatment. Additionally, a study is starting to see how this type of approach could be applied to adult couples in which one partner has anorexia nervosa.

Section 4.2

The Four Main Categories of Eating Disorders

Excerpted from "Eating Disorders," © 2010 A.D.A.M., Inc.
Reprinted with permission.

Introduction

Eating disorders are psychological problems marked by an obsession with food and weight. There are four general categories of eating disorders:

- Bulimia nervosa
- Anorexia nervosa
- Binge eating
- Eating disorders not otherwise specified

Bulimia Nervosa

Bulimia nervosa is more common than anorexia, and it usually begins early in adolescence. It is characterized by cycles of bingeing and purging, and typically takes the following pattern:

- Bulimia is often triggered when young women attempt restrictive diets, fail, and react by binge eating. (Binge eating involves consuming larger than normal amounts of food within a two-hour period.)

- In response to the binges, patients compensate, usually by purging, vomiting, using enemas, or taking laxatives, diet pills, or drugs to reduce fluids.

- Patients then revert to severe dieting, excessive exercise, or both. (Some patients with bulimia follow bingeing only with fasting and exercise. They are then considered to have nonpurging bulimia.)

- The cycle then swings back to bingeing and then to purging again.

- To be diagnosed with bulimia, however, a patient must binge and purge at least twice a week for three months.

- In some cases, the condition progresses to anorexia. Most people with bulimia, however, have a normal to high-normal body weight, although it may fluctuate by more than ten pounds because of the binge-purge cycle.

Anorexia Nervosa

The term "anorexia" literally means absence of appetite. Anorexia can be associated with medical conditions or medications that cause a loss of appetite. Anorexia nervosa, however, involves a psychological aversion to food that leads to a state of starvation and emaciation. In anorexia nervosa:

- At least 15 percent to as much as 60 percent of normal body weight is lost.

- The patient with anorexia nervosa has an intense fear of gaining weight, even when severely underweight.

- Individuals with anorexia nervosa have a distorted image of their own weight or shape and deny the serious health consequences of their low weight.

- Women with anorexia nervosa miss at least three consecutive menstrual periods. (Women can also be anorexic without this occurrence.) Patients with this condition are often characterized as anorexia restrictors or anorexic bulimic patients. Each type is equally prevalent.

- Anorexia restrictors reduce their weight by severe dieting.

- Anorexic bulimic patients maintain emaciation by purging. Although both types are serious, the bulimic type, which imposes additional stress on an undernourished body, is the more damaging.

Binge Eating (Binge Eating Disorder)

Bingeing without purging is characterized as compulsive overeating (binge eating) with the absence of bulimic behaviors, such as vomiting or laxative abuse (used to eliminate calories). Binge eating usually leads to becoming overweight.

To be diagnosed as a binge eater, a patient typically:

- consumes five thousand to fifteen thousand calories in one sitting;

28

- eats three meals a day plus frequent snacks;
- overeats continually throughout the day, rather than simply consuming large amounts of food during binges.

Treatment for binge eating is usually similar to treatment for bulimia. Since binge eating is often associated with obesity, it may also require weight and dietary management.

Eating Disorders Not Otherwise Specified

A fourth category called eating disorders not otherwise specified (EDNOS) is used to describe eating disorders not specifically defined as anorexia or bulimia. This category includes:

- infrequent binge-purge episodes (occurring less than twice a week or having such behavior for less than months);
- repeated chewing and spitting without swallowing large amounts of food;
- normal weight and anorexic behavior.

Such patients tend to be older at diagnosis. Although less serious than other eating disorders, these patients still face similar health problems, including a higher risk for fractures and other conditions.

Chapter 5

Binge Eating Disorder

Chapter Contents

Section 5.1

What Is Binge Eating Disorder?

Excerpted from "Binge Eating Disorder," Weight-Control Information Network, National Institute of Diabetes and Digestive and Kidney Diseases, National Institutes of Health, NIH Publication No. 04-3589, June 2008.

How do I know if I have binge eating disorder?

Most of us overeat from time to time, and some of us often feel we have eaten more than we should have. Eating a lot of food does not necessarily mean that you have binge eating disorder. Experts generally agree that most people with serious binge eating problems often eat an unusually large amount of food and feel their eating is out of control. People with binge eating disorder also may:

- eat much more quickly than usual during binge episodes;
- eat until they are uncomfortably full;
- eat large amounts of food even when they are not really hungry;
- eat alone because they are embarrassed about the amount of food they eat;
- feel disgusted, depressed, or guilty after overeating.

Binge eating also occurs in another eating disorder called bulimia nervosa. Persons with bulimia nervosa, however, usually purge, fast, or do strenuous exercise after they binge eat. Purging means vomiting or using a lot of diuretics (water pills) or laxatives to keep from gaining weight. Fasting is not eating for at least twenty-four hours. Strenuous exercise, in this case, means exercising for more than an hour just to keep from gaining weight after binge eating. Purging, fasting, and overexercising are dangerous ways to try to control your weight.

How common is binge eating disorder, and who is at risk?

Binge eating disorder is the most common eating disorder. It affects about 3 percent of all adults in the United States. People of any age can have binge eating disorder, but it is seen more often in adults age forty-six to fifty-five. Binge eating disorder is a little more common in women than in men; three women for every two men have it. The disorder affects blacks as often as whites, but it is not known how often it affects people in other ethnic groups.

Although most obese people do not have binge eating disorder, people with this problem are usually overweight or obese.[1] Binge eating disorder is more common in people who are severely obese. Normalweight people can also have the disorder.

People who are obese and have binge eating disorder often became overweight at a younger age than those without the disorder. They might also lose and gain weight more often, a process known as weight cycling or "yo-yo dieting."

What causes binge eating disorder?

No one knows for sure what causes binge eating disorder. As many as half of all people with binge eating disorder are depressed or have been depressed in the past. Whether depression causes binge eating disorder, or whether binge eating disorder causes depression, is not known.

It is also unclear if dieting and binge eating are related, although some people binge eat after dieting. In these cases, dieting means skipping meals, not eating enough food each day, or avoiding certain kinds of food. These are unhealthy ways to try to change your body shape and weight.

Studies suggest that people with binge eating disorder may have trouble handling some of their emotions. Many people who are binge eaters say that being angry, sad, bored, worried, or stressed can cause them to binge eat.

Certain behaviors and emotional problems are more common in people with binge eating disorder. These include abusing alcohol, acting quickly without thinking (impulsive behavior), not feeling in charge of themselves, not feeling a part of their communities, and not noticing and talking about their feelings.

Researchers are looking into how brain chemicals and metabolism (the way the body uses calories) affect binge eating disorder. Other research suggests that genes may be involved in binge eating, since the disorder often occurs in several members of the same family. This research is still in the early stages.

What are the complications of binge eating disorder?

People with binge eating disorder are usually very upset by their binge eating and may become depressed. Research has shown that people with binge eating disorder report more health problems, stress, trouble sleeping, and suicidal thoughts than do people without an eating disorder. Other complications from binge eating disorder could include joint pain, digestive problems, headache, muscle pain, and menstrual problems.

People with binge eating disorder often feel bad about themselves and may miss work, school, or social activities to binge eat.

Most people who binge eat, whether they are obese or not, feel ashamed and try to hide their problem. Often they become so good at hiding it that even close friends and family members do not know that their loved one binge eats.

How can people with binge eating disorder be helped?

People with binge eating disorder should get help from a healthcare professional such as a psychiatrist, psychologist, or clinical social worker. There are several different ways to treat binge eating disorder:

- Cognitive behavioral therapy teaches people how to keep track of their eating and change their unhealthy eating habits. It teaches them how to change the way they act in tough situations. It also helps them feel better about their body shape and weight.

- Interpersonal psychotherapy helps people look at their relationships with friends and family and make changes in problem areas.

- Drug therapy, such as antidepressants, may be helpful for some people.

The methods mentioned here seem to be equally helpful. Researchers are still trying to find the treatment that is the most helpful in controlling binge eating disorder. Combining drug and behavioral therapy has shown promising results for treating overweight and obese individuals with binge eating disorder. Drug therapy has been shown to benefit weight management and promote weight loss, while behavioral therapy has been shown to improve the psychological components of binge eating.

Other therapies being tried include dialectical behavior therapy, which helps people regulate their emotions; drug therapy with the anti-seizure medication topiramate; weight-loss surgery (bariatric surgery); exercise used alone or in combination with cognitive behavioral therapy; and self-help. Self-help books, videos, and groups have helped some people control their binge eating.

Am I alone?

If you think you might have binge eating disorder, it is important to know that you are not alone. Most people who have the disorder have tried but failed to control it on their own. You may want to get professional help. Talk to your healthcare provider about the type of help that may be best for you. The good news is that most people do well in treatment and can overcome binge eating.

Notes

1. The Clinical Guidelines on the Identification, Evaluation, and Treatment of Overweight and Obesity in Adults, published in 1998 by the National Heart, Lung, and Blood Institute, define overweight as a body mass index (BMI) of 25 to 29.9 and obesity as a BMI of 30 or more. BMI is calculated by dividing weight (in kilograms) by height (in meters) squared.

Section 5.2

Study Shows Binge Eating Disorder Is More Common than Other Eating Disorders

"First National Survey on Eating Disorders Finds Binge Eating More Common Than Other Eating Disorders," © 2007 McLean Hospital. Reprinted with permission.

The first national survey of individuals with eating disorders shows that binge eating disorder is more prevalent than either anorexia nervosa or bulimia nervosa. The study, conducted by researchers at Harvard-affiliated McLean Hospital, also calls binge eating disorder a "major public health burden" because of its direct link to severe obesity and other serious health effects. "For the first time, we have nationally representative data on eating disorders. These data clearly show that binge eating disorder is the most common eating disorder," says lead author James I. Hudson, MD, ScD, director of the Psychiatric

Epidemiology Research Program at McLean Hospital and professor of psychiatry at Harvard Medical School.

The study, published in the February 2007 issue of *Biological Psychiatry*, is based on data obtained over two years in the National Comorbidity Survey Replication (NCS-R), a survey of more than nine thousand people from across the United States about their mental health. Ronald C. Kessler, PhD, principal investigator of the NCS-R, and Eva Hiripi, of Harvard Medical School, and Harrison Pope Jr., MD, director of McLean Hospital's Biological Psychiatry Laboratory, are co-authors of the paper.

The survey found that 0.9 percent of women and 0.3 percent of men reported having anorexia nervosa at some point in their lives, and that 1.5 percent of women and 0.5 percent of men reported having bulimia nervosa. By contrast, binge eating disorder, a condition in which individuals experience frequent uncontrolled eating binges without purging, afflicts 3.5 percent of women and 2 percent of men at some point in their lives.

"Everybody knows about anorexia and bulimia; however, binge eating disorder affects more people, is often associated with severe obesity, and tends to persist longer," Hudson says. "The consequences of binge eating disorder can be serious—including obesity, diabetes, heart disease, high blood pressure, and stroke. It is imperative that health experts take notice of these findings."

The survey also found that the average lifetime duration of anorexia was 1.7 years, compared to 8.3 years for bulimia and 8.1 years for binge eating disorder. "Contrary to what people may believe, anorexia is not necessarily a chronic illness; in many cases, it runs its course and people get better without seeking treatment. So our survey suggests that for every one severe case [of anorexia], there may be many other milder cases."

The survey calls for further study of why some individuals with anorexia are able to recover more quickly and why others are crippled by the illness, say Hudson and Pope. "If we identified the factors that allowed people to recover from eating disorders quicker than others, then we might be better able to prevent the chronic, severe cases."

The findings, say Hudson and Pope, offer additional scientific support for including the diagnosis of binge eating disorder as an official psychiatric diagnosis in the next edition of the American Psychiatric Association's *Diagnostic and Statistical Manual of Mental Disorders*.

Chapter 6

Anorexia Nervosa

Introduction

People with anorexia have an extreme fear of gaining weight, which causes them to try to maintain a weight far less than normal. They will do almost anything to avoid gaining weight, including starving themselves or exercising too much. People with anorexia have a distorted body image—they think they are fat (even when they are extremely thin) and won't maintain a proper weight.

Anorexia is an emotional disorder that focuses on food, but it is actually an attempt to deal with perfectionism and a desire to control things by strictly regulating food and weight. People with anorexia often feel that their self-esteem is tied to how thin they are.

Anorexia is increasingly common, especially among young women in industrialized countries where cultural expectations encourage women to be thin. Fueled by popular fixations with thin and lean bodies, anorexia is also affecting a growing number of men, particularly athletes and those in the military.

Anorexia most commonly affects teens, as many as three in one hundred. Although anorexia seldom appears before puberty, associated mental conditions, such as depression and obsessive-compulsive behavior, are usually more severe when it does. Anorexia is often preceded by a traumatic event and is usually accompanied by other emotional problems. Anorexia is a life-threatening condition that can result in death from starvation, heart failure, electrolyte imbalance, or suicide.

It can be a chronic disease, one that you deal with over your lifetime. But treatment can help you develop a healthier lifestyle and avoid anorexia's complications.

Signs and Symptoms

The primary sign of anorexia nervosa is severe weight loss. People with anorexia may try to lose weight by severely limiting how much food they eat. They may also exercise excessively. Some people may engage in binging and purging, similar to bulimia. They may vomit after eating or take laxatives. At the same time, the person may insist that they are overweight.

Physical Signs

- Excessive weight loss
- Scanty or absent menstrual periods
- Thinning hair
- Dry skin
- Cold or swollen hands and feet
- Bloated or upset stomach
- Downy hair covering the body
- Low blood pressure
- Fatigue
- Abnormal heart rhythms
- Osteoporosis

Psychological and Behavioral Signs

- Distorted perception of self (insisting they are overweight when they are thin)
- Being preoccupied with food
- Refusing to eat
- Inability to remember things
- Refusing to acknowledge the seriousness of the illness
- Obsessive-compulsive behavior
- Depression

What to Watch For

- Skipping meals or making excises not to eat
- Eating only a few foods
- Refusing to eat in public
- Planning and preparing elaborate meals for others but not eating
- Constantly weighing themselves
- Ritually cutting food into tiny pieces
- Compulsive exercising

Causes

No one knows exactly what causes anorexia. Medical experts agree that several factors work together in a complex fashion to lead to the eating disorder. These may include:

- Severe trauma or emotional stress (such as the death of a loved one or sexual abuse) during puberty or prepuberty.
- Abnormalities in brain chemistry. Serotonin, a brain chemical that's involved in depression, may play a role.
- A cultural environment that puts a high value on thin or lean bodies.
- A tendency toward perfectionism, fear of being ridiculed or humiliated, a desire to always be perceived as being "good." A belief that being perfect is necessary in order to be loved.
- Family history of anorexia. About one-fifth of those with anorexia have a relative with an eating disorder.

Risk Factors

- Age and gender—anorexia is most common in teens and young adult women.
- Dieting.
- Weight gain.
- Unintentional weight loss.
- Puberty.
- Living in an industrialized country.

- Having depression, obsessive-compulsive disorder (OCD), or other anxiety disorders—OCD is present in up to two-thirds of people with anorexia. OCD associated with an eating disorder is often accompanied by a compulsive ritual around food (such as cutting it into tiny pieces).

- Participation in sports and professions that prize a lean body (such as dance, gymnastics, running, figure skating, horse racing, modeling, wrestling, acting).

- Difficulty dealing with stress (pessimism, tendency to worry, refusal to confront difficult or negative issues).

- History of sexual abuse or other traumatic event.

- Experiencing a big life change, such as moving or going to a new school.

Diagnosis

People with anorexia may think they are in control of their disease and don't want any help. But if you or a loved one is experiencing signs of anorexia, it's important to seek help. If you are a parent who suspects your child has anorexia, take your child to see the doctor immediately. If your doctor suspects anorexia, your doctor will order several laboratory tests as well as do a psychological evaluation. The SCOFF questionnaire, developed in Great Britain, is sometimes used when anorexia is suspected. A "yes" response to at least two of the following questions is a strong indicator of an eating disorder:

- S: "Do you feel sick because you feel full?"

- C: "Do you lose control over how much you eat?"

- O: "Have you lost more than thirteen pounds recently?"

- F: "Do you believe that you are fat when others say that you are thin?"

- F: "Does food and thoughts of food dominate your life?"

Lab tests may include:

- **Blood tests:** To look for signs of anemia, to check electrolytes, and to check liver and kidney function.

- **Electrocardiogram:** To look for abnormal heart rhythms.

- **Bone density test:** To check for osteoporosis.

If your doctor makes a diagnosis of anorexia, your doctor will likely ask you to work with a multidisciplinary team including a doctor, a psychologist or psychiatrist, and a registered dietitian.

Preventive Care

The most effective way to prevent anorexia is to develop healthy eating habits and a strong body image from an early age. Don't accept cultural values that place a premium on thin, perfect bodies. Make sure you and your children are educated about the life-threatening nature of anorexia.

For people who have already developed anorexia, the primary goal is to avoid relapse:

- Family and friends should be urged not to focus on the person's condition or on food or weight. Don't discuss anorexia at mealtimes, for example. Instead, devote mealtimes to social interaction and relaxation.

- Watch for signs of relapse. Careful and frequent monitoring of weight and other physical signs by your doctor can catch problems early.

- Cognitive behavioral therapy or other forms of psychotherapy can help the person develop coping skills and change unhealthy thought processes.

- Family therapy can help with any problems in the home that may contribute to the person's anorexia.

Treatment

The most successful treatment is a combination of psychotherapy, family therapy, and medication. It is important for the person with anorexia to be actively involved in their treatment. Many times the person with anorexia doesn't think they need any treatment. Even if they do, anorexia is a long-term challenge that may last a lifetime. People remain vulnerable to relapse when going through stressful periods of their lives.

A combination of treatments can give the person the medical, psychological, and practical support they need. Cognitive-behavioral therapy, along with antidepressants, can be an effective treatment for eating disorders. Complementary and alternative therapies may help with nutritional deficiencies.

If the person's life is in danger, hospitalization may be needed, particularly under the following circumstances:

- Continuing weight loss, in spite of outpatient treatment
- Body mass index (BMI) 30 percent below normal. The normal range is a BMI of 19–24. BMI is a measurement that takes into account a person's height and weight.
- Irregular heart rhythm
- Severe depression
- Suicidal tendencies
- Low potassium levels
- Low blood pressure

Even after some weight gain, many people with anorexia remain quite thin and risk of relapse is very high. Several social influences may make recovery difficult:

- Friends or family who admire how thin the person is
- Dance instructors or athletic coaches who put a premium on having a very lean body
- Denial on the part of parents or other family members
- The person's belief that extreme thinness is not only normal but also attractive, and that purging is the only way to avoid becoming overweight

Involving friends, family members, and others in the treatment can help deal with these issues.

Lifestyle

Treating anorexia nervosa involves major lifestyle changes:

- Establishing regular eating habits and a healthy diet
- Sticking with your treatment and meal plans
- Developing a support system and participating in a support group for help with stress and emotional issues
- Ignoring the urge to weigh yourself or check your appearance constantly
- Cutting back on exercise if obsessive exercise has been part of the disease. Once the person has gained weight, the doctor may set a controlled exercise program to help overall health.

Medications

There are no medications specifically approved to treat anorexia. However, antidepressants are often prescribed to treat depression that may accompany anorexia. Your doctor may also prescribe other drugs to help with OCD or anxiety. Medications, however, may not work alone and should be used in conjunction with a multidisciplinary approach that includes nutritional interventions and psychotherapy.

Selective serotonin reuptake inhibitors: These antidepressants are sometimes prescribed for people with anorexia. Fluoxetine (Prozac®) has been studied in people with anorexia and depression, with mixed results. In some early studies, it appeared to increase weight and improve mood over several months. But in another, it helped relieve symptoms of depression but did not affect the anorexia itself.

Recent studies indicate that the use of Prozac and other antidepressants may cause children and teenagers to have suicidal thoughts. Children who are taking these drugs must be monitored very carefully for signs of potential suicidal behavior.

People with anorexia may not be getting the essential nutrients their bodies need. Your healthcare provider may prescribe potassium or iron supplements, or other supplements to make up for any deficiency.

Cyproheptadine: An antihistamine that may stimulate appetite. In one study, using high doses of cyproheptadine hydrochloride decreased the number of days it took people with anorexia to gain an appropriate amount of weight.

Nutrition and Dietary Supplements

People with bulimia are more likely to have vitamin and mineral deficiencies, which can affect their health. Vitamin deficiencies can contribute to cognitive difficulties such as poor judgment or memory loss. Getting enough vitamins and minerals in your diet or through supplements can correct the problems.

Always tell your doctor about the herbs and supplements you are using or considering using, as some supplements may interfere with conventional treatments.

Following these nutritional tips may help overall health:

- Avoid caffeine, alcohol, and tobacco.
- Drink six to eight glasses of filtered water daily.

- Use quality protein sources—such as meat and eggs, whey, and vegetable protein shakes—as part of a balanced program aimed at gaining muscle mass and preventing wasting.

- Avoid refined sugars, such as candy and soft drinks.

Your doctor may suggest addressing nutritional deficiencies with the following supplements:

- A daily multivitamin, containing the antioxidant vitamins A, C, E, the B vitamins, and trace minerals, such as magnesium, calcium, zinc, phosphorus, copper, and selenium.

- Omega-3 fatty acids, such as fish oil, one to two capsules or one tablespoonful oil two to three times daily, to help decrease inflammation and improve immunity. Cold-water fish, such as salmon or halibut, are good sources; eat two servings of fish per week.

- Coenzyme Q10, 100–200 mg at bedtime, for antioxidant, immune, and muscular support.

- 5-hydroxytryptophan (5-HTP), 50 mg two to three times daily, for mood stabilization. Talk with your health care provider if you are on prescription medications before taking 5-HTP. Do not take 5-HTP if you are taking antidepressants.

- Creatine, 5–7 grams daily, when needed for muscle weakness and wasting.

- Probiotic supplement (containing *Lactobacillus acidophilus* among other strains), 5–10 billion CFUs (colony forming units) a day, for maintenance of gastrointestinal and immune health. Refrigerate probiotic supplements for best results.

- L-glutamine, 500–1,000 mg three times daily, for support of gastrointestinal health and immunity.

Herbs

Herbs are generally a safe way to strengthen and tone the body's systems. As with any therapy, you should work with your healthcare provider to get your problem diagnosed before starting any treatment. You may use herbs as dried extracts (capsules, powders, teas), glycerites (glycerine extracts), or tinctures (alcohol extracts). Unless otherwise indicated, you should make teas with one teaspoon herb per cup of hot water. Steep covered five to ten minutes for leaf or flowers, and ten to twenty minutes for roots. Drink two to four cups per day. You may use tinctures alone or in combination as noted:

- Ashwagandha (*Withania somnifera*) standardized extract, 450 mg one to two times daily, for general health benefits and stress.

- Fenugreek (*Trigonella foenum-graecum*), 250–500 mg two to three times daily, to stimulate appetite.

- Cayenne pepper (*Capsicum annuum*) standardized extract, 400 mg three times daily, for help with digestion.

- Milk thistle (*Silybum marianum*) seed standardized extract, 80–160 mg two to three times daily, for liver health.

- Catnip (*Nepeta spp.*), as a tea two to three times per day, to calm the nerves and soothe the digestive system.

Homeopathy

No scientific literature supports the use of homeopathy for bulimia. However, an experienced homeopath will consider your individual case and may recommend treatments to address both your underlying condition and any current symptoms.

Mind-Body Medicine

Cognitive behavioral therapy: Cognitive behavioral therapy is one of the most effective therapies for anorexia. In cognitive behavioral therapy, the person learns to replace negative, unrealistic thoughts and beliefs with positive, realistic ones. The person is also encouraged to acknowledge their fears and to develop new, healthier ways of solving problems.

Family therapy: In addition to individual therapy for someone who has anorexia, family therapy that involves parents and siblings is also recommended. Parents and other family members often have intense feelings of guilt and anxiety that they need to address. Family therapy is aimed, in part, at helping the parents or partner (in the case of an adult) understand the seriousness of this illness and the ways in which family patterns may contribute to it.

Hypnosis: Hypnosis may be helpful as part of an integrated treatment program for anorexia nervosa. Hypnosis may help the person strengthen both self-confidence and the ability to cope. That may result in healthier eating, improved body image, and greater self-esteem.

Biofeedback: Studies suggest that biofeedback may be helpful in reducing stress in people with anorexia.

Other Considerations

Pregnancy

Anorexia poses several potential problems for women who are pregnant or wish to become pregnant:

- Difficulty getting pregnant and carrying a pregnancy to term because of higher rates of infertility and spontaneous abortion
- Increased risk of low birth weight babies and birth defects
- Malnourishment (particularly calcium deficiency) as the fetus grows
- Increased risk of medical complications
- Increased risk of relapse triggered by the stress of pregnancy or parenthood

Prognosis and Complications

Medical complications associated with anorexia include:

- irregular heartbeat and heart attack;
- anemia, often related to lack of vitamin B_{12};
- low potassium, calcium, magnesium, and phosphate levels;
- increased cholesterol;
- hormonal changes (can lead to absence of menstrual periods, infertility, bone loss, and stunted growth);
- osteoporosis;
- seizures and numbness in hands and feet;
- disorganized thinking;
- death (suicide is responsible for 50 percent of fatalities associated with anorexia).

The outlook for people with anorexia is variable, with recovery often taking between four and seven years. There is also a high chance of relapse even after recovery. Long-term studies show that 50 to 70 percent of people recover from anorexia nervosa. However, 25 percent do not fully recover. Many, even after they are considered "cured," continue to show traits of anorexia, such as remaining very thin and striving for perfection.

Alternative Names

Eating disorders—anorexia

Supporting Research

Barabasz M. Efficacy of hypnotherapy in the treatment of eating disorders. *Int J Clin Exp Hypn*. 2007 Jul;55(3):318–35. Review.

Birmingham CL, Sidhu FK. Complementary and alternative medical treatments for anorexia nervosa: case report and review of the literature. *Eat Weight Disord*. 2007 Sep;12(3):e51–53. Review.

Escolar DM, Buyse G, Henricson E, et al. CINRG randomized controlled trial of creatine and glutamine in Duchenne muscular dystrophy. *Ann Neurol*. 2005;58(1):151–55.

Field T. Massage therapy effects. *Am Psychol*. 1998;53:1270–81.

Holman RT, Adams CE, Nelson RA, et al. Patients with anorexia nervosa demonstrate deficiencies of selected essential fatty acids, compensatory changes in nonessential fatty acids and decreased fluidity of plasma lipids. *J Nutr* 1995;125:901–7.

Kleifield EI, Wagner S, Halmi KA. Cognitive-behavioral treatment of anorexia nervosa. *Psychiatric Clin N Am*. 1996;19:715–37.

LaValle JB, Krinsky DL, Hawkins EB, et al. *Natural Therapeutics Pocket Guide*. Hudson, OH: LexiComp; 2000: 387–88.

Loeb KL, Walsh BT, Lock J, le Grange D, Jones J, Marcus S, Weaver J, Dobrow I. Open trial of family-based treatment for full and partial anorexia nervosa in adolescence: evidence of successful dissemination. *J Am Acad Child Adolesc Psychiatry*. 2007 Jul;46(7):792–800.

McNulty. Prevalence and contributing factors of eating disorder behaviors in active duty Navy men. *Mil Med*. 1997;162(11):753–58.

Moyano D, Sierra C, Brandi N, et al. Antioxidant status in anorexia nervosa. *Int J Eating Disord*. 1999;25:99–103.

Pop-Jordanova N. Psychological characteristics and biofeedback mitigation in preadolescents with eating disorders. *Ped Int*. 2000;42:76–81.

Rock CL, Vasantharajan S. Vitamin status of eating disorder patients: Relationship to clinical indices and effect of treatment. *Int J Eating Disord*. 1995;18:257–62.

Rotsein OD. Oxidants and antioxidant therapy. *Crit Care Clin*. 2001; 17(1):239–47.

Shay NF, Manigan HF. Neurobiology of zinc-influenced eating behavior. *J Nutr*. 2000;130:1493S–1499S.

Simopoulos AP. Omega-3 fatty acids in inflammation and autoimmune diseases. *J Am Coll Nutr*. 2002;21(6):495–505.

Wang HK. The therapeutic potential of flavonoids. *Expert Opin Investig Drugs*. 2000;9(9):2103–19.

Wheatland R. Alternative treatment considerations in anorexia nervosa. *Med Hypotheses*. 2002;59(6):710–15.

Williams PM, Goodie J, Motsinger CD. Treating eating disorders in primary care. *Am Fam Physician*. 2008 Jan 15;77(2):187–95.

Wiseman CV, Harris WA, Halmi KA. Eating disorders. *Medical Clin N Am*. 1998;82:145–59.

Wolfe BE, Metzger ED, Jimerson DC. Research update on serotonin function in bulimia nervosa and anorexia nervosa. *Psychopharmacol Bull*. 1997;33:345–54.

Yoon JH, Baek SJ. Molecular targets of dietary polyphenols with anti-inflammatory properties. *Yonsei Med J*. 2005;46(5):585–96.

Young D. The use of hypnotherapy in the treatment of eating disorders. *Contemporary Hypnosis*. 1995;12:148–53.

Chapter 7

Bulimia Nervosa

Introduction

Bulimia nervosa is an eating disorder in which a person binges and purges. The person may eat a lot of food at once and then try to get rid of the food by vomiting, using laxatives, or sometimes over-exercising. People with bulimia are preoccupied with their weight and body image. Bulimia is associated with depression and other psychiatric disorders and shares symptoms with anorexia nervosa, another major eating disorder. Because many individuals with bulimia can maintain a normal weight, they are able to keep their condition a secret for years. If not treated, bulimia can lead to nutritional deficiencies and even fatal complications.

Signs and Symptoms

Bulimia is often accompanied by the following signs and symptoms:

- Binge eating of high-carbohydrate foods, usually in secret
- Exercising for hours
- Eating until you are painfully full
- Going to the bathroom during meals
- Loss of control over eating, with guilt and shame

- Body weight that goes up and down
- Constipation, diarrhea, nausea, gas, abdominal pain
- Dehydration
- Irregular menstruation or lack of menstrual periods
- Damaged tooth enamel
- Bad breath
- Sore throat or mouth sores
- Depression

What Causes It?

No one knows what causes bulimia, although there are several theories. Bulimia may have a genetic component, and there is some evidence that women who have a sister or mother with bulimia are at higher risk of developing the condition. Families may put an overemphasis on achievement, or may be overly critical. Psychological factors may also be involved, including having low self-esteem, not being able to control impulsive behaviors, and having trouble expressing anger. Some people with bulimia may have a history of sexual abuse. People with bulimia may also experience depression, self-mutilation, substance abuse, and obsessive-compulsive behavior. Cultural pressures to appear thin contribute to the disorder, particularly among dancers and athletes.

Who's Most at Risk?

People with the following conditions or characteristics are at higher risk for developing bulimia:

- White, middle-class women (mostly teenagers and college students)
- People with a family history of mood disorders and substance abuse
- People with low self-esteem

What to Expect at Your Provider's Office

Often, people with bulimia are ashamed of their condition and do not seek help for many years. By then, their habits are deeply ingrained and harder to change. If you have symptoms of bulimia, you should see a doctor as soon as possible. The doctor should check for physical signs such as eroded tooth enamel and enlargement of the salivary glands, as well as signs of depression. Laboratory tests can reveal chemical changes caused by bingeing and purging. Your doctor or a mental health practitioner will do a psychological exam and ask about your feelings and your eating habits.

Treatment

Treatment Plan

The most successful treatment is a combination of psychotherapy, family therapy, and medication. It is important for the person with bulimia to be actively involved in their treatment.

Drug Therapies

Antidepressants are often prescribed for bulimia. The most common antidepressants prescribed are selective serotonin reuptake inhibitors (SSRIs). They include:

- fluoxetine (Prozac®);
- sertraline (Zoloft®);
- paroxetine (Paxil®);
- fluvoxamine (Luvox®).

Prozac is considered the drug of choice, although some studies suggest that other SSRIs, such as Luvox, may be even more effective.

Important note: Some studies indicate that the use of Prozac and other antidepressants may cause children and teenagers to have suicidal thoughts. Children who are taking these drugs must be monitored very carefully for signs of potential suicidal behavior.

People with bulimia may not be getting the essential nutrients their bodies need. Your healthcare provider may prescribe potassium or iron supplements, or other supplements to make up for any deficiency.

Complementary and Alternative Therapies

Psychotherapy is a cornerstone of bulimia treatment. Cognitive behavioral therapy, which teaches you to replace negative thoughts and behaviors with healthy ones, is often used. Other mind-body and stress-reduction techniques, such as yoga, tai chi, and meditation, may help you become more aware of your body and form a more positive body image. A six-week clinical trial showed that guided imagery helped people with bulimia reduce bingeing and vomiting, feel more able to comfort themselves, and improved feelings about their bodies and eating. More studies are needed to verify these findings and to determine if guided imagery has long-term benefits. Always tell your healthcare provider about the herbs and supplements you are using or considering using.

Nutrition and supplements: People with bulimia are more likely to have vitamin and mineral deficiencies, which can affect their health. Vitamin deficiencies can contribute to cognitive difficulties such as poor judgment or memory loss. Getting enough vitamins and minerals in your diet or through supplements can correct the problems.

Some natural therapies, including dietary supplements, may help general health and well-being.

Following these nutritional tips may help reduce symptoms:

- Avoid caffeine, alcohol, and tobacco.

- Drink six to eight glasses of filtered water daily.

- Use quality protein sources—such as organic meat and eggs, whey, and vegetable protein shakes—as part of a balanced program aimed at gaining muscle mass and preventing wasting.

- Avoid refined sugars, such as candy and soft drinks.

Your doctor may suggest addressing nutritional deficiencies with the following supplements:

- A daily multivitamin, containing the antioxidant vitamins A, C, E, the B vitamins, and trace minerals, such as magnesium, calcium, zinc, phosphorus, copper, and selenium.

- Omega-3 fatty acids, such as fish oil, one to two capsules or one tablespoonful oil two to three times daily, to help decrease inflammation and improve immunity. Cold-water fish, such as salmon or halibut, are good sources; eat two servings of fish per week.

- Coenzyme Q10, 100–200 mg at bedtime, for antioxidant, immune, and muscular support.

- 5-hydroxytryptophan (5-HTP), 50 mg two to three times daily, for mood stabilization. Talk with your healthcare provider if you are on prescription medications before taking 5-HTP. Do not take 5-HTP if you are taking antidepressants.

- Creatine, 5–7 grams daily, when needed for muscle weakness and wasting.

- Probiotic supplement (containing *Lactobacillus acidophilus* among other strains), 5–10 billion CFUs (colony forming units) a day, for maintenance of gastrointestinal and immune health. Refrigerate probiotic supplements for best results.

- L-glutamine, 500–1,000 mg three times daily, for support of gastrointestinal health and immunity.

Herbs: Herbs are generally a safe way to strengthen and tone the body's systems. As with any therapy, you should work with your healthcare provider to get your problem diagnosed before starting any treatment. You may use herbs as dried extracts (capsules, powders, teas), glycerites (glycerine extracts), or tinctures (alcohol extracts). Unless otherwise indicated, you should make teas with one teaspoon herb per cup of hot water. Steep covered five to ten minutes for leaf or flowers, and ten to twenty minutes for roots. Drink two to four cups per day. You may use tinctures alone or in combination as noted.

These herbs are not used to treat bulimia specifically, but may be helpful in maintaining overall health:

- Ashwagandha (*Withania somnifera*) standardized extract, 450 mg one to two times daily, for general health benefits and stress.

- Holy basil (*Ocimum sanctum*) standardized extract, 400 mg daily, for stress. You can also prepare teas from the plant.

- Milk thistle (*Silybum marianum*) seed standardized extract, 80–160 mg two to three times daily, for liver health.

- Grape seed (*Vitis vinifera*) standardized extract, 100–200 mg three times daily, for antioxidant effects, and heart and blood vessel protection.

- Catnip (*Nepeta spp.*), as a tea two to three times per day, to calm the nerves and soothe the digestive system.

Homeopathy: No scientific literature supports the use of homeopathy for bulimia. However, an experienced homeopath will consider your individual case and may recommend treatments to address both your underlying condition and any current symptoms.

Acupuncture: No scientific literature supports the use of acupuncture for bulimia. However, a trained acupuncturist may be able to recommend acupuncture treatments to support your overall health. Many inpatient treatment centers that focus on eating disorders include acupuncture in their overall treatment plan. Studies have found that acupuncture can be helpful in treating addictive behaviors and anxiety in general, which can help people with bulimia who are in recovery.

Massage: Therapeutic massage can be an effective part of a bulimia treatment plan. In one study, adolescent women with bulimia were randomly assigned either to receive massage therapy for five weeks or to participate in a control group (not receiving massage therapy). The twenty-four women receiving massage improved immediately, while bulimia in women in the control group did not improve. Women in the massage group were less anxious and depressed right after their initial massages. They also had better scores on the Eating Disorder Inventory, which helps healthcare providers assess psychological and behavioral traits in eating disorders.

Prognosis/Possible Complications

Many people with bulimia relapse after treatment and need ongoing care. Possible complications from repeated bingeing and purging include problems with the esophagus, stomach, heart, lungs, muscles, or pancreas. People with suicidal thoughts or severe symptoms may need to be hospitalized. Women with bulimia may find pregnancy emotionally difficult because of the changes in body shape that occur. The mother's poor nutritional health can affect the baby. Women who have stopped menstruating because of bulimia will be unable to become pregnant.

Following Up

Because bulimia is usually a long-term disease, a healthcare provider will need to check the person's weight, exercise habits, and physical and mental health periodically.

Alternative Names

Eating disorders—bulimia

Supporting Research

Barabasz M. Efficacy of hypnotherapy in the treatment of eating disorders. *Int J Clin Exp Hypn*. 2007 Jul;55(3):318–35. Review.

Becker AE, Grinspoon SK, Klibanski A, Herzog DB. Current concepts: eating disorders. *N Engl J Med*. 1999;340:1092–98.

Dambro MR, ed. *Griffith's 5 Minute Clinical Consult*. Baltimore, Md: Lippincott Williams & Wilkins; 1999:160–61.

Esplen MJ, Garfinkel PE, Olmsted M, Gallop RM, Kennedy S. A randomized controlled trial of guided imagery in bulimia nervosa. *Psychol Med*. 1998;28(6):1347–57.

Field T, Schanberg S, Kuhn C, et al. Bulimic adolescents benefit from massage therapy. *Adolescence*. 1998;33(131):555–63.

Fauci AS, Braunwald E, Isselbacher KJ, et al, eds. *Harrison's Principles of Internal Medicine*. 17th ed. New York, NY: McGraw-Hill; 2008.

Hamilton EM, Gropper SA. *The Biochemistry of Human Nutrition: A Desk Reference*. New York, NY: West Publishing Company; 1987:278–79.

Holman RT, Adams CE, Nelson RA, et al. Patients with anorexia nervosa demonstrate deficiencies of selected essential fatty acids, compensatory changes in nonessential fatty acids and decreased fluidity of plasma lipids. *J Nutr* 1995;125:901–7.

Humphries L, Vivian B, Stuart M, McClain CJ. Zinc deficiency and eating disorders. *J Clin Psychiatry*. 1989;50:456–59.

Kronenberg, HM ed. *Williams Textbook of Endocrinology*. 11th ed. Philadelphia, Pa: W.B. Saunders; 2008.

Krysanski VL, Ferraro FR. Review of controlled psychotherapy treatment trials for binge eating disorder. *Psychol Rep*. 2008 Apr;102(2):339–68. Review.

Laessle RG, Beumont PJV, Butow P, et al. A comparison of nutritional management with stress management in the treatment of bulimia nervosa. *Br J Psychiatry*. 1991;159:250–61.

LaValle JB, Krinsky DL, Hawkins EB, et al. *Natural Therapeutics Pocket Guide*. Hudson, OH: LexiComp; 2000: 387–88.

McClain CJ, Humphries LL, Hill KK, Nickl NJ. Gastrointestinal and nutritional aspects of eating disorders. *J Am Coll Nutr*. 1993;12(4):466–74.

Mooney J. Management of eating disorders. *J Naturopathic Med*. 1997;7(1):114–18.

Moyano D, Sierra C, Brandi N, et al. Antioxidant status in anorexia nervosa. *Int J Eating Disord*. 1999;25:99–103.

Pop-Jordanova N. Psychological characteristics and biofeedback mitigation in preadolescents with eating disorders. *Pediatr Int*. 2000;42:76–81.

Rock CL, Vasantharajan S. Vitamin status of eating disorder patients: Relationship to clinical indices and effect of treatment. *Int J Eating Disord*. 1995;18:257–62.

Rotsein OD. Oxidants and antioxidant therapy. *Crit Care Clin*. 2001;17(1):239–47.

Schauss A, Costin C. Zinc as a nutrient in the treatment of eating disorders. *Am J Nat Med*. 1997;4(10):8–13.

Simopoulos AP. Omega-3 fatty acids in inflammation and autoimmune diseases. *J Am Coll Nutr*. 2002;21(6):495–505.

Smith KA, Fairburn CG, Cowen PJ. Symptomatic relapse in bulimia nervosa following acute tryptophan depletion. *Arch Gen Psychiatry*. 1999;56:171–76.

Ullman D. *The Consumer's Guide to Homeopathy*. New York, NY: Tarcher/Putnam; 1995.

Wang HK. The therapeutic potential of flavonoids. *Expert Opin Investig Drugs*. 2000;9(9):2103–19.

Wheatland R. Alternative treatment considerations in anorexia nervosa. *Med Hypotheses*. 2002;59(6):710–15.

Williams PM, Goodie J, Motsinger CD. Treating eating disorders in primary care. *Am Fam Physician*. 2008 Jan 15;77(2):187–95. Review.

Wiseman CV, Harris WA, Halmi KA. Eating disorders. *Medical Clin N Am*. 1998;82:145–59.

Wolfe BE, Metzger ED, Jimerson DC. Research update on serotonin function in bulimia nervosa and anorexia nervosa. *Psychopharmacol Bull*. 1997;33:345–54.

Yoon JH, Baek SJ. Molecular targets of dietary polyphenols with anti-inflammatory properties. *Yonsei Med J*. 2005;46(5):585–96.

Young D. The use of hypnotherapy in the treatment of eating disorders. *Contemporary Hypnosis*. 1995;12:148–53.

Chapter 8

Diet Pill, Diuretic, Ipecac, and Laxative Abuse

Laxatives

Laxative abuse is defined as a use (or overuse) of laxatives over a long period of time, and used a means of weight control. Laxative abuse is most common among bulimics (although not exclusive) as a way of purging. There are two main types of laxatives, stimulant laxatives and bulk-forming laxatives. Stimulant laxatives irritate the colon to induce bowel movements (and are not recommended for use greater than one week) and bulk-forming laxatives add mass and volume to the bowel movement. Continual overstimulation of the intestines from laxative abuse can eventually cause the bowels to become nonresponsive. Laxatives *do not* help you lose weight.

Reasons for laxative abuse are as follows:

- To get rid of food before it can be properly digested. In reality, it doesn't really happen. The body already absorbs all the nutrients and calories from the food before it is excreted. Laxatives work near the lower end of the bowel, and do not alter the way that food (and calories) are absorbed by the body.

- They become addictive. The sufferer is aware that these are no weight loss benefits, but still continues to take them.

"Abusive Substances," © 2005 Alliance for Eating Disorders Awareness. Reprinted with permission. For additional information, visit www.eating disordersinfo.org. Reviewed by David A. Cooke, M.D., October 2010.

- A method of coping with stress, anger, feelings of rejection, etc.
- A psychological safety net to fall back on if other methods of weight loss fail.

Over a period of time, laxatives lose their effectiveness and actually start working against you. Some of the adverse side effects of laxative abuse include:

- *severe* abdominal pain and cramping;
- diarrhea (which can occur while sleeping in extreme abuse situations);
- dehydration;
- stomach ulcers;
- constipation;
- fluid retention/bloating (especially in your hands, feet, ankles, face, and stomach);
- development of blood in stools, which leads to anemia;
- renal stones;
- severe electrolyte, fluid, and mineral imbalances;
- fatigue and lethargy;
- malabsorption, which can cause deformed bone development;
- death.

Diuretics

Diuretics come in a pill form, as do stimulant laxatives, and they are used to rid the body of fluid. They act on the kidneys to increase the flow of urine. They are *not* intended for weight loss. Actually, it only reduces the amount of water in the body, and water in the body is vital for the appropriate functioning of all systems. Anorexics, bulimics, and some binge eaters use them as a "quick fix," an attempt to control weight, or to lose weight. However, if diuretics are misused, there is a high risk of developing several serious side effects.

Some adverse side effects of diuretic abuse include:

- headaches;
- dizziness;
- dehydration;

- muscle weakness;
- potassium deficiency;
- electrolyte imbalance;
- kidney damage;
- cardiac arrhythmia;
- heart palpitations;
- fluid retention;
- nausea;
- death.

Diet Pills

Both prescription and over-the-counter (OTC) diet pills are one of the most dangerous and unhealthy ways to lose weight. The scariest aspect of OTC diet pills is that they are readily available in grocery stores, pharmacies, gas stations, health food stores, etc. to everyone, including children and teens. Similar to other addictions, individuals will start to take the pills as recommended, but will completely start abusing them and become dependent on them. Natural (herbal) diet pills are just as dangerous and are not regulated by the Food and Drug Administration.

Some adverse side effects of diet pill abuse include:

- headaches;
- heart palpitations;
- dizziness;
- vomiting;
- shallow breathing;
- blurred vision;
- hallucinations;
- convulsions/seizures;
- fatigue;
- chest pains;
- high blood pressure.

Ipecac Abuse

Ipecac syrup is meant for use in cases of accidental poisoning, as a last resort. Ipecac induces vomiting by chemically irritating the stomach lining and stimulating the area of the brain that controls vomiting. The affects of ipecac syrup, however, are worse (and more traumatic) than purging alone. It literally eats away at your throat and stomach tissue. *Abuse of this is deadly!*

Some adverse side effects of ipecac abuse include:

- electrolyte abnormalities;
- dehydration;
- high blood pressure;
- blackouts;
- irreversible damage to the muscles of the heart;
- seizures;
- shock;
- respiratory complications;
- hemorrhaging;
- cardiac arrest;
- death.

Compulsive Exercise

Contrary to popular belief, there is such a thing as too much exercise. Compulsive exercise is another way to "purge" calories, and can be as dangerous as anorexia and bulimia. The main goal when an individual is suffering from compulsive exercise can be burning calories, relieving the guilt from eating/binging, or to give them the permission to eat. The exercise may give the person a sense of control, power, and self-respect. Most overexercise is done *in secret* and away from prying eyes, and can also be a form of punishment.

Signs and symptoms:

- Working out with an injury or if the individual is sick.

- The individual may feel tremendously guilty/seriously depressed if they cannot exercise.

- Finding time, no matter at what expense, to do the exercise (i.e., missing work, skipping school, missing parties, hiding in the bathroom, and skipping appointments).

- Not giving himself/herself any "rest days", or "recovery days" between workouts.

- Working at out hours at a time, beyond what can be considered safe or healthy.

There are serious side effects associated with compulsive overexercise:

- Dehydration

- Fatigue

- Injuries such as shin splints, strains and sprains, cartilage and ligament damage, and stress fractures

- Fractured bones

- Osteoporosis

- Degenerative arthritis

- Amenorrhea

- Reproductive problems

- Heart problems

Chapter 9

Female Athlete Triad

Hannah joined the track team her freshman year and trained hard to become a lean, strong sprinter. When her coach told her losing a few pounds would improve her performance, she immediately started counting calories and increased the duration of her workouts. She was too busy with practices and meets to notice that her period had stopped—she was more worried about the stress fracture in her ankle slowing her down.

Although Hannah thinks her intense training and disciplined diet are helping her performance, they may actually be hurting her—and her health.

What Is Female Athlete Triad?

Sports and exercise are part of a balanced, healthy lifestyle. People who play sports are healthier; get better grades; are less likely to experience depression; and use alcohol, cigarettes, and drugs less frequently than people who aren't athletes. But for some girls, not balancing the needs of their bodies and their sports can have major consequences.

Some girls who play sports or exercise intensely are at risk for a problem called female athlete triad. Female athlete triad is a combination

"Female Athlete Triad," February 2010, reprinted with permission from www.kidshealth.org. Copyright © 2010 The Nemours Foundation. This information was provided by KidsHealth, one of the largest resources online for medically reviewed health information written for parents, kids, and teens. For more articles like this one, visit www.KidsHealth.org, or www.TeensHealth.org.

of three conditions: disordered eating, amenorrhea, and osteoporosis. A female athlete can have one, two, or all three parts of the triad.

Triad Factor #1: Disordered Eating

Most girls with female athlete triad try to lose weight as a way to improve their athletic performance. The disordered eating that accompanies female athlete triad can range from avoiding certain types of food the athlete thinks are "bad" (such as foods containing fat) to serious eating disorders like anorexia nervosa or bulimia nervosa.

Triad Factor #2: Amenorrhea

Exercising intensely and not eating enough calories can lead to decreases in estrogen, the hormone that helps to regulate the menstrual cycle. As a result, a girl's periods may become irregular or stop altogether. Of course, it's normal for teens to occasionally miss periods, especially in the first year. A missed period does not automatically mean female athlete triad. It could mean something else is going on, like pregnancy or a medical condition. If you are having sex and miss your period, talk to your doctor.

Some girls who participate intensively in sports may never even get their first period because they've been training so hard. Others may have had periods, but once they increase their training and change their eating habits, their periods may stop.

Triad Factor #3: Osteoporosis

Low estrogen levels and poor nutrition, especially low calcium intake, can lead to osteoporosis, the third aspect of the triad. Osteoporosis is a weakening of the bones due to the loss of bone density and improper bone formation. This condition can ruin a female athlete's career because it may lead to stress fractures and other injuries.

Usually, the teen years are a time when girls should be building up their bone mass to their highest levels—called peak bone mass. Not getting enough calcium now can also have a lasting effect on how strong a woman's bones are later in life.

Who Gets Female Athlete Triad?

Many girls have concerns about the size and shape of their bodies. But being a highly competitive athlete and participating in a sport that requires you to train extra hard can increase that worry.

Girls with female athlete triad often care so much about their sports that they would do almost anything to improve their performance. Martial arts and rowing are examples of sports that classify athletes by weight class, so focusing on weight becomes an important part of the training program and can put a girl at risk for disordered eating.

Participation in sports where a thin appearance is valued can also put a girl at risk for female athlete triad. Sports such as gymnastics, figure skating, diving, and ballet are examples of sports that value a thin, lean body shape. Some athletes may even be told by coaches or judges that losing weight would improve their scores.

Even in sports where body size and shape aren't as important, such as distance running and cross-country skiing, girls may be pressured by teammates, parents, partners, and coaches who mistakenly believe that "losing just a few pounds" could improve their performance.

The truth is, losing those few pounds generally doesn't improve performance at all. People who are fit and active enough to compete in sports generally have more muscle than fat, so it's the muscle that gets starved when a girl cuts back on food. Plus, if a girl loses weight when she doesn't need to, it interferes with healthy body processes such as menstruation and bone development.

In addition, for some competitive female athletes, problems such as low self-esteem, a tendency toward perfectionism, and family stress place them at risk for disordered eating.

What Are the Signs and Symptoms?

If a girl has risk factors for female athlete triad, she may already be experiencing some symptoms and signs of the disorder, such as:

- weight loss;
- no periods or irregular periods;
- fatigue and decreased ability to concentrate;
- stress fractures (fractures that occur even if a person hasn't had a significant injury);
- muscle injuries.

Girls with female athlete triad often have signs and symptoms of eating disorders, such as:

- continued dieting in spite of weight loss;
- preoccupation with food and weight;
- frequent trips to the bathroom during and after meals;

- using laxatives;

- brittle hair or nails;

- dental cavities because in girls with bulimia tooth enamel is worn away by frequent vomiting;

- sensitivity to cold;

- low heart rate and blood pressure;

- heart irregularities and chest pain.

How Doctors Help

An extensive physical examination is a crucial part of diagnosing female athlete triad. A doctor who thinks a girl has female athlete triad will probably ask questions about her periods, her nutrition and exercise habits, any medications she takes, and her feelings about her body. This is called the medical history.

Poor nutrition can also affect the body in many ways, so a doctor might order blood tests to check for anemia and other problems associated with the triad. The doctor also will check for medical reasons why a girl may be losing weight and missing her periods. Because osteoporosis can put someone at higher risk for bone fractures, the doctor may also request tests to measure bone density.

Doctors don't work alone to help a girl with female athlete triad. Coaches, parents, physical therapists, pediatricians and adolescent medicine specialists, nutritionists and dietitians, and mental health specialists can all work together to treat the physical and emotional problems that a girl with female athlete triad faces.

It might be tempting to shrug off several months of missed periods, but getting help right away is important. In the short term, female athlete triad may lead to muscle weakness, stress fractures, and reduced physical performance. Over the long term, it can cause bone weakness, long-term effects on the reproductive system, and heart problems.

A girl who is recovering from female athlete triad might work with a dietitian to help reach and maintain a healthy weight while eating enough calories and nutrients for health and good athletic performance. Depending on how much the girl is exercising, she may have to reduce the length of her workouts. Talking to a psychologist or therapist can help her deal with depression, pressure from coaches or family members, or low self-esteem and can help her find ways to deal with her problems other than restricting food intake or exercising excessively.

Some girls may need to take hormones to supply their bodies with estrogen to help prevent further bone loss. Calcium and vitamin D supplementation can also help when someone has bone loss as the result of female athlete triad.

What If I Think Someone I Know Has It?

It's tempting to ignore female athlete triad and hope it goes away. But it requires help from a doctor and other health professionals. If a friend, sister, or teammate has signs and symptoms of female athlete triad, discuss your concerns with her and encourage her to seek treatment. If she refuses, you may need to mention your concern to a parent, coach, teacher, or school nurse.

You might worry about seeming nosy when you ask questions about a friend's health, but you're not: Your concern is a sign that you're a caring friend. Lending an ear may be just what your friend needs.

Tips for Female Athletes

Here are a few tips to help teen athletes stay on top of their physical condition:

- Keep track of your periods. It's easy to forget when you had your last visit from Aunt Flo, so keep a calendar in your gym bag and mark down when your period starts and stops and if the bleeding is particularly heavy or light. That way, if you start missing periods, you'll know right away and you'll have accurate information to give to your doctor.

- Don't skip meals or snacks. If you're constantly on the go between school, practice, and competitions you may be tempted to skip meals and snacks to save time. But eating now will improve performance later, so stock your locker or bag with quick and easy favorites such as bagels, string cheese, unsalted nuts and seeds, raw vegetables, granola bars, and fruit.

- Visit a dietitian or nutritionist who works with teen athletes. He or she can help you get your dietary game plan into gear and find out if you're getting enough key nutrients such as iron, calcium, and protein. And if you need supplements, a nutritionist can recommend the best choices.

- Do it for you. Pressure from teammates, parents, or coaches can turn a fun activity into a nightmare. If you're not enjoying your

67

sport, make a change. Remember: It's your body and your life. You—not your coach or teammates—will have to live with any damage you do to your body now.

Chapter 10

Orthorexia

Those who are obsessed with healthy eating may be suffering from "orthorcxia nervosa," a term which means literally "fixation on righteous eating." Orthorexia starts out as an innocent attempt to eat more healthfully, but the orthorexic becomes fixated on food quality and purity. They become more and more consumed with what and how much to eat, and how to deal with "slip-ups." An iron-clad will is needed to maintain this rigid eating style. Every day is a day to eat right, be "good," rise above others in dietary prowess, and self-punish if temptation wins (usually stricter eating, fasts, and exercise). Self-esteem becomes wrapped up in the purity of their diet and they often feel superior to others, especially in regard to food intake.

Eventually food choices become so restrictive, with both variety and calories, that health suffers—an ironic twist for a person so completely dedicated to healthy eating. Eventually, the obsession with healthy eating can crowd out other activities and interests, impair relationships, and become physically dangerous.

Is Orthorexia an Eating Disorder?

Orthorexia is a term coined by Steven Bratman, M.D., to describe his own experience with food and eating. It is not an officially recognized disorder, but is similar to other eating disorders—those with

"Orthorexia Nervosa," © 2006 National Eating Disorders Association. For more information visit www.NationalEatingDisorders.org. Reviewed by David A. Cooke, M.D., FACP, September 2010.

anorexia nervosa or bulimia nervosa obsess about calories and weight while orthorexics obsess about healthy eating (not about being "thin" and losing weight).

Why Does Someone Get Orthorexia?

Orthorexia appears to be motivated by health, but there are underlying motivations, which can include safety from poor health, compulsion for complete control, escape from fears, wanting to be thin, improving self-esteem, searching for spirituality through food, and using food to create an identity.

Do I Have Orthorexia?

Consider the following questions. The more "yes" responses, the more likely you are dealing with orthorexia:

- Do you wish that occasionally you could just eat and not worry about food quality?
- Do you ever wish you could spend less time on food and more time on living and loving?
- Does it sound beyond your ability to eat a meal prepared with love by someone else—one single meal—and not try to control what is served?
- Are you constantly looking for the ways foods are unhealthy for you?
- Do love, joy, play, and creativity take a backseat to having the perfect diet?
- Do you feel guilt or self-loathing when you stray from your diet?
- Do you feel in control when you eat the correct diet?
- Have you positioned yourself on a nutritional pedestal and wonder how others can possibly eat the food they eat?

So What's the Big Deal?

The diet of the orthorexic can actually be unhealthy, with the nutritional problems dependent on the specific diet the person has imposed upon him- or herself. Social problems are more obvious. An orthorexic may be socially isolated, often because they plan their life around food. They may have little room in life for anything other than thinking about and planning food intake. Orthorexics lose the ability to eat intuitively—to know when they are hungry, how much they need, and when they are full. The orthorexic never learns how to eat naturally and is destined to keep "falling off the wagon" and thus feeling shameful, similar to any other diet mentality.

When Orthorexia Becomes All Consuming

Dr. Bratman, who went through orthorexia, states "I pursued wellness through healthy eating for years, but gradually I began to sense that something was going wrong. The poetry of my life was disappearing. My ability to carry on normal conversations was hindered by intrusive thoughts of food. The need to obtain meals free of meat, fat, and artificial chemicals had put nearly all social forms of eating beyond my reach. I was lonely and obsessed. . . . I found it terribly difficult to free myself. I had been seduced by righteous eating. The problem of my life's meaning had been transferred inexorably to food, and I could not reclaim it." (Source: www.orthorexia.com)

Are You Telling Me It's Unhealthy to Follow a Healthy Diet?

Following a healthy diet does not mean you are orthorexic, and nothing is wrong with eating healthfully. Unless, however, (1) it is taking up an inordinate amount of time and attention in your life; (2) deviating from that diet is met with guilt and self-loathing; and/or (3) it is used to avoid life issues.

What Is the Treatment for Orthorexia?

Society pushes healthy eating and thinness, so it is easy for many to not realize how problematic this behavior can become. Even more difficult is that the person doing the healthy eating can hide behind the thought that they are simply eating well (and that others do not). Further complicating treatment is the fact that motivation behind orthorexia is multifaceted. First, the orthorexic must admit there is a problem, then identify what caused the obsession. They must also become more flexible and less dogmatic with their eating. There will be deeper emotional issues, and working through them will make the transition to normal eating easier.

While orthorexia is not a condition your doctor will diagnose, recovery can require professional help. A practitioner skilled at treating those with eating disorders is the best choice. This chapter can be used to help the professional understand more about orthorexia.

Recovery

The recovered orthorexic will still eat healthfully, but there will be a different understanding of what healthy eating is. They will realize that food will not make them a better person and that basing their self-esteem on the quality of their diet is irrational. Their identity will shift from "the person who eats health food" to a broader definition of who they are—a person who loves, who works, who is fun. They will find that while food is important, it is one small aspect of life and, often, there are things that are more important!

Reference

The Orthorexia Home Page. (2003). Retrieved February 8, 2006, from http://www.orthorexia.com.

Chapter 11

Pica and Rumination Disorder

Chapter Contents

Section 11.1

Pica

Many young kids put nonfood items in their mouths at one time or another. They're naturally curious about their environment and might, for instance, eat some dirt out of the sandbox.

Kids with pica, however, go beyond this innocent exploration of their surroundings. As many as 25 to 30 percent of kids (and 20 percent of those seen in mental health clinics) have the eating disorder pica, which is characterized by persistent and compulsive cravings (lasting one month or longer) to eat nonfood items.

About Pica

The word *pica* comes from the Latin word for magpie, a bird known for its large and indiscriminate appetite.

Pica is most common in people with developmental disabilities, including autism and mental retardation, and in children between the ages of two and three. Although kids younger than eighteen to twenty-four months can try to eat nonfood items, it isn't necessarily considered abnormal at that age.

Pica is also a behavior that may surface in children who've had a brain injury affecting their development. It can also be a problem for some pregnant women, as well as people with epilepsy.

People with pica frequently crave and consume nonfood items such as:

- dirt;
- clay;
- paint chips;
- plaster;
- chalk;
- cornstarch;
- laundry starch;
- baking soda;
- coffee grounds;
- cigarette ashes;
- burnt match heads;
- cigarette butts;

- feces;
- ice;
- glue;
- hair;
- buttons;
- paper;
- sand;
- toothpaste;
- soap.

Although consumption of some items may be harmless, pica is considered to be a serious eating disorder that can sometimes result in serious health problems such as lead poisoning and iron-deficiency anemia.

Signs of Pica

Look for these warning signs that your child may have pica:

- Repetitive consumption of nonfood items, despite efforts to restrict it, for a period of at least one month or longer.

- The behavior is considered inappropriate for your child's age or developmental stage (older than eighteen to twenty-four months).

- The behavior is not part of a cultural, ethnic, or religious practice.

Why Do Some People Eat Nonfood Items?

The specific causes of pica are unknown, but certain conditions and situations can increase a person's risk for pica:

- Nutritional deficiencies, such as iron or zinc, that may trigger specific cravings (however, the nonfood items craved usually don't supply the minerals lacking in the person's body)

- Dieting—people who diet may attempt to ease hunger by eating nonfood substances to get a feeling of fullness

- Malnutrition, especially in underdeveloped countries, where people with pica most commonly eat soil or clay

- Cultural factors—in families, religions, or groups in which eating nonfood substances is a learned practice

- Parental neglect, lack of supervision, or food deprivation—often seen in children living in poverty

- Developmental problems, such as mental retardation, autism, other developmental disabilities, or brain abnormalities

- Mental health conditions, such as obsessive-compulsive disorder (OCD) and schizophrenia

- Pregnancy, but it's been suggested that pica during pregnancy occurs more frequently in women who exhibited similar practices during their childhood or before pregnancy or who have a history of pica in their family

Theories about what causes pica abound. One is that a nutritional deficiency, such as iron deficiency, can trigger specific cravings. Evidence supports that at least some pica cases are a response to dietary deficiency—nutritional deficiencies often are associated with pica and their correction often improves symptoms. Some pregnant women, for example, will stop eating nonfood items after being treated for iron-deficiency anemia, a common condition among pregnant women with pica.

However, not everyone responds when a nutritional deficiency is corrected, which may be a consequence of pica rather than the cause, and some people with pica don't have a documented nutritional deficiency.

Known as geophagia, eating earth substances such as clay or dirt is a form of pica that can cause iron deficiency. One theory to explain pica is that in some cultures, eating clay or dirt may help relieve nausea (and therefore, morning sickness), control diarrhea, increase salivation, remove toxins, and alter odor or taste perception.

Some people claim to enjoy the taste and texture of dirt or clay, and eat it as part of a daily habit (much like smoking is a daily routine for others). And some psychological theories explain pica as a behavioral response to stress or an indication that the individual has an oral fixation (is comforted by having things in his or her mouth).

Another explanation is that pica is a cultural feature of certain religious rituals, folk medicine, and magical beliefs. For example, some people in various cultures believe that eating dirt will help them incorporate magical spirits into their bodies.

None of these theories, though, explains every form of pica. A doctor must treat each case individually to try to understand what's causing the condition.

When to Call the Doctor

If your child is at risk for pica, talk to your doctor. If your child has consumed a harmful substance, seek medical care immediately. If you think your child has ingested something poisonous, call Poison Control at (800) 222-1222.

A child who continues to consume nonfood items may be at risk for serious health problems, including:

- lead poisoning (from eating paint chips in older buildings with lead-based paint);

- bowel problems (from consuming indigestible substances like hair, cloth, etc.);

- intestinal obstruction or perforation (from eating objects that could get lodged in the intestines);

- dental injury (from eating hard substances that could harm the teeth);

- parasitic infections (from eating dirt or feces).

Medical emergencies and death can occur if the craved substance is toxic or contaminated with lead or mercury, or if the item forms an indigestible mass blocking the intestines. Pica involving lead-containing substances during pregnancy may be associated with an increase in both maternal and fetal lead levels.

What Will the Doctor Do?

Your doctor will play an important role in helping you manage and prevent pica-related behaviors, educating you on teaching your child about acceptable and unacceptable food substances. The doctor will also work with you to find ways to restrict the nonfood items your child craves (i.e., using child-safety locks and high shelving, and keeping household chemicals and medications out of reach). Some kids require behavioral intervention and families may need to work with a psychologist or other mental health professional.

Depending on a child's age and developmental stage, doctors will work with kids to teach them ways to eat more appropriately. Medication may also be prescribed if pica is associated with significant behavioral problems not responding to behavioral treatments.

Your doctor may check for anemia or other nutritional deficiencies, if indicated. A child who has ingested a potentially harmful substance, such as lead, will be screened for lead and other toxic substances and might undergo stool testing for parasites. In some cases, x-rays or other imaging may be helpful to identify what was eaten or to look for bowel problems, such as an obstruction.

Fortunately, pica is usually a temporary condition that improves as kids get older or following pregnancy. But for individuals with developmental or mental health issues, pica can be a more prolonged concern.

Following treatment, if your child's pica behavior continues beyond several weeks despite attempts to intervene, contact your doctor again for additional treatment. Remember that patience is key in treating pica because it can take time for some kids to stop wanting to eat nonfood items.

Section 11.2

Rumination Disorder

Rumination disorder is a condition in which a person keeps bringing up food from the stomach into the mouth (regurgitation) and re-chewing the food.

Causes

Rumination disorder usually starts after age three months, following a period of normal digestion. It occurs in infants and is rare in children and teenagers. The cause is often unknown. Certain problems, such as lack of stimulation of the infant, neglect, and high-stress family situations, have been associated with the disorder.

Rumination disorder may also occur in adults.

Symptoms

- Repeatedly bringing up (regurgitating) food
- Repeatedly re-chewing food

Symptoms must go on for at least one month to fit the definition of rumination disorder.

People do not appear to be upset, retching, or disgusted when they bring up food. It may appear to cause pleasure.

Exams and Tests

The healthcare provider must first rule out physical causes, such as hiatal hernia and pyloric stenosis. These conditions can be mistaken for rumination disorder.

Rumination disorder can cause malnutrition. The following lab tests can measure how severe the malnutrition is and determine what nutrients need to be increased:

- Blood test for anemia

- Endocrine—hormone functions
- Serum electrolytes

Treatment

Rumination disorder is treated with behavioral techniques. One treatment associates bad consequences with rumination and good consequences with more appropriate behavior (mild aversive training).

Other techniques include improving the environment (if there is abuse or neglect) and counseling the parents.

Outlook (Prognosis)

In some cases rumination disorder will disappear on its own, and the child will go back to eating normally without treatment. In other cases, treatment is necessary.

Possible Complications

- Failure to thrive
- Lowered resistance to disease
- Malnutrition

When to Contact a Medical Professional

Call your healthcare provider if your baby appears to be repeatedly spitting up, vomiting, or re-chewing food.

Prevention

There is no known prevention. However, normal stimulation and healthy parent-child relationships may help reduce the odds of rumination disorder.

References

Boris NW, Dalton R. Vegetative disorders. In: Kliegman RM, Behrman RE, Jenson HB, Stanton BF, eds. *Nelson Textbook of Pediatrics*. 18th ed. Philadelphia, Pa: Saunders Elsevier;2007:chap 22.

Chapter 12

Sleep Eating

Overview

Sleep eating is a sleep-related disorder, although some specialists consider it to be a combination of a sleep and an eating disorder. It is a relatively rare and little known condition that is gaining recognition in sleep medicine. Other names for sleep eating are sleep-related eating (disorder), nocturnal sleep-related eating disorder (NS-RED), and sleep-eating syndrome.

Sleep eating is characterized by sleepwalking and excessive nocturnal overeating (compulsive hyperphagia). Sleep eaters are comparable to sleepwalkers in many ways: they are at risk for self-injury during an episode, they may (or may not) experience excessive daytime sleepiness, and they are usually emotionally distressed, tired, angry, or anxious. Sleep eaters are also at risk for the same health complications as compulsive overeaters, with the added dangers of sleepwalking. Common concerns include excessive weight gain, daytime sleepiness, choking while eating, sleep disruption, and injury from cooking or preparing food such as from knives, utensils, or hot cooking surfaces. There is also the potential for starting a fire.

As with sleepwalkers, sleep eaters are unaware and unconscious of their behavior. If there is any memory of the episode, it is usually sketchy. A sleep eater will roam the house, particularly the kitchen,

"Sleep Eating," © 2000 Talk About Sleep (www.talkaboutsleep.com). Reprinted with permission. Editor's note added by David A. Cooke, M.D., FACP, September 2010.

and may eat large quantities of food (as well as non-food items). In the morning, sleep eaters have no recollection of the episode. However, in many cases there are clues to their behavior. One woman woke up with a stomachache and chocolate smeared on her face and hands. Candy wrappers littered the kitchen floor. The next morning her husband informed her that she had been eating during the night. She was shocked and distressed because she had no recollection of the event.

As in the case described above, food consumed by sleep eaters tends to be either high sugar or high fat. Odd combinations of foods, such as potato chips dipped in peanut butter or butter smeared on hotdogs, as well as non-food items, have been reported. Oddly, one person was discovered cutting a bar of soap into slices and then eating it as if it were a slice of cheese!

Sleep eating is classified as a parasomnia. It is a rare version of sleepwalking, which is an arousal disorder. In 1968, Roger Broughton published a paper in *Science* (159: 1070–78) that outlined the major features of arousal disorders. They are:

- abnormal behavior that occurs during an arousal from slow wave sleep;
- the absence of awareness during the episode;
- automatic and repetitive motor activity;
- slow reaction time and reduced sensitivity to environment;
- difficulty in waking despite vigorous attempts;
- no memory of the episode in the morning (retrograde amnesia); and
- no or little dream recall associated with the event.

How Common Is Sleep Eating?

The actual number of sleep-eating sufferers is unknown; however, it is estimated that 1 to 3 percent of the population is affected by sleep eating. A higher percentage of persons with eating disorders, as many as 10 to 15 percent, are affected. For this reason, sleep eating is more common in younger women. Symptoms typically begin in the late twenties. Episodes may reoccur, in combination with a stressful situation, or an episode may occur only once or twice. Additionally, many parasomnias seem to run in families, which may indicate that sleep eating is genetically linked.

When Should I See a Doctor?

In many cases, sleep eating is the outward sign of an underlying problem. Many sufferers are overweight and dieting. When their control is diminished by sleep, these individuals binge at night to satisfy their hunger. Some sleep eaters have histories of alcoholism, drug abuse, or a primary sleep disorder, such as sleepwalking, restless legs syndrome, or sleep apnea. An article in *Sleep* (October 1991: 14(5): 419–31) suggested that sleep eating is directly linked to the onset of another medical problem.

Because sleep eating occurs in people that are usually dieting and emotionally distressed, attempts at weight loss may be unsuccessful and cause even more stress. Compounded with the dangers of sleepwalking, compulsive eating while asleep is a sleep disorder that results in weight gain, disrupted sleep, and daytime sleepiness. As these consequences of sleep eating impact daily living, the necessity of seeing a healthcare professional becomes more important.

Parasomnias are complex and often serious in nature. If you think you suffer from sleep eating, consult with your physician or a healthcare professional who can refer you to a sleep disorders treatment center. It is strongly recommended that a sleep specialist carry out the diagnosis and treatment. Medical or psychological evaluation should also be investigated.

How Is Sleep Eating Treated?

The first step in treating any sleep disorder is to ascertain any underlying causes. As with most parasomnias, sleep eating is usually the result of an underlying problem, which may include another sleep disorder, prescription drug abuse, nicotine withdrawal, chronic autoimmune hepatitis, encephalitis (or hypothalmic injury), or acute stress (*Sleep* 1991 Oct; 14(5): 419–31).

It is important to keep in mind that throughout life, people experience varying patterns of sleep and nutrition during positive and negative situations. Problems with eating are defined as overeating or not eating enough. Problems with sleeping can be simplified with two symptoms, too much or not enough sleep. Medical attention is required for abnormal behaviors in either or both areas.

For some people who have been diagnosed with sleep eating, interventions without the use of medications have proven helpful. Courses on stress management, group or one-on-one counseling with a therapist, or self-confidence training may alleviate the stress and anxiety that leads to nighttime bingeing. Although considered an alternative treatment, hypnosis may be an option for some sleep eaters. A change in diet that includes avoiding certain foods and eating at specified times of the day, as well as reducing the intake of caffeine or alcohol, may be therapeutic. Professional advice may also suggest avoiding certain medications.

If the underlying problem is diagnosed as sleepwalking, medications in the benzodiazepine family have had some success. In sleepwalkers, this class of drugs reduces motor activity during sleep. Another class of drug found to be effective for sleep eaters has been the dopaminergic agents such as Sinemet® (carbidopa plus levodopa) and Mirapex® (pramipexole dihydrochloride).

Night Eating: Another Disorder of Sleep and Eating

A similar sleep-related eating disorder has also been clinically described. It is different from sleep eating in that the individual is awake during episodes of nocturnal bingeing. This disorder has many names: nocturnal eating (or drinking) syndrome, nighttime hunger, nocturnal eating, night eating or drinking (syndrome), or the "Dagwood" syndrome. Affected individuals are physically unable to sleep without food intake.

The *Merck Manual* lists night eating under the heading obesity. It states that the disorder "consists of morning anorexia, excessive ingestion of food in the evening, and insomnia." Because night eating is associated with increased weight gain as well as insomnia, this may cause the individual stress, anxiety, or depression.

Night eating or drinking may occur once or many times during the night. It is diagnosed when 50 percent or more of an individual's diet is consumed between sleeping hours. Unlike sleep eaters, this person will eat foods that are similar to his/her normal diet.

People who are night eaters typically avoid food until noon or later, eat small portions frequently when they do eat, and binge in the evening. They are usually overweight and in adults, overly stressed or anxious. They will also complain of not being able to maintain sleep or not being able to initiate sleep. For night eaters, the urge to eat is an abnormal need, rather than true hunger, according to an article in *Sleep* by Italian researchers (September 1997; 20(9): 734–38).

Night eaters/drinkers are usually children, although the disorder can occur in adults. For children, eating or drinking at night is a conditioned behavior. This is a common occurrence for babies, but most infants can sleep the entire night by the age of six months. Sleep disturbance can persist to an older age if the child is allowed a bottle or drinks throughout the night. An older child may consistently wake up during the night and ask for a drink or something to eat and refuse to return to bed until the snack is consumed. In this case, the caregiver should identify actual need versus repeated requests.

According to the International Classification of Sleep Disorders, night eating is characterized as a dyssomnia (as opposed to sleep eating, which is considered a parasomnia). A dyssomnia is a disorder of sleep or wakefulness in which insomnia or excessive daytime sleepiness daytime sleepiness is a complaint. Within the heading of dyssomnia, night eating is classified as an extrinsic sleep disorder, which means that it originates, develops, or is caused by an external source. Eating or drinking at night is usually a conditioned, conscious behavior; although it is a disorder, in many cases night eating is not caused by a psychological or medical condition.

Night eating may arise because of an ulcer, by dieting during the day, by undue stress, or by a routine expectation (conditioned behavior). Hypoglycemia, or low blood sugar, has also been proposed as possible cause of nighttime bingeing in some people. This can be determined by a glucose tolerance test.

How Is Night Eating Treated?

For children, treatment of this disorder mainly involves the caregiver. For a young child, weaning from the breast, bottle, or drinks during the night is essential. The adult should evaluate if the request for food or drink is based on real need. If the demand is false, the adult should deny the request. Eventually, waking up with the urge for food or drink will be eliminated.

For an adult, it is important to first recognize that the behavior is not normal. (If the pattern of eating at night has been persistent for a long time, a night eater may only complain of insomnia and weight gain.) Secondly, a night eater should schedule an appointment with a physician. Night eating may be the result of a medical condition or hypoglycemia, both of which can be treated. If not, the habit of eating in the middle of the night can be broken with behavior modification and/or stress reduction. Eating frequent small meals during the day beginning in the morning, reducing carbohydrate intake, and increasing protein intake before bedtime are diet patterns that may help. Protein metabolizes slowly and will stabilize blood sugar levels during sleep. Contrary to protein, sugary snacks raise the blood sugar quickly, then cause it to plunge. So, avoid sweet foods before bedtime.

Night eaters who have conquered their uncontrollable need for nocturnal food or drink often sleep equally as well or better than before they started night eating.

Notes from the Health Reference Series *Medical Editor*

Over the past decade, an association between the popular sleeping medication zolpidem (Ambien®) has been recognized. Sleep eating will emerge for the first time in some patients when they take this medication and typically improve if the medication is stopped. It is possible that other sleeping medications may have the same effect.

There have also been developments in the treatment of sleep eating and night eating. For sleep eating, the antidepressant medication Wellbutrin® (bupropion) has been reported to be effective. Several studies have reported that the antidepressant Zoloft® (sertraline) is effective for night eating. The antiseizure drug Topamax® (topiramate) has been reported to be effective for both sleep eating and night eating.

Chapter 13

Eating Disorder Not Otherwise Specified (EDNOS)

What is eating disorder not otherwise specified (EDNOS)?

The *Diagnostic and Statistical Manual—4th Edition* (*DSM-IV*) recognizes two distinct eating disorder types, anorexia nervosa and bulimia nervosa. If a person is struggling with eating disorder thoughts, feelings, or behaviors, but does not have all the symptoms of anorexia or bulimia, that person may be diagnosed with eating disorder not otherwise specified (EDNOS). The following section lists examples of how an individual may have a profound eating problem and not have anorexia nervosa or bulimia nervosa:

- A female patient could meet all of the diagnostic criteria for anorexia nervosa except she is still having her periods.

- A person could meet all of the diagnostic criteria for anorexia nervosa except that, despite significant weight loss, the individual's current weight is in the normal range.

- A person could meet all of the diagnostic criteria for bulimia nervosa except that the binge eating and inappropriate compensatory mechanisms occur at a frequency of less than twice a week or for duration of less than three months.

- The person could use inappropriate compensatory behavior by an individual of normal body weight after eating small amounts of food (e.g., self-induced vomiting after the consumption of two cookies). This variant is often called purging disorder.

- The person could repeatedly chew and spit out, but not swallow, large amounts of food.

- Binge-eating disorder is also officially an EDNOS category: recurrent episodes of binge eating in the absence of the regular use of inappropriate compensatory behaviors characteristic of bulimia nervosa.

The examples provided above illustrate the variety of ways disordered eating can look when a person has EDNOS, but this list of examples does not provide a complete picture of the many different ways that eating disorder symptoms can occur.

The "not otherwise specified" label often suggests to people that these disorders are not as important, as serious, or as common as anorexia or bulimia nervosa. This is not true. Far more individuals suffer from EDNOS than from bulimia and anorexia combined, and the risks associated with having EDNOS are often just as profound as with anorexia or bulimia because many people with EDNOS engage in the same risky, damaging behaviors seen in other eating disorders.

Individuals with EDNOS who are losing weight and restricting their caloric intake often report the same fears and obsessions as patients with anorexia. They may be overly driven to be thin, have very disturbed body image, restrict their caloric intake to unnatural and unhealthy limits, and may eventually suffer the same psychological, physiological, and social consequences of anorexic people. Those who binge, purge, or binge and purge typically report the same concerns as people with bulimia, namely, that they feel they need to purge to control their weight, that they are afraid of getting out of control with their eating, and that binging and/or purging often turn into a very addictive, yet ineffective coping strategy that they feel they cannot do without. In all meaningful ways, people with EDNOS are very similar to those with anorexia or bulimia, and are just as likely to require extensive, specialized, multidisciplinary treatment.

Who develops EDNOS?

EDNOS typically begins in adolescence or early adulthood although it can occur at any time throughout the lifespan. Like anorexia nervosa and bulimia, EDNOS is far more common in females; however, among those individuals whose primary symptom is binge eating, the number of males and females is more even. Because EDNOS has not been studied as extensively as anorexia and bulimia, it is harder to gauge an exact prevalence, but estimates suggest that EDNOS accounts for almost three-quarters of all community-treated eating disorder cases.

What are the common signs of EDNOS?

Signs of EDNOS are the same signs you would look for in anorexia and bulimia nervosa. Constant concern about food and weight is a primary sign, as are behaviors designed to restrict eating or compensate for eating (such as exercise or purging). For individuals who binge, most notable is the disappearance of large amounts of food, long periods of eating, or noticeable blocks of time when the individual is alone. Individuals who restrict often find the need to eat by the end of the day and the urge is so strong that it results in a binge. This binge can lead to guilt and shame that leads to purging, which may prompt the individual to promise to "do better tomorrow" by restricting. Cycles like this are consistent with EDNOS and bulimia, and can become very intractable if not addressed. Characteristically, these individuals have many rules about food—e.g., good foods, bad foods—and can be entrenched in these rules and particular thinking patterns. This preoccupation and these behaviors allow the person to shift their focus from painful feelings and reduce tension and anxiety perpetuating the need for these behaviors appropriately.

Are there any serious medical complications?

Individuals with EDNOS are at risk for many of the medical complications of anorexia or bulimia, depending on the symptoms they have. Those who binge and purge run risks similar to bulimia in that they can severely damage their bodies. Electrolyte imbalance and dehydration can occur and may cause cardiac complications and, occasionally, sudden death. In rare instances, binge eating can cause the stomach to rupture, and purging can result in heart failure due to the loss of vital minerals like potassium. Persons with EDNOS who are restricting may have low blood pressure, slower heart rate, disruption of hormones and bone growth, and significant mental and emotional disturbance.

Do we know what causes EDNOS?

As with other eating disorders that have been more widely studied, the cause of EDNOS is most likely a combination of environmental and biological factors that contribute to the development and expression of these disorders. While each individual may feel that they developed these behaviors "on their own" they are often amazed to find that other people have the same obsessions, irrational fears, and self-loathing. They are not alone, and they are not to blame for having this problem.

Is treatment available for persons with EDNOS?

Unfortunately, treatment studies specifically for EDNOS are rare. Cognitive-behavioral therapy, either in a group setting or individual therapy session, has been shown to benefit many people with bulimia and would logically be applicable to those with EDNOS who binge or purge. It focuses on self-monitoring of eating and purging behaviors as well as changing the distorted thinking patterns associated with the disorder. Cognitive-behavioral therapy is often combined with nutritional counseling and/or antidepressant medications such as fluoxetine (Prozac®).

Treatment plans should be adjusted to meet the needs of the individual concerned, but usually a comprehensive treatment plan involving a variety of experts and approaches is best. It is important to take an approach that involves developing support for the person with an eating disorder from the family environment or within the patient's community environment (support groups or other socially supportive environments).

What about prevention?

Prevention research is increasing as scientists study the known "risk factors" for these disorders. Given that EDNOS and other eating disorders are multi-determined and often affect young people, there is preliminary information on the role and extent such factors as self-esteem, resilience, family interactions, peer pressure, the media, and dieting might play in its development. Eating disorders and body image are commonly seen as a problem affecting women, but men are also touched by media influence. Steroid abuse and body image to create the strong, cut male physique results in many short- and long-term effects, but falls under the radar in terms of indicating distorted body image and eating disorders. Advocacy groups are also engaged in prevention through efforts such as removing damaging articles from teen magazines on "dieting" and the importance of being thin.

Chapter 14

Disorders Often Accompanying Eating Disorders

Chapter Contents

Section 14.1

Body Dysmorphic Disorder

"Body Dysmorphic Disorder," November 2007, reprinted with permission from www.kidshealth.org. Copyright © 2009 The Nemours Foundation. This information was provided by KidsHealth, one of the largest resources online for medically reviewed health information written for parents, kids, and teens. For more articles like this one, visit www.KidsHealth.org, or www.TeensHealth.org.

Focusing on Appearance

Most of us spend time in front of the mirror checking our appearance. Some people spend more time than others, but taking care of our bodies and being interested in our appearance is natural.

How we feel about our appearance is part of our body image and self-image. Lots of people have some kind of dissatisfaction with their bodies. This can be especially true during the teen years when our bodies and appearance go through lots of changes.

Although many people feel dissatisfied with some aspect of their appearance, these concerns usually don't constantly occupy their thoughts or cause them to feel tormented. But for some people, concerns about appearance become quite extreme and upsetting.

Some people become so focused on imagined or minor imperfections in their looks that they can't seem to stop checking or obsessing about their appearance. Being constantly preoccupied and upset about body imperfections or appearance flaws is called body dysmorphic disorder.

What Is Body Dysmorphic Disorder?

Body dysmorphic disorder (BDD) is a condition that involves obsessions, which are distressing thoughts that repeatedly intrude into a person's awareness. With BDD, the distressing thoughts are about perceived appearance flaws.

People with BDD might focus on what they think is a facial flaw, but they can also worry about other body parts, such as short legs, breast size, or body shape. Just as people with eating disorders obsess about their weight, people with BDD become obsessed over an aspect of their appearance. People with BDD may worry their hair is thin, their face is scarred, their eyes aren't exactly the same size, their nose is too big, or their lips are too thin.

BDD has been called "imagined ugliness" because the appearance issues the person is obsessing about usually are so small that others don't even notice them. Or, if others do notice them, they consider them minor. But for a person with BDD, the concerns feel very real, because the obsessive thoughts distort and magnify any tiny imperfection.

Because of the distorted body image caused by BDD, a person might believe that he or she is too horribly ugly or disfigured to be seen.

Behaviors That Are Part of BDD

Besides obsessions, BDD also involves compulsions and avoidance behaviors.

A compulsion is something a person does to try to relieve the tension caused by the obsessive thoughts. For example, someone with obsessive thoughts that her nose is horribly ugly might check her appearance in the mirror, apply makeup, or ask someone many times a day whether her nose looks ugly. These types of checking, fixing, and asking are compulsions.

A person with obsessions usually feels a strong or irresistible urge to do compulsions because they can provide temporary relief from the terrible distress. To someone with obsessions, compulsions seem like the only way to escape bad feelings caused by bad thoughts. Compulsive actions often are repeated many times a day, taking up lots of a person's time and energy.

Avoidance behaviors are also a part of BDD. A person might stay home or cover up to avoid being seen by others. Avoidance behaviors also include things like not participating in class or socializing, or avoiding mirrors.

With BDD, a pattern of obsessive thoughts, compulsive actions, and avoidance sets in. Even though the checking, fixing, asking, and avoiding seem to relieve terrible feelings, the relief is just temporary. In reality, the more a person performs compulsions or avoids things, the stronger the pattern of obsessions, compulsions, and avoidance becomes.

After a while, it takes more and more compulsions to relieve the distress caused by the bad thoughts. A person with BDD doesn't want to be preoccupied with these thoughts and behaviors, but with BDD it can seem impossible to break the pattern.

What Causes BDD?

Although the exact cause of BDD is still unclear, experts believe it is related to problems with serotonin, one of the brain's chemical neurotransmitters. Poor regulation of serotonin also plays a role in obsessive compulsive disorder (OCD) and other anxiety disorders, as well as depression.

Some people may be more prone to problems with serotonin balance, including those with family members who have problems with anxiety or depression. This may help explain why some people develop BDD but others don't.

Cultural messages can also play a role in BDD by reinforcing a person's concerns about appearance. Critical messages or unkind teasing about appearance as someone is growing up may also contribute to a person's sensitivity to BDD. But while cultural messages, criticism, and teasing might harm somebody's body image, these things alone usually do not result in BDD.

It's hard to know exactly how common BDD is because not many people with BDD are willing to talk about their concerns or seek help. But compared with people who feel somewhat dissatisfied with their appearance, very few people have true BDD. BDD usually begins in the teen years, and if it's not treated, can continue into adulthood.

How BDD Can Affect a Person's Life

Sometimes people with BDD feel ashamed and keep their concerns secret. They may think that others will consider them vain or superficial.

Sometimes other people become annoyed or irritated with somebody's obsessions and compulsions about appearance. They don't understand BDD or what the person is going through. As a result, people with BDD may feel misunderstood, unfairly judged, or alone. Because they avoid contact with others, they may have few friends or activities to enjoy.

It's extremely upsetting to be tormented by thoughts about appearance imperfections. These thoughts intrude into a person's awareness throughout the day and are hard to ignore. People with mild to moderate symptoms of BDD usually spend a great deal of time grooming themselves in the morning. Throughout the day, they may frequently check their appearance in mirrors or windows. In addition, they may repeatedly seek reassurance from people around them that they look OK.

Although people with mild BDD usually continue to go to school, the obsessions can interfere with their daily lives. For example, someone might measure or examine the "flawed" body part repeatedly or spend large sums of money and time on makeup to cover the problem. Some people with BDD hide from others, and avoid going places because of fear of being seen. Spending so much time and energy on appearance concerns robs a person of pleasure and happiness, and of opportunities for fun and socializing.

People with severe symptoms may drop out of school, quit their jobs, or refuse to leave their homes. Many people with BDD also develop depression. People with the most severe BDD may even consider or attempt suicide.

Many people with BDD seek the help of a dermatologist or cosmetic surgeon to try to correct appearance flaws. But dermatology treatments or plastic surgery don't change the BDD. People with BDD who find cosmetic surgeons willing to perform surgery are often not satisfied with the results. They may find that even though their appearance has changed, the obsessive thinking is still present, and they begin to focus on some other imperfection.

Getting Help for BDD

If you or someone you know has BDD, the first step is recognizing what might be causing the distress. Many times, people with BDD are so focused on their appearance that they believe the answer lies in correcting how they look, not with their thoughts.

The real problem with BDD lies in the obsessions and compulsions, which are distorting a person's body image, making that person feel ugly. Because people with BDD believe what they are perceiving is true and accurate, sometimes the most challenging part of overcoming the disorder is being open to new ideas about what might help.

BDD can be treated by an experienced mental health professional. Usually, the treatment involves a type of talk therapy called cognitive-behavioral therapy. This approach helps to correct the pattern that's causing the body image distortion and the extreme distress.

In cognitive-behavioral therapy, a therapist helps a person to examine and change faulty beliefs, resist compulsive behaviors, and face stressful situations that trigger appearance concerns. Sometimes doctors prescribe medication along with the talk therapy.

Treatment for BDD takes time, hard work, and patience. It helps if a person has the support of a friend or loved one. If someone with BDD is also dealing with depression, anxiety, feeling isolated or alone, or other life situations, the therapy can address those issues, too.

Body dysmorphic disorder, like other obsessions, can interfere with a person's life, robbing it of pleasure and draining energy. An experienced psychologist or psychiatrist who is knowledgeable about BDD can help break the grip of the disorder so that a person can fully enjoy life.

Section 14.2

Compulsive Exercise

Melissa has been a track fanatic since she was twelve years old. She has run the mile in meets in junior high and high school, constantly improving her times and winning several medals. Best of all, Melissa truly loves her sport.

Recently, however, Melissa's parents have noticed a change in their daughter. She used to return tired but happy from practice and relax with her family, but now she's hardly home for fifteen minutes before she heads out for another run on her own. On many days, she gets up to run before school. When she's unable to squeeze in extra runs, she becomes irritable and anxious. And she no longer talks about how much fun track is, just how many miles she has to run today and how many more she should run tomorrow.

Melissa is living proof that even though exercise has many positive benefits, too much can be harmful. Teens, like Melissa, who exercise compulsively are at risk for both physical and psychological problems.

What Is Compulsive Exercise?

Compulsive exercise (also called obligatory exercise and anorexia athletica) is best defined by an exercise addict's frame of mind: He or she no longer chooses to exercise but feels compelled to do so and struggles with guilt and anxiety if he or she doesn't work out. Injury, illness, an outing with friends, bad weather—none of these will deter those who compulsively exercise. In a sense, exercising takes over a compulsive exerciser's life because he or she plans life around it.

Of course, it's nearly impossible to draw a clear line dividing a healthy amount of exercise from too much. The government's 2005 dietary guidelines, published by the U.S. Department of Agriculture

(USDA) and the U.S. Department of Health and Human Services (HHS), recommend at least sixty minutes of physical activity for kids and teens on most—if not all—days of the week.

Experts say that repeatedly exercising beyond the requirements for good health is an indicator of compulsive behavior, but because different amounts of exercise are appropriate for different people, this definition covers a range of activity levels. However, several workouts a day, every day, is overdoing it for almost anyone.

Much like with eating disorders, many people who engage in compulsive exercise do so to feel more in control of their lives, and the majority of them are female. They often define their self-worth through their athletic performance and try to deal with emotions like anger or depression by pushing their bodies to the limit. In sticking to a rigorous workout schedule, they seek a sense of power to help them cope with low self-esteem.

Although compulsive exercising doesn't have to accompany an eating disorder, the two often go hand in hand. In anorexia nervosa, the excessive workouts usually begin as a means to control weight and become more and more extreme. As the person's rate of activity increases, the amount he or she eats may also decrease. A person with bulimia may also use exercise as a way to compensate for binge eating.

Compulsive exercise behavior can also grow out of student athletes' demanding practice schedules and their quest to excel. Pressure, both external (from coaches, peers, or parents) and internal, can drive the athlete to go too far to be the best. He or she ends up believing that just one more workout will make the difference between first and second place . . . then keeps adding more workouts.

Eventually, compulsive exercising can breed other compulsive behavior, from strict dieting to obsessive thoughts about perceived flaws. Exercise addicts may keep detailed journals about their exercise schedules and obsess about improving themselves. Unfortunately, these behaviors often compound each other, trapping the person in a downward spiral of negative thinking and low self-esteem.

Why Is Exercising Too Much a Bad Thing?

We all know that regular exercise is an important part of a healthy lifestyle. But few people realize that too much can cause physical and psychological harm:

- Excessive exercise can damage tendons, ligaments, bones, cartilage, and joints, and when minor injuries aren't allowed to heal, they often result in long-term damage. Instead of building muscle, too much exercise actually destroys muscle mass, especially if the body isn't getting enough nutrition, forcing it to break down muscle for energy.

- Girls who exercise compulsively may disrupt the balance of hormones in their bodies. This can change their menstrual cycles (some girls lose their periods altogether, a condition known as amenorrhea) and increase the risk of premature bone loss (a condition known as osteoporosis). And of course, working their bodies so hard leads to exhaustion and constant fatigue.

- An even more serious risk is the stress that excessive exercise can place on the heart, particularly when someone is also engaging in unhealthy weight loss behaviors such as restricting intake, vomiting, and using diet pills or supplements. In extreme cases, the combination of anorexia and compulsive exercise can be fatal.

- Psychologically, exercise addicts are often plagued by anxiety and depression. They may have a negative image of themselves and feel worthless. Their social and academic lives may suffer as they withdraw from friends and family to fixate on exercise. Even if they want to succeed in school or in relationships, working out always comes first, so they end up skipping homework or missing out on time spent with friends.

Warning Signs

A child may be exercising compulsively if he or she:

- won't skip a workout, even if tired, sick, or injured;
- doesn't enjoy exercise sessions, but feels obligated to do them;
- seems anxious or guilty when missing even one workout;
- does miss one workout and exercises twice as long the next time;
- is constantly preoccupied with his or her weight and exercise routine
- doesn't like to sit still or relax because of worry that not enough calories are being burnt;
- has lost a significant amount of weight;
- exercises more after eating more;
- skips seeing friends, gives up activities, and abandons responsibilities to make more time for exercise;

- seems to base self-worth on the number of workouts completed and the effort put into training;

- is never satisfied with his or her own physical achievements.

It's important, too, to recognize the types of athletes who are more prone to compulsive exercise because their sports place a particular emphasis on being thin. Ice skaters, gymnasts, wrestlers, and dancers can feel even more pressure than most athletes to keep their weight down and their body toned. Runners also frequently fall into a cycle of obsessive workouts.

Getting Professional Help

If you recognize two or more warning signs of compulsive exercise in your child, call your doctor to discuss your concerns. After evaluating your child, the doctor may recommend medical treatment and/or other therapy. Because compulsive exercise is so often linked to an eating disorder, a community agency that focuses on treating these disorders might be able to offer advice or referrals. Extreme cases may require hospitalization to get a child's weight back up to a safe range.

Treating a compulsion to exercise is never a quick-fix process—it may take several months or even years. But with time and effort, kids can get back on the road to good health. Therapy can help improve self-esteem and body image, as well as teach them how to deal with emotions. Sessions with a nutritionist can help develop healthy eating habits. Once they know what to watch out for, kids will be better equipped to steer clear of unsafe exercise and eating patterns.

Ways to Help at Home

Parents can do a lot to help a child overcome a compulsion to exercise:

- Involve kids in preparing nutritious meals.

- Combine activity and fun by going for a hike or a bike ride together as a family.

- Be a good body image role model. In other words, don't fixate on your own physical flaws, as that just teaches kids that it's normal to dislike what they see in the mirror.

- Never criticize another family member's weight or body shape, even if you're just kidding around. Such remarks might seem harmless, but they can leave a lasting impression on kids or teens struggling to define and accept themselves.

- Examine whether you're putting too much pressure on your kids to excel, particularly in a sport (because some teens turn to exercise to cope with pressure). Take a look at where kids might be feeling too much pressure. Help them put it in perspective and find other ways to cope.

Most important, just be there with constant support. Point out all of your child's great qualities that have nothing to do with how much he or she works out—small daily doses of encouragement and praise can help improve self-esteem. If you teach kids to be proud of the challenges they've faced and not just the first-place ribbons they've won, they will likely be much happier and healthier kids now and in the long run.

Part Two

Risk Factors for Eating Disorders

Chapter 15

Who Develops Eating Disorders?

Chapter Contents

Section 15.1

Factors that Increase Risk for Eating Disorders

Excerpted from "Eating Disorders," © 2010 A.D.A.M., Inc.
Reprinted with permission.

In the United States, about seven million females and one million males suffer from eating disorders.

Age

Eating disorders occur most often in adolescents and young adults. However, they are becoming increasingly prevalent among young children. Eating disorders are more difficult to identify in young children because they less commonly suspected.

Gender

Eating disorders occur predominantly among girls and women. About 90 to 95 percent of patients with anorexia nervosa, and about 80 percent of patients with bulimia nervosa, are female.

Race and Ethnicity

Most studies of individuals with eating disorders have focused on Caucasian middle-class females. However, eating disorders can affect people of all races and socioeconomic levels.

Personality Disorders

People with eating disorders tend to share similar personality and behavioral traits, including low self-esteem, dependency, and problems with self-direction. Specific psychiatric personality disorders may put people at higher risk for eating disorders.

Avoidant Personalities

Some studies indicate that many patients with anorexia nervosa have avoidant personalities. This personality disorder is characterized by:

- being a perfectionist;

- being emotionally and sexually inhibited;

- having less of a fantasy life than people with bulimia or those without an eating disorder;

- being perceived as always being "good," not being rebellious;

- being terrified of being ridiculed or criticized or of feeling humiliated.

People with anorexia are extremely sensitive to failure, and any criticism, no matter how slight, reinforces their own belief that they are "no good."

Obsessive-Compulsive Personality

Obsessive-compulsive personality defines certain character traits (being a perfectionist, morally rigid, or preoccupied with rules and order). This personality disorder has been strongly associated with a higher risk for anorexia. These traits should not be confused with the anxiety disorder called obsessive-compulsive disorder (OCD), although they may increase the risk for this disorder.

Borderline Personalities

Borderline personality disorder (BPD) is associated with self-destructive and impulsive behaviors. People with BPD tend to have other co-existing mental health problems, including eating disorders.

Narcissistic Personalities

People with narcissistic personalities tend to:

- have an inability to soothe oneself;

- have an inability to empathize with others;

- have a need for admiration;

- be hypersensitive to criticism or defeat.

Accompanying Mental Health Disorders

Many patients with eating disorders experience depression and anxiety disorders. It is not clear if these disorders, particularly obsessive-compulsive disorder (OCD), cause the eating disorders, increase susceptibility to them, or share common biologic causes.

Obsessive-Compulsive Disorder (OCD)

Obsessive-compulsive disorder is an anxiety disorder that may occur in up to two-thirds of patients with anorexia and up to a third of patients with bulimia. Some doctors believe that eating disorders are variants of OCD. Women with anorexia and OCD may become obsessed with exercise, dieting, and food. They often develop compulsive rituals (weighing every bit of food, cutting it into tiny pieces, or putting it into tiny containers).

Other Anxiety Disorders

Other anxiety disorders associated with both bulimia and anorexia include:

- **Phobias:** Phobias often precede the onset of the eating disorder. Social phobias, in which a person is fearful about being humiliated in public, are common in both types of eating disorders.

- **Panic disorder:** Panic disorder often follows the onset of an eating disorder. It is characterized by periodic attacks of anxiety or terror (panic attacks).

- **Post-traumatic stress disorder:** Some patients with serious eating disorders report a past traumatic event (such as sexual, physical, or emotional abuse), and exhibit symptoms of post-traumatic stress disorder (PTSD)—an anxiety disorder that occurs in response to life-threatening circumstances.

Depression

Depression is common in anorexia and bulimia. Major depression is unlikely to be a cause of eating disorders, however, because treating and relieving depression rarely cures an eating disorder. In addition, depression often improves after anorexic patients begin to gain weight.

Being Overweight

Extreme eating disorder behaviors, including use of diet pills, laxatives, diuretics, and vomiting, are reported more often in overweight than normal weight teenagers.

Body Image Disorders

Body Dysmorphic Disorder

Body dysmorphic disorder (BDD) involves a distorted view of one's body that is caused by social, psychologic, or possibly biologic factors. It is often associated with anorexia or bulimia, but it can also occur without any eating disorder. As part of obsessive thinking, some people with BDD may obsess about a perceived deformity in one area of their body.

Muscle Dysmorphia

Muscle dysmorphia is a form of body dysmorphic disorder in which the obsession involves musculature and muscle mass. It tends to occur in men who perceive themselves as being underdeveloped or "puny," which results in excessive bodybuilding, preoccupation with diet, and social problems.

Excessive Physical Activity

Highly competitive athletes are often perfectionists, a trait common among people with eating disorders.

Female Athletes

Excessive exercise is associated with many cases of anorexia (and, to a lesser degree, bulimia). In young female athletes, exercise and low body weight postpone puberty, allowing them to retain a muscular boyish shape without the normal accumulation of fatty tissues in breasts and hips that may blunt their competitive edge. Many coaches and teachers compound the problem by overstressing calorie counting and loss of body fat.

In response, people who are vulnerable to such criticism may feel compelled to strictly diet and lose weight. The term "female athlete triad" is a common and serious disorder that affects young female athletes and dancers. It includes:

- eating disorders, including anorexia;
- amenorrhea (absent or irregular menstruation);
- osteoporosis (bone loss, which is related to low weight).

Male Athletes

Male wrestlers and lightweight rowers are also at risk for excessive dieting. Many high school wrestlers use a method called weight-cutting for rapid weight loss. This process involves food restriction and fluid depletion by using steam rooms, saunas, laxatives, and diuretics. Although male athletes are more apt to resume normal eating patterns once competition ends, studies show that the body fat levels of many wrestlers are still well below their peers during off-season and are often as low as 3 percent during wrestling season.

Diabetes or Other Chronic Diseases

Eating disorders may be more common in teenagers with chronic illness, such as diabetes or asthma. They are particularly serious problems for people with either type 1 or type 2 diabetes:

- Binge eating (without purging) is most common in type 2 diabetes and, in fact, the obesity it causes may even trigger this diabetes in some people.

- Both bulimia and anorexia are common among young people with type 1 diabetes. The combination of diabetes and an eating disorder can have serious health consequences. Some women with diabetes often omit or underuse insulin in order to control weight.

Early Puberty

There appears to be a greater risk for eating disorders and other emotional problems for girls who undergo early menarche and puberty, when the pressures experienced by all adolescents are intensified by experiencing these early physical changes, including normal increased body fat.

Section 15.2

Why Are Women Diagnosed with Eating Disorders More Often Than Men?

"Men, Women, and Eating Disorders," © 2009 Cleveland Center for Eating Disorders (www.eatingdisorderscleveland.org). Reprinted with permission.

Why are eating disorders primarily diagnosed in women over men? From one angle is answer is obvious, many more women than men present for eating disorder treatment. The National Institute of Mental Health suggests that 5 to 15 percent of individuals diagnosed with anorexia or bulimia will be male. Of clients diagnosed with binge eating disorder, 35 percent will be male. But does this really mean that eating disorders are more common in women? Nobody really knows. There are multiple reasons for this confusion:

- **The *DSM IV*:** In the diagnostic manual, the criteria for anorexia is gender biased so that it is relatively certain that more women than men will carry this diagnosis. The *DSM* specifically references the absence or delay of menses as one of the criteria for the identification of anorexia in presenting clients. This may therefore decrease the likelihood that a male will meet the criteria for a diagnosis. Similarly, the criteria for bulimia nervosa speaks of compensatory behaviors such as laxative usage, diuretics, and enemas that are generally marketed more directly toward women. The diagnostic criteria do not include the abuse of muscle building agents, thermogenics, or other agents typically used by men obsessed with body size and shape.

- **Social factors:** The image of a person with an eating disorder in our common culture is most commonly portrayed by the thin young woman with anorexia. For men with anorexia, this likely increases both the shame and stigma associated with the disease and makes them less likely to present for treatment. This stereotype also affects patients with bulimia, which is more commonly diagnosed than anorexia. Because of this misconception, individuals with bulimia may feel their eating disorder is invisible, and may therefore be less likely to present for treatment.

- **Environmentally supporting factors:** Men have a multitude of "acceptable" body types in our culture. This ideal ranges from hyper-thin male models, to Brad Pitt, to hyper-muscular Hulk Hogans. In general, women must adhere only to the thin female ideal. Therefore the social support for eating disorders in women may be significantly higher than for men.

These reasons are not exhaustive and the fact is that we truly do not have a definite answer as to why more women than men present for treatment. What we do know is that this issue requires much more research. Figuring out why so many more women present for treatment than men may help us understand how eating disorders are triggered and thus how to prevent them.

Chapter 16

Eating Disorders in Youth and Young Adults

Chapter Contents

Section 16.1

Eating Disorders in Young Children

"When Very Young Kids Have Eating Disorders" by Abigail H. Natenshon, MA, LCSW, GCFP. © 2010. Reprinted with permission. Abigail H. Natenshon has been a psychotherapist specializing in eating disorders for four decades. As the director of Eating Disorder Specialists of Illinois: a Clinic Without Walls, she has authored two books, *When Your Child Has an Eating Disorder: a Step-by-Step Workbook for Parents and Caregivers* and *Doing What Works: an Integrative System for the Treatment of Eating Disorders from Diagnosis to Recovery*. Natenshon, who is also a Guild Certified Feldenkrais Practitioner, hosts three informative web sites, including www.empoweredparents.com, www.empoweredkidZ.com, and www.treatingeatingdisorders.com.

Although anorexia nervosa typically appears during adolescence, a disturbing number of cases have been appearing in young children as early as age seven or eight. In young children, eating disorders are significantly associated with depression as well as obsessive-compulsive symptomatology. According to Dr. Barton J. Blinder, a Mayo Clinic study of six hundred anorexic patients of all ages found that 3 percent were prepubescent anorexics.

"Young children are challenging to diagnose, as only 38 percent meet the criteria for anorexia nervosa. For example, children with poor growth in height as a result of malnutrition may have an 'expected' weight that is falsely low; amenorrhea as a criterion for anorexia does not apply to young girls (or boys); younger children present at a lower percentage of ideal body weight and lose weight more rapidly." (Natenshon, 2009, p.128) In a suite101.com article (Ellison, January 2000) entitled "Childhood Anorexia," Dr. Blinder argues that a 15 percent weight loss, rather than the usual 25, should be a criterion for diagnosis. Childhood-onset anorexia can delay puberty, physical growth, and breast development. A warning sign of an eating disorder in a young child that is more common than food restriction is a child's inability to control and regulate his or her eating.

It is important that parents learn to distinguish the difference between a clinical eating disorder and other highly prevalent forms of eating dysfunction in infants and small children. These might include selective eating disorder or picky eating syndrome, whose origins stem from sensory integration disturbances which lead to an aversion to certain tastes and textures in the mouth (research has shown that for some taste buds, vegetables take on a distinctly metallic taste.) More severe, neurologically based feeding disorders are often the result of trauma (choking) or early tube feeding and typically accompany other syndromes such as autistic spectrum disorder. Pediatricians invariably fail to acknowledge or diagnose the less extreme eating dysfunctions, as most children with picky eating habits tend to be of normal weight and do not present with physiological problems. The current "wisdom" is that these aversions, which affect approximately 30 percent of children, represent benign preference or immaturity that will be outgrown; the growing number of picky eating adults refutes this prognosis. Children with picky eating syndrome and more severe feeding dysfunctions may suffer stunted growth, poor bone development, sociability problems, and overweight in adulthood; intolerant of new foods, these individuals invariably have difficulty adapting to novelty and change in other life spheres, as well.

Parents are clearly not the cause of their child's eating disorder, with the possible exception of those who have been physically or sexually abusive to their child. The origin of these disorders lies in gene clusters, in temperament, in a family history of eating disorders, addictions, mood disorders, etc. Parents, however, are largely responsible for educating their child about what healthy eating is, and for shaping a child's healthy eating lifestyle. Parents who are themselves preoccupied with body image and weight gain, who are fearful or rigid about their own approach to food and cooking, and/or who do not prepare family meals on a regular basis in the effort to foster a healthy eating lifestyle in their children could possibly increase the ranks of childhood anorexics in those instances where there is a genetic propensity for the onset of an eating disorder. At the very least, such parents might foster disordered eating habits, which could eventually morph into a clinical eating disorder where there is genetic susceptibility. Dr. W. Stewart Agras cited a study that showed that children of anorexic mothers were already more depressed, whiny, and eating dysfunctional by age five.

Enlightened parents who are good communicators and sensitive to the child's developmental needs and concerns can do a great deal to detect early signs, preventing the onset of a clinical eating disorder, or nipping the problem in the bud.

What parents can do:

- If there is a concern that a child may be restricting certain foods, food groups, or portion sizes, it is wise to first consult a medical doctor to rule out physiological problems.

- Create a healthy eating lifestyle at home and expect your child to comply with the family's eating patterns. Offer your child healthy foods, prepare or oversee at least three nourishing meals a day, and be sure to eat those meals together with your child and family as often as possible. Your child learns by imitating your behaviors. As nourishing as a family dinner is the sharing and camaraderie that accompanies it.

- Never skip meals. Remember that breakfast is the most important meal of the day. Know what healthy eating is, that it involves eating three meals daily . . . diverse, balanced and nutritious meals, consisting of all the food groups and consumed without fear. Healthy eating is not fat-free eating.

- Keep your own lifestyle active and expect your child to do the same. If children are too sedentary, turn off the television and encourage a walk with the dog or biking to the library.

- Spend quality time with your child. Listen to what they say and to how they feel. Know what their concerns are.

- Encourage your child to become aware of her feelings and to express them freely. Communicating through the use of words diminishes the odds that anxious feelings will be expressed through food-abusing behaviors.

- Be aware that girls typically reach puberty as young as age nine. Explain to them that it is normal (and essential) that they gain weight at the onset of puberty in order to stimulate a healthfully functioning reproductive system that will allow them to bear their own children one day.

- Become aware of your own personal attitudes about eating, body image, and weight control. Do you encourage your son to eat so that he can grow big and strong, yet caution your daughter against becoming fat?

- Never force your child to "clean her plate," giving her a sense of not being in control of her own food. The parent should determine the menu and the child should determine the amounts of food consumed.

- Do not criticize your own or your child's weight, shape, or size.

- Don't tolerate casual derogatory comments about other people's weight and physical appearance. Children take to heart and personalize what you say.

- Be aware of how your responses to your child's problem may be affecting your child's behavior and feelings.

- Beware of your child's sudden decision to become vegetarian, particularly if very young. More often than not, the underlying motives may be weight loss, and result in a less than healthy eating lifestyle in the child who does not understand the complexities of healthy and balanced vegetarian eating, of creating proteins, etc.

Remember that too much of a good thing is no longer a good thing. Don't allow your child to overdo athletics or dance activities; to shop too much or to watch TV or Facebook too much; to talk on the phone or play video games too much; to eat too much or too little, to study too much or too little, to sleep too much or too little, etc. Moderation and balance in life reflects a healthy lifestyle.

If your child is engaged in competitive sports, be aware that food restriction, the use of hormones, and extreme workouts are not uncommon practices for participants in certain of these sports. Stay involved as parents, and aware of what the coach or teacher is asking of the team and of your child; always be prepared to intervene where you believe requests may have become extreme or unhealthy. A study (Davison, Earnest, Birch, "Participation in Aesthetic Sports," *International Journal of Eating Disorders*, April 2002 pp. 315–16) demonstrates that in comparison to girls who participated in non-aesthetic sports or no sports, girls who participated in aesthetic sports reported higher weight concerns at ages five and seven.

If you believe a problem exists, be certain to seek out expert professional help. When children are young, you may consider consultation with a therapist or nutritionist first, before bringing in the child. There is a tremendous amount of good that can come of parents making changes within the family system; in some instances, that alone might be enough to adjust whatever might be troubling your child.

Reference

Natenshon, Abigail MA, LCSW, GCFP, *Doing What Works: an Integrative System for the Treatment of Eating Disorders from Diagnosis to Recovery* (Washington, D.C.: NASW Press, 2009).

Section 16.2

Eating Disorders and Adolescents: Research Facts and Findings

"Eating Disorders and Adolescents," Research Facts & Findings, November 2006, by Richard Kreipe, M.D., University of Rochester School of Medicine. Reprinted with permission from the author and the Cornell University Family Life Development Center. Reviewed by David A. Cooke, M.D., FACP, September 2010.

An Internet search of "eating disorders" yields fifteen million websites and almost twenty thousand images. Stories about eating disorders among popular performers also regularly appear in the press and TV. As is often true, when there is a large amount of easily accessed information there is also a large amount of misinformation. The purpose of this section is to inform readers about the facts and recent and emerging research findings about eating disorders. First, the what (definitions), how (behaviors related to eating disorders), who (affected individuals), when (developmental stages), and why (causes and risk factors) will be discussed. Then, some key points about prevention and treatment will be reviewed. Next, recent and emerging research findings will be described. Finally, an innovative system of care being developed in New York State under the leadership of the Department of Health will be shared.

What Are Eating Disorders?

In restrictive anorexia nervosa (AN), a person severely restricts caloric intake, and often exercises excessively because of an overwhelming desire to lose weight. In bulimia nervosa (BN), a person is afraid of gaining weight, but ingests large amounts in a brief period (binges), then tries to rid the body of the effects of these extra calories by fasting, vomiting, exercising, or using laxatives immediately afterward. Most people with an eating disorder do not fit neatly into either of these categories and are said to have an eating disorder, not otherwise specified (ED-NOS), popularly called "disordered eating."

How Do Adolescents with Eating Disorders Behave?

The best way to understand how adolescents with an eating disorder might behave is to put one's self in their shoes. Imagine believing that losing weight is the only way that you can achieve a sense of mastery in your life. Things are happening all around and within your own life that seem out of your control. Also imagine that you have always been a perfectionist, but have never really felt very good about yourself—regardless of praise that you get from others. Finally, you are surrounded by "you can never be too thin" messages from a variety of sources. This might be the situation for a person with AN. What do you do? You might: stop eating breakfast, schedule a class during lunch, eliminate snacks, exercise every way possible, and keep busy. However, when these behaviors become extreme or numerous and affect every organ system, including your brain, you end up feeling worse, not better, and assume that you just need to lose more weight to feel better about yourself.

Likewise, imagine that you have an intense fear of obesity, but lack the "will power" to limit calories on a consistent basis, the motivation to exercise regularly, and the ability to control impulses or sad moods. You also find comfort eating large amounts of high-calorie foods, but doing so only makes you feel worse. So, you do things to rid your body of calories. Although harmful, these things are less frightening than gaining weight, and may even make you feel less guilty or sad. This might be the situation for a person with BN. You might end up not eating breakfast or lunch because you want to lose weight, but then come home from school, feeling lonely or sad and eat a donut. You start feeling better eating donuts and before you know it, you've eaten the whole box. This makes you feel guilty and ashamed, and the only thing you can think of is to vomit before anyone else gets home. Your brother arrives home a few minutes later, goes to the pantry, and starts yelling at you because all the donuts are gone. Embarrassment, sadness, and anger cause you to vow to never binge and vomit again, but you know deep in your heart that you will, because you are trapped in an addictive cycle, and don't see any way out of the pattern.

Who Are Affected by Eating Disorders?

The Academy for Eating Disorders (AED) reports that among late adolescent and young adult females, at least 10 percent have symptoms of eating disorders and those with BN outnumber those with AN by at least two to one. Although the stereotype for eating disorders is a white adolescent or young adult female living in the suburbs, males get eating disorders, as do older women (who often have a chronic form starting in adolescence), and people of color. Some individuals seem to be particularly at-risk, however, including models, those with a family member who has/had an eating disorder (see research findings), or anyone who places an undue emphasis on thinness or avoiding obesity, such as athletes who follow diet, appearance, size, or weight requirements for their sport. For example, the National Eating Disorders Association (NEDA) cites a study of college athletes, in which more than one-third of females reported attitudes and symptoms placing them at risk for AN. The "female athlete triad" (low weight, loss of menstrual periods, and weakened bones [osteoporosis]) even has its own website for professionals (www.femaleathletetriad.org). Although eating disorders occur in an individual, it is essential to recognize that the illness affects the family, school, workplace, and community in which the person lives.

When Do Eating Disorders Appear?

Eating disorders typically are first diagnosed between ten to twenty years of age, with AN generally occurring appearing thirteen to seventeen, and BN tending to emerge fifteen to nineteen. However, developmental issues are probably more important than chronologic age, so they can occur in childhood through adulthood. That is, issues related to puberty (see research findings), autonomy, identity, and relationships often seem to trigger the illness. Sheila MacLeod (MacLeod, 1987) noted that an eating disorder is actually "a last ditch effort" to gain control over feelings of low self-esteem and ineffectiveness that precede dieting by months to years.

Why Do Eating Disorders Develop?

Simply put, there is no single cause for an eating disorder. They are complex illnesses with multiple causes that require treatment across a number of domains. Eating disorders are better considered as "developmental" rather than "mental" problems. This acknowledges the depth and breadth of systems that are affected, and minimizes the stigma still associated with psychological disorders. As NEDA notes, "Eating disorders are illnesses, not choices." Dr. Jean Kilbourne, author of *Can't Buy My Love: How Advertising Changes the Way We Think and Feel* (2000), addresses the powerful influence of advertising, but notes that media and marketing are not the sole causes of eating disorders.

How to Prevent and Treat Eating Disorders?

The basic principles of prevention cited by NEDA include: (1) eating disorders are serious and complex problems that should not be simplified as "anorexia is just a plea for attention," or "bulimia is just an addiction to food." Eating disorders arise from a variety of physical, emotional, social, and familial issues, all of which need to be addressed for effective prevention and treatment; (2) eating disorders should not be framed as a "woman's problem" or "something for the girls"; (3) prevention efforts will fail, or encourage disordered eating, if they concentrate solely on warning the public about the signs, symptoms, and dangers of eating disorders. Efforts should address: (a) our cultural obsession with slenderness as a physical, psychological, and moral issue, (b) stereotypic gender roles, and (c) developing self-esteem and self-respect in a variety of areas (school, work, community service, hobbies) that transcend physical appearance. In her book, *I'm Like, SO Fat!*, Dr. Dianne Neumark-Sztainer (2004) notes that prevention messages should be directed not only at eating disorders, or the more common concern of obesity. She argues for a positive approach emphasizing the benefits of healthy eating and physical activity.

Once an eating disorder occurs, holistic treatment is necessary by professionals addressing the medical, nutritional, and psychosocial needs of the adolescent and the family. Therefore, a team approach is generally used. Newer evidence refutes previously held beliefs about parents being the cause of eating disorders and research now shows that parents have an essential role in helping their teenager restore weight, as the first step toward recovery. Two books for consumers about the positive role of parents in treatment are the internationally acclaimed *Help Your Teenager Beat an Eating Disorder* (Lock & leGrange, 2004) and *A Stranger at the Table* (Haltom, C 2004) written by a practicing psychologist in Ithaca, New York. Medications like Prozac® can be helpful to treat the binge eating and vomiting associated with BN, but the most important "medicine" is healthy eating balanced with enjoyable exercise. Treatment may need to continue for two years or more.

Recent and Emerging Research

Recent studies have increased our understanding of why and when eating disorders tend to emerge as they do. First, international, multi-center studies suggest that genetic factors play a role in the development of AN more than BN (Bulik, et al 2005, Bacanu et al 2005). However, genes do not simply cause eating disorders. Instead, the increased risk appears to be related to a vulnerability to depression and/or anxiety, for which genetic factors are widely accepted (Kaye et al 2004). This should not be interpreted as parents who have a personal or family history of depression or anxiety "giving" their child an eating disorder, nor as the inevitability of developing an eating disorder if a person is depressed or anxious.

Second, Kelly Klump's group has found evidence that genes are expressed differently in girls who are early in puberty compared to those who are more physically mature (Klump et al 2006), and hypothesize that the female brain begins to respond to hormones at puberty and that estrogen activates the genes contributing to disordered eating in vulnerable girls. Finally, this hypothesis is based on recent findings that genes, though fixed at birth, vary in their expression, depending on complex environmental factors (Bulik 2005). Thus, both the why and when of eating disorders appear to be linked as biological factors which interact with environmental influences, in a classic ecological dynamic. This exciting line of research will undoubtedly continue to enlighten our approach to eating disorders.

Closely related to these recent studies is emerging research focused on imaging brain function for patients with eating disorders. The most promising technique in this regard is functional magnetic resonance imaging (fMRI), which localizes brain activity in anatomically distinct areas of the brain, including activity associated with specific neurotransmitters, such as serotonin (Kaye et al 2005). Studies using fMRI to detail brain activity associated with specific behaviors and symptoms are underway, and in combination with genetic studies, will help improve the treatment of these conditions.

Comprehensive Care Centers for Eating Disorders (CCCED)

Based on legislation spearheaded by New York State (NYS), Senator Joseph Bruno, and funding from the NYS Department of Health, three CCCEDs have been established to develop an integrated system of care that will assure access to consistent, evidence based treatment through a network of professionals. In addition this legislation will fund community outreach, education of consumers and professionals, and multi-center research to determine the effectiveness of various treatments for eating disorders.

References

Bacanu SA. Bulik CM. Klump KL. Fichter MM. Halmi KA. Keel P. Kaplan AS. Mitchell JE. Rotondo A. Strober M. Treasure J. Woodside DB. Sonpar VA. Xie W. Bergen AW. Berrettini WH. Kaye WH. Devlin B. Linkage analysis of anorexia and bulimia nervosa cohorts using selected behavioral phenotypes as quantitative traits or covariates. *American Journal of Medical Genetics*. Part B, Neuropsychiatric Genetics: the Official Publication of the International Society of Psychiatric Genetics. 139(1):61–68, 2005.

Bulik CM. Bacanu SA. Klump KL. Fichter MM. Halmi KA. Keel P. Kaplan AS. Mitchell JE. Rotondo A. Strober M. Treasure J. Woodside DB. Sonpar VA. Xie W. Bergen AW. Berrettini WH. Kaye WH. Devlin B. Selection of eating-disorder phenotypes for linkage analysis. *American Journal of Medical Genetics*. Part B, Neuropsychiatric Genetics: the Official Publication of the International Society of Psychiatric Genetics. 139(1):81-7, 2005.

Bulik CM. Exploring the gene-environment nexus in eating disorders. *Journal of Psychiatry & Neuroscience*. 30(5):335–39, 2005.

Haltom, CA. *Stranger at the Table: Dealing with Your Child's Eating Disorder* Ronjon Publishing: Denton, TX 2004

Kaye WH. Bulik CM. Thornton L. Barbarich N. Masters K. Comorbidity of anxiety disorders with anorexia and bulimia nervosa. *American Journal of Psychiatry*. 161(12):2215–21, 2004 Dec.

Kaye WH. Frank GK. Bailer UF. Henry SE. Meltzer CC. Price JC. Mathis CA. Wagner A. Serotonin alterations in anorexia and bulimia nervosa: new insights from imaging studies. *Physiology & Behavior*. 85(1):73–81, 2005.

Kilbourne, J. *Can't Buy My Love: How Advertising Changes the Way We Think and Feel*. Simon & Schuster, Inc. 2000.

Klump KL. Gobrogge KL. Perkins PS. Thorne D. Sisk CL. Marc Breedlove S. Preliminary evidence that gonadal hormones organize and activate disordered eating. *Psychological Medicine*. 36(4):539–46, 2006.

Lock, J. leGrange D. *Help Your Teenager Beat an Eating Disorder*. Guilford Press, 2004.

MacLeod, S. *Art of Starvation*. Random House, 1987.

Newmark-Sztainer, D. *I'm, Like, SO Fat!: Helping Your Teen Make Healthy Choices About Eating and Exercise in a Weight-Obsessed World*. New York, NY, The Guilford Press, 2005.

Section 16.3

Eating Disorders: Information for Adults Who Care about Teens

"Eating Disorders: Information for Adults Who Care about Teens,"
reprinted with permission from the Washington Department of Health.
Reviewed by David A. Cooke, M.D., FACP, September 2010.

What's It All About?

Eating disorders are serious mental and physical health problems for teens. Young people may develop unhealthy eating habits as a way of coping with the pressures of adolescence. The development of an eating disorder involves many complex factors including personality and genetics as well as the family, social and cultural environment of the adolescent. Eating disorders are most common among adolescent girls but the number of adolescent boys affected with eating disorders is rising.

Concerns about body size and weight may begin as early as eight years old, laying the groundwork for unhealthy eating habits with devastating consequences. Two types of eating disorders are anorexia and bulimia. Anorexia involves an intense fear of gaining weight, even though the person is underweight. Bulimia involves repeated binge eating followed by vomiting, misuse of laxatives, or other behaviors to prevent weight gain.

What Are the Details?

- Approximately 1 out of 100 adolescent girls develop anorexia nervosa and 2 to 5 out of every 100 adolescent girls develop bulimia.

- An estimated 10 percent of people with eating disorders are male.

- Among Washington students who are not overweight, about half of the girls and 1 in 7 boys in eighth, tenth, and twelfth grade say they are trying to lose weight.

- According to the 2002 Washington State Healthy Youth Survey, 15 to 20 percent of girls in eighth, tenth, and twelfth grade report engaging in risky dieting behavior, including fasting, using diet pills or powders without a doctor's prescription, vomiting, or taking laxatives to lose weight, in the past month.

Why Does It Matter?

- Low self-esteem, poor coping skills, childhood physical or sexual abuse, and early sexual maturation may place teens at increased risk for eating disorders.

- The percentage of young people diagnosed with an eating disorder may seem low, but dangerous eating behaviors that may lead to eating disorders are much more widespread.

- Eating disorders may begin with poor eating behaviors at early ages.

- Some researchers link troublesome eating patterns to increased pressures on women by the mass media, fashion, and diet industry to pursue thinness.

Health Consequences: Now and Later

Eating disorders are one of the deadliest mental illnesses.

Short-term health consequences may include altered growth, abnormal brain structure, decreased bone strength, delayed sexual maturation, the absence of periods in girls, infertility, hair loss, tooth loss and decay, increased infections, low blood pressure, internal organ damage, and irregular heartbeat, which may lead to heart attacks.

Long-term consequences, even after treatment, may include short stature, weak bones, a decrease in brain cells, increased blood pressure and cholesterol, gall bladder disease, osteoporosis, diabetes, heart disease, and certain types of cancer in adults.

Eating disorders are also related to other risk behaviors, such as failure to meet goals for education and income, substance abuse, delinquency, unprotected sexual activity, and suicide attempts.

What Can I Do?

Here are some eating disorders prevention tips adapted from Dr. Michael Levine:

- Be aware of troublesome eating behaviors that may develop into eating disorders.

- Learn about eating disorders and share what you know with teens. Help avoid mistaken attitudes about food, body shape, and eating disorders.

- Discourage the idea that a particular diet, weight, or body size will lead to happiness.

- Challenge the belief that thinness is great and that body fat or weight gain is horrible.

- Talk positively about the kinds of foods teens should eat. Avoid categorizing foods as "good or safe" vs. "bad or dangerous." We all need a variety of foods.

- Talk positively about body image. Avoid making judgments based on body weight or shape. Discard the idea that body weight reflects character or value.

- Talk function over form. Encourage all family members to focus on all the positive things the body can do and discourage an emphasis on body shape and size.

- Provide teens clear messages that you value them, no matter what their size or shape.

- Be critical of the media's messages about self-esteem and body image.

- If you think someone has an eating disorder, express your concerns in a forthright, caring manner. Gently but firmly encourage the person to seek trained professional help.

- Exercise for fun and fitness—not to burn calories—get your teen involved in lifelong recreational sports such as swimming, jogging, hiking, and canoeing.

- Teens learn from the way you talk about yourself and your body. Talk about yourself with respect and appreciation.

What Causes Eating Disorders?

The cause of eating disorders is unknown but some major risk factors include the following:

- Low self-esteem and feelings of helplessness.

- A history of sexual, emotional, or physical abuse.

- Family history and environment that includes regular discussions about dieting and physical appearance, weight-related teasing, or involvement in a profession that emphasizes thinness.

- Personal or family history of obesity, drug abuse, or depression.

Tools to Protect Teens

Certain habits and skills will promote a healthy outlook on eating and physical fitness, and help teens manage the stresses of adolescence:

- Healthy eating habits protect teens from associating shame or guilt with eating.

- Support and counseling help address mental health issues.

- Healthy involvement in sports and exercise protects teens by improving self-esteem.

Section 16.4

Eating Disorders among College Students

"Eating Disorders in College Students," by David A. Cooke, M.D., FACP,
© 2010 Omnigraphics, Inc.

Eating disorders are common among college students. As in other settings, women represent the overwhelming majority of college students with eating disorders. One study reported that 70 to 94 percent of female college students desire to lose weight, which was a much higher proportion than were classified overweight or obese. Estimates vary, but evidence suggests that 8 to 20 percent of female college students can be classified as suffering from eating disorders, and as many as 60 percent may have some disordered eating behaviors. There is less data on male college students with eating disorders, but some believe it to be greatly underdiagnosed; some studies have concluded that 5 to 20 percent of male college students are affected.

Why are college students so prone to eating disorders? There has been some debate regarding whether eating disorders are actually more common in college students than other groups. Some studies indicate that disordered eating patterns typically begin in high school. Most population studies of eating disorders have been done in college students, so it is possible this has biased perceptions of the problem. Nevertheless, it is clear that a large number of college students do suffer from eating disorders.

There are a number of reasons why college students might be more likely to develop eating disorders. Most college students are in their teens and early twenties, which is a peak age group for the first appearance of eating disorders. College is a time of major transition for young people. For many, it is the first time they have lived away from home and family. College students also have more control over their food choices and exercise habits than they may have at home. There are new social pressures associated with being exposed to a different group of peers, and for some, the pressure to "fit in" may be stronger than they are accustomed to. Eating disorders are associated with smoking and other substance abuse disorders, and these issues often first present in the college age demographic.

There may be other factors as well. Specific personality styles seem to predict eating disorders. College-bound students tend to be high academic achievers, and a number of studies have shown correlations between perfectionist traits and subsequent development of eating disorders. Some studies have also linked eating disorders to poor intellectual flexibility, and the broader range of choices available to college students may be a stressor for those who are less resilient. Depression and anxiety are quite common among young adults and college students. While most people with mood disorders do not have eating disorders, having a mood disorder greatly increased the odds of developing an eating disorder.

One study has linked the so-called "freshman fifteen" to eating disorders in college students. Experts debate whether the "freshman fifteen" weight gain phenomenon actually exists; not all studies have shown that college freshmen typically gain weight. Nevertheless, belief in it is widespread among college students. The study results suggest these concerns can lead to preoccupation with weight and weight gain, and provide a push toward developing eating disorders.

While all of the above may have some role in the development of eating disorders, a great deal remains unknown as to why some people develop eating disorders and others do not. Some studies suggest that there may be hereditary elements involved, but it is likely that there is rarely, if ever, a single reason why a given person is afflicted by an eating disorder.

Diagnosis of eating disorders is not always straightforward. While binging, purging, and extreme weight loss are obvious clues, many college students do not reveal them. Binging and purging is often done secretively, and friends and family may not notice surprisingly large weight changes. College students often present with indirect symptoms of eating disorders. Fatigue, swollen glands, sore throat, dental problems, and broken blood vessels in the eyes may be primary complaints.

Because eating disorders in college students are common and underdiagnosed, a number of colleges have created programs to provide education, diagnosis, and treatment services to affected students. Many student counseling services are now more attuned to eating disorder problems, and are more likely to identify them in students who seek care for other reasons.

For individual students, treatment is typically similar to other eating disorder populations. Outpatient therapy is usually preferred in college students, if the disease severity allows for it and resources are available. Individual and group psychological counseling is often helpful in addressing psychological factors that promote eating disorders. For bulimia sufferers, certain classes of antidepressants have been reported to improve symptoms. Anorexia nervosa tends to be more resistant to medication treatment, but it may be appropriate for some individuals.

The high number of affected and at-risk college students has lead to broader screening and intervention efforts for broad college populations. While a number of preventive approaches have been tried, it is less clear how successful they are. One review of published literature found that programs that focused on education, cognitive behavioral therapy, and psycho-educational therapy were not particularly effective. However, the review found that programs based on a "dissonance" approach, which aim to promote more realistic body images and standards of attractiveness, were more successful. Programs focusing on improvement of self-esteem in college students may be effective, but more data is needed. "Media literacy" interventions, which aim to counter images and standards in mass media, may also be of some benefit.

A number of computer-based interventions have been tried for eating disorders in college students. This approach may have some advantages, as it provides for greater anonymity, and college students tend to be fairly computer-literate. Some programs have used CD-based or online structured therapy exercises. Others have used online eating, exercise and behavior logs, as well as email support programs. Positive results have generally been reported, and this area deserves further study.

In summary, eating disorders are common in college students, and generally under-recognized. In addition to students who meet criteria for eating disorders, there is a large pool of others who are at risk for developing them. Treatment is available, but it requires recognition of the problem and willingness of sufferers to seek it. Broad college population interventions may be useful, but it is still not clear which strategies are most effective for this problem.

Chapter 17

Eating Disorders in Men

Chapter Contents

Section 17.1

How Eating Disorders Affect Males

When we think of eating disorders, we rarely picture a man working out obsessively, starving himself to look lean, or wanting to emulate celebrities on magazine covers.

For years, eating disorders have been viewed as a "white woman's disease." And estimates of male eating disorders told a similar story: while the majority of women suffered from eating disorders, only about 10 percent of men did.

Recent research, however, paints a different, bigger picture: more men are suffering from eating disorders than previously thought. Out of three thousand people with anorexia and bulimia, 25 percent were men (and 40 percent had binge eating disorder), according to a Harvard study.

What Distinguishes Men with Eating Disorders from Their Female Counterparts?

Symptoms: The diagnostic criteria for anorexia, for instance, focus on women, which is evident in its hallmark symptoms of amenorrhea (the absence of menstruation) and fear of fatness. Though some men do exhibit a fear of fat, others typically want to be muscular (particularly their chest and arms), obsess over attaining a low body fat percentage, and focus their efforts on excelling at a sport (which prompts some to abuse steroids and exercise excessively).

Instead of engaging in traditional compensatory behaviors like vomiting or abusing laxatives, men instead are more likely to exercise compulsively (as cited in Weltzin, Weisensel, Franczyk, Burnett, Klitz & Bean, 2005).

Images and ideals: For decades, women have been inundated with unrealistic, thin images in magazines, movies, ads, and other media outlets. And now, men are also feeling the pressure for physical perfection, surrounded by unattainable images of muscular physiques, six-pack abs, bulging biceps, and lean bodies.

But, in contrast to women, where the images are one size fits all (thin is always in), men have a variety of images to emulate, psychiatrist Arnold Andersen, M.D., told the *Wall Street Journal*: "Some want to be wiry like Mick Jagger; some want to be lean like David Beckham, and some want to be really buff and bulked, like Arnold Schwarzenegger."

Interestingly, reports that wiry images are contributing to eating disorders have prompted one fashion show to ban thin male models with a body mass index (BMI) below 19 or 26- and 28-inch waists, the United Kingdom's *Telegraph* reported.

Dieting: Men might diet for different reasons than women, including (as cited in Greenberg & Schoen, 2008):

- to prevent weight gain (many eating disordered men were overweight as kids).

- to excel in sports. According to an article on CBS News: "Athletes whose weight is crucial to their performance—jockeys, wrestlers, distance runners and gymnasts—have a higher incidence of eating disorders. [Co-author of *Making Weight*] Cohn said they can develop bad habits when weight loss is seen as a requirement of the sport."

- to avoid health complications.

- to improve appearance after childhood teasing.

- for their jobs. Dr. Andersen told *The Washington Post*: "Other patients include men who began dieting to meet job requirements—and couldn't stop. 'We've had a number of military people like colonels,' said Andersen, who was formerly on the staffs of Johns Hopkins Hospital and the National Institutes of Health. 'The military is very strict, and they're afraid they're going to get chucked out' or fail to win a promotion if they don't lose weight to meet certain requirements."

Not surprisingly, these differences make it harder for professionals to diagnose eating disorders in men. And, oftentimes men are unaware that they're suffering from an eating disorder in the first place.

In Homosexual Men

Eating disorders are more prevalent in gay and bisexual men than in heterosexual men (Feldman & Meyer, 2007), though one expert attributes the higher prevalence to a greater likelihood to seek treatment.

131

Either way, some have pointed to the increased emphasis on physical attractiveness in gay communities as a contributing factor, whereas others view participation in these communities as protection against eating disorders (as cited in Feldman et. al, 2007).

Why Now?

Unfortunately, we can't confirm the reasons behind this increase in male eating disorders. It's uncertain whether more men are actually developing eating disorders today or if more men are coming forward.

Barriers to Treatment

- **Stigma:** Since eating disorders are known as a woman's disease, men might be embarrassed to seek treatment, worried that they'd be seen as less of a man.

- **Services:** Because male eating disorders have only recently received attention, many treatment centers don't have separate services that treat men.

References

Feldman, M.B. & Meyer, I.A. (2007). Eating disorders in diverse lesbian, gay, and bisexual populations. *International Journal of Eating Disorders*, 40 (3), 218–26.

Greenberg, S.T. & Schoen, E.G. (2008). Males and eating disorders: Gender-based therapy for eating disorder recovery. *Professional Psychology: Research and Practice*, 39 (4), 464–71.

Weltzin, T.E., Weisensel, N., Franczyk, D., Burnett, K., Klitz, C. & Bean P. (2005). Eating disorders in men: Update. *Journal of Men's Health & Gender*, 2 (2), 186–91.

Section 17.2

Strategies for Prevention and Early Intervention in Male Eating Disorders

"Strategies for Prevention and Early Intervention of Male Eating Disorders," © 2005 National Eating Disorders Association. For more information, visit www.NationalEatingDisorders.org. Reviewed by David A. Cooke, M.D., FACP, September 2010.

Recognize that eating disorders do not discriminate on the basis of gender. Men can and do develop eating disorders.

Learn about eating disorders and know the warning signs. Become aware of your community resources (treatment centers, self-help groups, etc.). Consider implementing an Eating Concerns Support Group in a school, hospital, or community setting to provide interested young men with an opportunity to learn more about eating disorders and to receive support. Encourage young men to seek professional help if necessary.

Understand that athletic activities or professions that necessitate weight restriction (e.g., gymnastics, track, swimming, wrestling, rowing) put males at risk for developing eating disorders. Male wrestlers, for example, present with a higher rate of eating disorders than the general male population (Andersen, 1995). Coaches need to be aware of and disallow any excessive weight control or body building measures employed by their young male athletes.

Talk with young men about the ways in which cultural attitudes regarding ideal male body shape, masculinity, and sexuality are shaped by the media. Assist young men in expanding their idea of "masculinity" to include such characteristics as caring, nurturing, and cooperation. Encourage male involvement in traditional "nonmasculine" activities such as shopping, laundry, and cooking.

Demonstrate respect for gay men, and men who display personality traits or who are involved in professions that stretch the limits of traditional masculinity; e.g., men who dress colorfully, dancers, skaters, etc.

Never emphasize body size or shape as an indication of a young man's worth or identity as a man. Value the person on the "inside" and help him to establish a sense of control in his life through self-knowledge and expression rather than trying to obtain control through dieting or other eating disordered behaviors.

Confront others who tease men who do not meet traditional cultural expectations for masculinity. Confront anyone who tries to motivate or "toughen up" young men by verbally attacking their masculinity; e.g., calling names such as "sissy" or "wimp."

Listen carefully to a young man's thoughts and feelings, take his pain seriously, allow him to become who he is.

Validate a young man's strivings for independence and encourage him to develop all aspects of his personality, not only those that family and/or culture find acceptable. Respect a person's need for space, privacy, and boundaries. Be careful about being overprotective. Allow him to exercise control and make his own decisions whenever possible, including control over what and how much he eats, how he looks, and how much he weighs.

Understand the crucial role of the father and other male influences in the prevention of eating disorders. Find ways to connect young men with healthy male role models.

Chapter 18

Eating Disorders in Pregnancy

Eating disorders (EDs) are complex disorders. However, the complexity increases when women are struggling with eating disorders while pregnant—a time when the lives of two people are at stake: Mom and baby.

"Pregorexia" is the current fashionable phrase for this situation. The term, coined by the media, is not a diagnosed medical condition, but rather a clever descriptive name of a condition that can be life threatening to both a pregnant mom and her unborn child.

What Is Pregorexia?

Pregorexia refers to any woman who is engaging in ED behaviors while pregnant. These behaviors might include restriction of calories, overexercise, bingeing and purging, or abuse of laxatives or diet pills. Any of these unhealthy behaviors is used by the mom-to-be to control her weight gain and body size.

Most women who are in recovery or in an active phase of the ED struggle with fears related to pregnancy weight gain. Yet, pregnancy can be a time when an ED goes into remission because the mom feels she can let go of the behaviors in order to provide for the health of her baby.

"Pregorexia Starves Mom and Baby," by Maggie Baumann, M.A., *Eating Disorders Recovery Today*, Summer 2009, Volume 7, Number 3. © 2009 Gürze Books. Reprinted with permission.

However, in the case of someone who is experiencing pregorexia, the thoughts and behaviors of the ED are stronger than her will to properly care for herself and her baby. The pressure to be thin, even during pregnancy, can be overwhelming.

Dangers for Mom

Pregorexia can cause a number of medical and psychological complications for a mother during and after pregnancy, including:

- miscarriage;
- poor nutrition;
- dehydration;
- cardiac irregularities;
- premature births;
- labor complications including Caesarean delivery;
- difficulties with nursing;
- pregnancy and/or postpartum depression.

Calorie restriction during pregnancy affects both the mother and baby. To insure the health of the fetus, the baby's nutritional needs are biologically primary, often at the expense of the mother. For example, if only a limited amount of calcium is ingested, it first goes to the growing baby and the mom may get little or none, putting her at greater risk for development of osteoporosis.

Dangers for Baby

Experts suggest that behaviors such as purging, restricting, and use of laxatives or diuretics on a regular basis can be harmful to a developing fetus and may lead to abnormalities. Studies report complications can affect both the baby before birth and the growing child years after birth.

Risks to fetus and infant include:

- intrauterine growth retardation (poor fetal growth);
- low birth weight;
- premature birth;
- low APGAR scores;
- respiratory distress;

- feeding difficulties;

- neurological defects due to oxygen deprivation resulting from mom's excessive exercise;

- attention deficit hyperactivity disorder (ADHD).

Potential Causes

A number of factors can lead to the development of pregorexia, many of which are the same as those that underlie the development of an eating disorder during another time of life, such as a history of trauma, neglect, excessive dieting, and poor coping skills. Genetics also plays a factor, as does individual temperament, which includes traits such as perfectionism and anxiety.

Still some specific contributors that occur for a woman during pregnancy include:

- a prior history of an ED;

- increased body image issues due to pregnancy weight gain;

- ambivalence of being a new mom and its lifelong responsibilities;

- relationship difficulties with partner due to pending parenthood;

- societal pressure to be thin, even during pregnancy.

Illustrating this last point are the increasing numbers of celebrity pregnancies chronicled in the media. We marvel at how trim and fit they remain, sometimes barely showing their "baby bumps." Then we watch them quickly regain their pre-pregnancy shape, often within weeks post-delivery. Falsely touted as a "good" thing to which all of us should aspire, these stories actually place tremendous pressure on women who are already struggling with body image issues as a result of their ED.

Warning Signs

Someone with pregorexia may show some of the following warning signs:

- Preoccupation with the number on the scale and weight gain

- Exercising excessively

- Highly critical of her body

- Minimal weight gain

- Smaller than average "baby bump"
- Dieting
- Signs of depression

Steps to Ensure a Healthy Pregnancy

It's important for women to resolve any eating disorder behaviors well before conception. However, if you have an ED and become pregnant, you can take these steps to safeguard your health and your baby's:

- Abstain from any disordered eating, including restricting intake or bingeing and purging.

- Be proactive in disclosing your ED history with your obstetrician.

- Per obstetrician's guidance, ensure proper weight gain during pregnancy. New guidelines from the Institute of Medicine recommend that women of normal weight should gain approximately twenty-five to thirty-five pounds during pregnancy. If the woman is underweight at the time of conception, the weight gain suggested is forty to fifty pounds or more, depending on the patient.

- If needed, recruit a team of specialists to work with you during pregnancy, including an obstetrician, therapist, nutritionist, and psychiatrist, as needed, all of whom are experienced in treating EDs.

Call For Action

If you, or someone you know, is struggling with pregorexia, seek out help immediately from medical specialists who are experienced in treating women with eating disorders. It's imperative that the obstetrician is informed because pregnant women with EDs require "high risk" obstetrical care. The heath of both baby and mom depends on it.

Chapter 19

Eating Disorders in Older Adults

Chapter Contents

Section 19.1

Elder Eating Disorders: A Surprising New Challenge

"Elder Eating Disorders: Surprising New Challenge,"
by Juliann Schaeffer, *Aging Well*, © 2009 Great Valley Publishing Co.
Reprinted with permission.

Anorexia nervosa, bulimia, and binge eating. Previously associated primarily with the younger set—preteens and teens—such eating disorders have unfortunately expanded to affect more individuals in midlife and beyond, as older age proves to be no barrier for disordered eating practices.

"To date, eating disorders have always been considered an illness of young people, predominantly females," says Vivian Hanson Meehan, president and founder of the National Association of Anorexia Nervosa and Associated Disorders (ANAD), an internationally recognized authority in the eating disorders field. Holly Grishkat, Ph.D., site director of the Renfrew Center in Radnor, Pennsylvania, who also runs the facility's Thirty-Something and Beyond program, adds, "The 'new' face of eating disorders is younger, older, and more diverse. We are seeing the emergence of eating disorders in preadolescents, women over thirty, and in people regardless of race, gender, religion, sexual orientation, and socioeconomic status."

Even though eating disorders have pushed their way into the lives of older adults, Grishkat says they often surface early. "I think eating disorders are still primarily a disease of the youth, as most midlife women with eating disorders developed the problem prior to the age of eighteen. Many of those women are just now reaching out for treatment," she says. "So while it may look like they are emerging later in life, most eating disordered women have been suffering since adolescence. The difference is that we are now working with women who have had the disorder for ten, twenty, and thirty years rather than the adolescents who may have a much shorter experience with these disorders. After thirty years, the eating disorder has become almost a personality characteristic for these women, as many of them define themselves by the eating disorder."

Grishkat says that women in midlife or older are currently part of the largest group of "new" sufferers of eating disorders seen at the facility but due to a lack of research data, it's difficult to say whether the prevalence of eating disorders in older women is increasing. "We do get them," she says of patients over the age of fifty. "I currently have a woman in my Thirty-Something and Beyond Group who is age fifty-eight. I have experienced both a sixty-four-year-old and a seventy-two-year-old in treatment at the residential facility. I believe seventy-two years old is the oldest that we have treated so far at Renfrew," she says, admitting that more data on the prevalence of eating disorders in older adults is sorely needed.

Meehan, head of ANAD, a nonprofit organization dedicated to alleviating eating disorders, acknowledges the difficulty of defining the level of prevalence of eating disorders in older adults. "I know several women who have developed anorexia nervosa after they have had children and the children are older," she says. She recounts the stories of two women she encountered who suffered from eating disorders in older age.

"In the case of one woman—this was probably the oldest woman I know who came into treatment—she had either eight or twelve children. She kept very busy; all of her children were grown, and all had graduated from college with degrees of one sort or another. It was her children who insisted that she come into therapy, but she was worried about her husband's [health], as he was older than she was. While he was still alive, she refused to go into treatment. Her husband died [some time after] and then she decided to go into treatment because of the pressure from her kids, but she didn't stay more than three days. Her children's pushing for her to have treatment didn't seem to matter. There was also a big question as to how long she had actually had an eating disorder because none of her family had remembered her as anything but thin. Whether or not she had the eating disorder when they were younger was unclear, but she did not receive treatment, to my knowledge, and steadfastly refused any treatment for a long time.

"[Another older woman] was very unwilling to get treatment, and her husband and doctor colluded and lied to her and told her that she was going into the hospital just for an interview at his office in the hospital. Then when she got into the hospital, she was admitted. She was very unhappy about it and couldn't make up her mind to stay, was talked into staying a day or so, and then decided that since she was there, she'd stay a little longer. She ended up staying and going through the entire treatment and recovering."

Types of Eating Disorders

According to Grishkat, the women who come to the Renfrew Center residential facility fall evenly into three diagnoses, regardless of age: anorexia, bulimia, and eating disorder not otherwise specified.

Meehan believes that the diagnoses of eating disorder types fall evenly across the spectrum in older adults, but she notes that the patients she's known have mostly exhibited anorexia nervosa. "Now that may be because it's easy to see when a person is getting thin, very thin, and maintains their thinness over great protestations, whereas bulimics are so good at hiding it," she says. "I remember a husband who reported that he never knew that his wife had an eating disorder, and I think they had been married for something like fifteen years. One day, he came home from work early because he wasn't feeling well, and as he entered the kitchen, he saw his wife vomiting into the sink."

After the husband confronted his wife, she denied the vomiting. "He said he wanted to believe her, but that he actually couldn't. He began to put two and two together, but she was adamant about denying her illness all through that period where he was trying to get her into treatment. I don't know if she ever did go into treatment or go into treatment successfully," Meehan recounts.

Older adults suffering from eating disorders fall mainly into the following three categories:

- Those who have suffered from an eating disorder in the past and went untreated

- Those whose eating disorder went into remission and resurfaced later in life

- Those whose disorder emerged later in life

Grishkat says the majority of women who suffer from later-life eating disorders have actually been dealing with them from a much younger age. "The largest of the three categories are those women who have had an eating disorder their entire lives," she notes, adding that this category is followed by that including women who had eating disorders when they were young, that went into remission and reemerged later in life because of some stressor.

"The smallest group includes those who have only recently developed an eating disorder. Even with this group, when we look more closely at the history of these women, most of them have had some type of disordered eating throughout most of their lives, although it may not have risen to the point of a formal eating disorder diagnosis," Grishkat explains.

Triggers for Disordered Eating

While some triggers of eating disorders may look similar for younger vs. older patients, there are some definite differences as the stressors in life change as one gets older. "The triggers differ for younger vs. older women in that older women are dealing a lot more with issues of loss and grieving," says Grishkat. "Younger women's issues tend to focus more on transitions. Regardless of when you develop an eating disorder, the one common trigger is stress of some sort. The stressors just change with age. So while younger, the women may have been dealing with the transition from high school to college or from childhood to adulthood, older women's stressors include such things as empty nest, divorce, loss of parents, widowhood, retirement, chronic illness/disability, death of an adult child, and growing old/facing mortality."

Additional triggers for older adults dealing with eating disorders can include lack of enthusiasm for life; attempts to get attention from family members; protest against living conditions, such as in a nursing home; economic hardship; and medical problems.

Meehan says certain medical circumstances can also bring on an eating disorder in older adults. She recalls one woman who she believes began disordered eating practices quite unintentionally: "I remember once I was at a college health fair, and an older woman walked in and said that she wanted to take the eating attitudes test. [After taking it,] she scored very high, and so I started asking her questions about what was going on in her life. She said that she had recently (about two years [previously]) been diagnosed with a heart attack and that [healthcare professionals] began telling her that she had to be very careful with her diet and make sure that she ate the right things. She got very anxious, and she didn't know what to eat or how she should eat and began eating less than she should. She began losing weight, and she talked to the doctors about it but they didn't seem to know [that she had a problem].

"Now whether she had fully explained to the doctors all of her fears, I don't know," Meehan continues. "But the fact is that she was scared to death because she was afraid that she was going to die if she didn't eat the right things. And she had a hard time figuring out what were the right things. So, I don't think she had an eating disorder early on in her life; I think this developed sometime later. When she developed a heart attack, she was concerned that this was going to be it. So for her, it was fear that maintained and perhaps increased her eating disorder."

As Grishkat says, "Eating disorders are never about weight, food, numbers, etc., but they are a way of coping with something else that the person finds extremely difficult to express, feel, or control. In this way, the role of the eating disorder is much like alcohol for an alcoholic. Both serve the same purpose—to avoid, numb, and cope. So, if as an adolescent the person learned that this was an effective way of coping, we wouldn't find it unusual that they might revert back to this unhealthy coping mechanism to deal with later life stressors, particularly if the person has never learned other, healthier ways of coping."

Signs, Symptoms, and Treatment

It can be difficult to identify or diagnose an eating disorder in older adults, Grishkat says. But the following signs can be clues to later-life disordered eating:

- Significant change in weight (up or down) over a relatively short period of time
- Changes in behavior such as disappearing after a meal or using the restroom after eating something
- Boxes of laxatives, diet pills, or diuretics
- Desire to eat in the bedroom alone rather than eating with family or spouse
- Missing food
- Sensitivity to cold
- Excessive hair loss, dental damage, or heart or gastrointestinal problems

"Not all patients have all of the symptoms," Meehan acknowledges. She also notes that eating disorders often occur co-morbidly with depression or other types of anxiety disorders, so these can also serve as clues to possible problems.

A lack of sufficient treatment options that provide programming for midlife and older women could be a deterrent to later-life women getting into treatment, according to Grishkat. "Many fear being put into groups with adolescents and young adults with whom they cannot relate because they are at such a different place in their lives. Additionally, these women tend to experience more shame and self-blame around their eating disorders and feel they should be the role models for the younger girls rather than sitting in a group as one of them. We have also found in our experience that when the younger women and [older] women are treated together, the older women tend to take on a motherly role with the younger women and focus their energies on taking care of others rather than caring for themselves," she says.

In a study conducted by ANAD, 86 percent of participants reported the onset of their eating disorder occurred by the age of twenty, but only 50 percent reported being cured. "This is one reason why we find large numbers of women and men in their thirties, forties, fifties, and beyond suffering from these illnesses," says Meehan. But on a slightly more positive note, Grishkat says she has noticed that most of the older women she has treated tend to be very determined in their pursuit for health and wellness. "They dedicate themselves to the treatment and have many motivators that the younger women don't have—i.e., children, a family, aging, etc. As a result, these women tend to do well in treatment."

Hope and Help

Meehan holds out hope for the possibility of recovery for older women dealing with eating disorders. "If older women seek treatment and join support groups through organizations like ANAD, they can recover and go on to lead healthy and productive lives," she says, noting that sometimes healthcare professionals or family members need to get creative in getting older women into treatment.

In the realm of helping older adults suffering from an eating disorder, Grishkat says the advice crosses the age divide. "Women should know that there is treatment out there for them—women of any age," she says.

Section 19.2

Identifying Eating Disorders in the Elderly

"Is It an Eating Disorder?" © 2009 Eating Disorders Foundation of Victoria. Reprinted with permission. For additional information and resources, visit www.eatingdisorders.org.au.

Many older people experience problems with eating which may be classified as "disordered eating" or "eating distress" and these may be a result of physical or emotional issues in a person's life. It is important to note that an eating disorder is a mental illness which originates as a coping mechanism to deal with overwhelming internal and/or external issues. It is not uncommon for middle-aged or older people to experience a loss in appetite due to physical health concerns—if this type of food refusal takes place without psychological factors such as a pursuit of thinness, avoidance of normal weight, or body image distortion, it would most likely not be diagnosed as an eating disorder. Below are a few reasons why a decrease in appetite may take place, which are not independently classified as an eating disorder:

- An undiscovered illness or infection can cause loss of appetite—reflux, gastrointestinal problems.

- Some medications cause loss of appetite, others cause stomach upset or pain that discourages eating.

- Missing or decaying teeth make it difficult to eat, similarly poorly fitting dentures may cause pain and difficulty with food consumption.

- Poor memory may lead to confusion over whether one has eaten and result in missed meals.

- Lack of energy and/or motivation for grocery shopping and food preparation can discourage eating.

- Poverty is a problem for many seniors and some may not have the financial means to buy food, particularly of nutritious value.

- Depression is often associated with decreased appetite, as are associated feelings of loneliness and lack of meaningful connections with other people.

Regardless, these factors are very important to address as there are many physical, mental, and emotional consequences that can accompany a marked decrease in appetite and resulting nutrient deficiency for older people. Please consult your doctor if this is the case.

Chapter 20

Eating Disorders in Athletes

Chapter Contents

Section 20.1

Athletes and Eating Disorders: What Coaches, Parents, and Teammates Need to Know

"Athletes and Eating Disorders: What Coaches, Parents, and Teammates Need to Know,"© 2005 National Eating Disorders Association. For more information, visit www.NationalEatingDisorders.org. Reviewed by David A. Cooke, M.D., FACP, October 2010.

Involvement in organized sports can offer many benefits, such as improved self esteem and body image and encouragement for individuals to remain active throughout their lives. Athletic competition, however, can also cause severe psychological and physical stress. When the pressures of athletic competition are added to an existing cultural emphasis on thinness, the risks increase for athletes to develop disordered eating. In a study of Division 1 National Collegiate Athletic Association (NCAA) athletes, over one-third of female athletes reported attitudes and symptoms placing them at risk for anorexia nervosa. Though most athletes with eating disorders are female, male athletes are also at risk—especially those competing in sports that tend to place an emphasis on the athlete's diet, appearance, size, and weight requirements, such as wrestling, bodybuilding, crew, running, and football.

Risk Factors for Athletes

- Sports that emphasize appearance or weight requirements. For example: gymnastics, diving, bodybuilding, or wrestling—e.g., wrestlers trying to "make weight."

- Sports that focus on the individual rather than the entire team. For example: gymnastics, running, figure skating, dance, or diving, versus teams sports like basketball or soccer.

- Endurance sports such as track and field/running, swimming.

- Inaccurate belief that lower body weight will improve performance.

- Training for a sport since childhood or being an elite athlete.

- Low self-esteem; family dysfunction; families with eating disorders; chronic dieting; history of physical or sexual abuse; peer, family, and cultural pressures to be thin; and other traumatic life experiences.

- Coaches who focus only on success and performance rather than on the athlete as a whole person.

Three factors have been thought to contribute to the odds that a person will be dissatisfied with his or her body: social influences, performance anxiety, and the athlete's self-appraisal.

Protective Factors for Athletes

- Positive, person-oriented coaching style rather than negative, performance oriented coaching style.

- Social influence and support from teammates with healthy attitudes toward size and shape.

- Coaches who emphasize factors that contribute to personal success such as motivation and enthusiasm rather than body weight or shape.

Female Athlete Triad

The female athlete triad includes (1) disordered eating, (2) loss of menstrual periods, and (3) osteoporosis (loss of calcium resulting in weak bones). The lack of nutrition resulting from disordered eating can cause the loss of several or more consecutive periods. This in turn leads to calcium and bone loss, putting the athlete at greatly increased risk for stress fractures of the bones. Each of these conditions is a medical concern. Together they create serious health risks that may be life threatening. While any female athlete can develop the triad, adolescent girls are most at risk because of the active biological changes and growth spurts, peer and social pressures, and rapidly changing life circumstances that go along with the teenage years. Males may develop similar syndromes.

Section 20.2

Identifying Eating Disorders in Athletes

"Eating Disorders among Athletes," © 2001 The Ohio State University
Extension (http://ohioline.osu.edu/). Reprinted with permission.
Reviewed by David A. Cooke, MD, FACP, October 2010.

Some athletes spend hours of intense training for their sport while
practicing dangerous eating patterns in an attempt to lose weight. This
practice often leads to eating disorders among athletes. This section
will give signs and symptoms of eating disorders. Parents, coaches, and
trainers need to recognize athletes with disordered eating patterns
and refer them to appropriate resources.

Athletes at greatest risk include gymnasts, dancers, wrestlers, swim-
mers, figure skaters, and participants in any sport that emphasizes
weight control. The eating disorders anorexia nervosa and bulimia
nervosa are considered to be psychological and behavioral disorders
that may develop into potentially life-threatening weight loss. Sometimes an eating disorder occurs along with such things as anxiety or
pain and the eating disorder is used as a way to cope.

Females are most susceptible to eating disorders which may be
brought on by social pressure to be thin or parental pressure to succeed. Persons with eating disorders feel the need to gain control over
their lives through dieting or refusing to eat.

Signs and Symptoms

Anorexia

- Significant weight loss
- Hyperactivity, depression, or moodiness
- Distorted body image (believe they are fat even when very thin)
- Loss of menstrual periods for at least three cycles
- Growth of fine, downy hair on body
- Feeling cold much of the time
- Excessive exercise

- Restricted food intake
- Obsessive-compulsive behavior

Bulimia

- Consume large amounts of food within a specific time period, usually less than two hours
- Binges are followed by vomiting
- Secretly eating food
- Dependent on laxatives, diuretics or diet pills, excessive exercise
- Swollen salivary glands
- Dental problems caused by acid on teeth
- Feeling ashamed and depressed about eating habits

Even though these eating disorders are considered to be psychological and behavioral, if identified early, treatment is more easily handled. The athletes will give clues that a problem exists. Adults in charge need to keep their eyes and ears open to these clues.

Watch for the following clues to help you identify an eating disorder:

- Hearing the athlete repeatedly express concerns about being overweight, when in fact his or her weight is below average.
- The athlete expresses fears of becoming obese. These fears do not diminish, even after the athlete has lost weight.
- Refusal by the athlete to maintain a minimal normal weight that is consistent with the athlete's weight.
- Observing the athlete consume large amounts of food and then promptly head to the bathroom. When the athlete returns, he or she continues to eat additional large portions of food. A pattern of this particular behavior indicates a problem might exist.
- Bloodshot eyes, especially after the athlete has made a trip to the bathroom.
- Wide fluctuations in weight over a short period of time.
- The athlete may complain of lightheadedness or disequilibrium which cannot be accounted for by other medical causes.
- The odor of vomit in the toilet, sink, shower, or even wastebasket.

- The athlete wears bulky clothes to hide thinness and complains of being cold.

- The athlete may refuse to eat in public or with his or her friends.

If you are a parent or a coach who suspects an athlete is experiencing an eating disorder, express your concern to the individual very carefully. Do not accuse the athlete of being anorexic or bulimic. Remember the disorder is more than an eating problem. Eating disorders generally reflect an inability to cope with life's day-to-day stresses. Instead, express concern about the athlete's health and energy. Do not discuss weight or eating habits.

Don't expect athletes to readily admit that they have an eating disorder, but be supportive, patient, consistent, and concerned. Listen to what they say with empathy and be able to offer a list of places and sources that can offer professional help.

Realize that you alone cannot solve the problems of eating disorders. It is a complex situation that has more to do with life than it has to do with food. Food just happens to be the factor the athlete is able to control. The athlete needs to be assured that there will be no criticism for admitting to an eating disorder. Patience is also a key word. The healing process may take a long time, but it can occur.

Resources

Clark, N. (1990). *Sports Nutrition Guidebook, Eating to Fuel Your Active Lifestyle.* Champaign, Illinois: Human Kinetics.

Frissell, S., & Harney, P. (1998). *Eating Disorders and Weight Control.* Springfield, N.J.: Enslow.

Smith, N. J., & Worthington-Roberts, B. (1989). *Food for Sport.* Palo Alto, California: Bull Publishing.

Thompson, C. (1996). Athletes and Eating Disorders. http://www.mirror-mirror.org/athlete.htm.

Section 20.3

Preventing Eating Disorders in Athletes: Tips for Coaches

"Tips for Coaches: Preventing Eating Disorders in Athletes," © 2005 National Eating Disorders Association. For more information, visit www.National EatingDisorders.org. Reviewed by David A. Cooke, M.D., FACP, October 2010.

1. Take warning signs and eating disordered behaviors seriously! Cardiac arrest and suicide are the leading causes of death for people with eating disorders.

2. If an athlete is chronically dieting or exhibits mildly abnormal eating, refer to a health professional with eating disorder expertise. Early detection increases the likelihood of successful treatment; left untreated the problem may progress to an eating disorder.

3. Deemphasize weight by not weighing athletes and eliminate comments about weight. Instead, focus on areas in which athletes have more control in order to improve performance. For example, focus on strength and physical conditioning, as well as the mental and emotional components of performance. There is no risk in improving mental and emotional capacities.

4. Don't assume that reducing body fat or weight will enhance performance. While weight loss or a reduction in body fat can lead to improved performance, studies show this does not apply to all athletes. It is not uncommon for individuals attempting to lose weight to develop eating disorder symptoms. Performance should not be at the expense of the athlete's health.

5. Instruct coaches and trainers to recognize signs and symptoms of eating disorders and understand their role in prevention. Those with eating problems often hide their symptoms to avoid calling attention to them. They are often ashamed and aware that the behavior is abnormal.

6. Provide athletes with accurate information regarding weight, weight loss, body composition, nutrition, and sports

performance to reduce misinformation and to challenge unhealthy practices. Be aware of local professionals who will help
educate the athletes.

7. Emphasize the health risks of low weight, especially for female
athletes with menstrual irregularities or amenorrhea. The athlete should be referred for medical assessments in these cases.

8. Understand why weight is such a sensitive and personal issue
for many women. Eliminate derogatory comments or behaviors
about weight—no matter how slight. If there is concern about
an athlete's weight, the athlete should be referred for an assessment to a professional skilled in diagnosing and treating
eating disorders.

9. Do not automatically curtail athletic participation if an athlete
is found to have eating problems, unless warranted by a medical condition. Consider the athlete's health, physical and emotional safety, and self-image when making decisions regarding
an athlete's level of participation in his/her sport.

10. Coaches and trainers should explore their own values and attitudes regarding weight, dieting, and body image, and how their
values and attitudes may inadvertently affect their athletes.
They should understand their role in promoting a positive self-
image and self-esteem in their athletes.

Chapter 21

Eating Disorders among Other Specific Populations

Chapter Contents

Section 21.1

Eating Disorders among Gays, Lesbians, and Bisexuals

"Eating Disorders among Gays, Lesbians, and Bisexuals,"
Eating Disorders Review, November/December 2007, Volume 18, Number 6.
© 2007 Gurze Books. Reprinted with permission.

Although anorexia nervosa and bulimia nervosa are reported primarily among women, men make up from 5 to 20 percent of patients with eating disorders. Studies also suggest that a disproportionate number of these men are gay or bisexual. In both community and clinical samples of men with eating disorders, from 14 to 42 percent are gay or bisexual (in contrast to about 3 percent of the U.S. male population). Numerous studies have found that, compared with heterosexual men, gay men have more behavioral symptoms indicative of eating disorders. In one study, the proportion of gay and bisexual men with symptoms related to eating disorders was ten times higher than among heterosexual men (*J Soc Clin Psychol*. 2000;19:240).

A Community Study

Matthew B. Feldman, Ph.D., and Ilan H. Meyer, Ph.D., recently interviewed 524 gay, lesbian, or bisexual men and women who were recruited from various New York City community venues, including bookstores, coffee shops, and social groups. The respondents were equally divided among men, women, whites, blacks, and Hispanics. A heterosexual comparison group included 65 white men and 63 white women. Diagnoses were made using the computer-assisted personal interview version 19 of the World Mental Health Composite International Diagnostic Interview, a fully structured measure used in the National Co-morbidity Study. The authors assessed the presence of both lifetime and current (twelve months) eating disorders, including full syndrome anorexia nervosa, bulimia nervosa, and binge eating disorder. This was the first study to assess *Diagnostic and Statistical Manual* (DSM) diagnostic categories rather than using measures indicative of eating disorders in community-based ethnically and racially diverse populations.

Higher Incidence Found among Members of Gay Clubs

Compared with heterosexual men, gay and bisexual men had a significantly higher prevalence of lifetime full-syndrome bulimia, subclinical bulimia, and any other subclinical eating disorders. There were no significant differences between heterosexual women and lesbians and bisexual women in the prevalence of any eating disorders. The incidence of eating disorders among lesbians and bisexual women was comparable to that found in heterosexual women.

Gay men who participated in a gay recreational organization or group had a significantly higher prevalence of current subclinical eating disorders, including anorexia, bulimia, and/or binge eating disorder. Other results, however, did not show the same pattern. For example, men who were members of gyms, whether the gym had a primarily gay clientele or not, did not differ from respondents who were not gym members. Similarly, the authors did not find any association between the prevalence of current eating disorders and the number and percentage of lesbian-gay-bisexual-affiliated groups and organizations where the respondents were members.

Younger Men and Women More Likely to Have Subclinical Bulimia

Younger lesbian, gay, and bisexual men and women, or those from eighteen to twenty years of age, were more likely to have subclinical bulimia compared with older participants, or those thirty to fifty-nine years of age. The authors theorize that this pattern may be due to a cohort effect that suggests that the younger generation of men and women are more vulnerable to sociocultural messages about appearance. The finding that black and Latino gays, lesbians, and bisexuals have a prevalence of eating disorders at least as high as do whites has not been evaluated because racial/ethnicity has not yet been studied, according to the authors.

Younger Patients Are at Higher Risk

The findings suggest that clinicians and public health practitioners working with gay and bisexual men need to be aware of the clinical signs of eating disorders, and should be especially attentive to younger gay/lesbian/bisexual clients, who are at increased risk. They should also avoid commonly held conventions that lesbian and bisexual women are less vulnerable to developing eating disorders than are heterosexual women. Similarly, the authors note that racial and ethnic minorities are no less vulnerable to these disorders than are whites.

Section 21.2

Eating Disorders in Minority Populations

"Multicultural Issues and Eating Disorders,"
by Jacquelyn Ekern, MS, LPC. © 2010 Eating Disorder Hope
(www.eatingdisorderhope.com).
Reprinted with permission.

Abstract

Eating disorders amongst Caucasian, African American, Native American, Asian, and Pacific Islanders are reviewed considering the values, cultural norms, and mores of these groups as they face acculturation into the United States. Cultural influences, physiology, and psychology are also examined in light of their contribution to cross-cultural eating disorders. Treatment options and techniques are discussed, such as: cognitive behavior therapy, locus of control, and the stages of the counseling relationship as applied to clients struggling with eating disorders.

Multicultural Issues in Eating Disorders

Anorexia nervosa and bulimia nervosa are composed of complex etiologies of developmental, social, and biological processes. How these various factors interact and influence an individual to develop an eating disorder continues to be researched. There is limited evidence that cultural factors are the primary contributor to these disorders. This can be observed in all industrialized countries, where dieting and emphasis on thinness are highly valued (Kaye,W. & Strober, M., 1999). The more a woman, of any ethnicity, rejects her own heritage and identifies with the European American mainstream culture, the more likely that she will prefer a thinner body type and show more signs of an eating disorder (Meshreki, L. & Hansen, C., 2004). Further, when women of all races base their evaluation of their self upon what is considered the culturally ideal body, the incidence of eating disorders increases (Jung, J. & Lennon, S., 2003).

Hispanic Women

Among Hispanic Americans, having an overweight body does not necessarily reflect negatively upon the individual. The determining factor, to the Hispanic mindset, is whether the state of being overweight is the individual's fault or not. For example, if an overweight individual continually overeats and does not exercise, they are more likely to be blamed for their weight and stigmatized. However, if the individual is perceived as fat, through no fault of their own, it is likely to not be judged negatively.

A 1996 study conducted by Christian Crandall and Rebecca Martinez compared attitudes regarding weight amongst students from the United States and Mexico. The United States is considered to be the most individualistic culture in the world. The culture of the United States values independence and fosters the belief that individuals are responsible for the results in their lives (Grogan, S., 1999). Whereas Mexico offers a culture that values interdependence and connection; emphasizing external influences on behavior. Crandall and Martinez predicted and found that Mexican students, in general, did not blame the individual for being overweight and did not see it as a matter of lack of personal control. The Mexican students also were less likely to stigmatize someone for being overweight or support anti-fat attitudes. While students of the United States viewed being overweight as a sign of weak willpower and the fault of the individual. Crandall and Martinez contend that anti-fat attitudes reflect the pervasive Western ideology that individuals determine their own fate (Grogan, S., 1999).

Asian Women

Research shows that white women are more likely to feel fat and diet than are Asian American women. However, because of increasing global acceptance of dominant white socio-cultural values regarding body weight and image, increasingly more Asian Americans and other cultural groups are developing greater dissatisfaction with their weight (Grogan, S., 1999). More Japanese women are expressing dissatisfaction with their bodies and weight—almost to the level of American women (Mukai, Kambara, & Sasaki, 1998).

Some qualitative studies have shown that Chinese women view seeking treatment for an eating disorder as reflecting individual weakness. Even if the disorder is more than the individual can handle, they remain unlikely to pursue treatment (Lai Bovenkerk, 2001; Leung et al., 1978).

Asian Americans value loyalty to family and deference to authority. Sharing personal problems with others may bring shame upon the family. The family can often be threatening to the self-esteem of an Asian individual, instead of supportive. For example, a female Asian American might be experiencing significant marital and financial problems, but she would not likely speak to anyone, including her family, about her struggles. She believes that others, particularly her family, will lose respect for her if she is unable to solve her problems herself. She may feel greater depression because of her secrecy (Chiu, M., 2002).

The Asian culture values self-reliance and maintaining the honor of the family. Therefore, medical and psychological treatments designed to meet the needs of Asian women should strive to avoid blaming or emphasizing that the eating disorder is the result of any personal deficiencies in the individual or the family (Chiu, M., 2002). Sensitivity toward protecting the pride of the family is important with the Asian culture. Offering anonymous hotlines and websites that inform consumers of treatment options would allow this group to explore treatment and information regarding the eating disorder without fearing that they will bring shame upon themselves or the family. Leaving the choice up to the Asian client of whether or not to more publicly seek out treatment is also important with this group (Sharma and Aradhana, 2000).

The Chinese culture is based upon the teachings of Confucianism and Taoism. The social order of Chinese society is structured upon harmonious interpersonal relationships amongst families. These harmonious relationships are maintained by avoiding conflict; using nonconfrontational language, self-discipline, self-restraint, indirect expression of disapproval, and allowing others to save face (Chen, 2002). Chinese families commonly deny any familial problems, and will blame individual problems, such as anorexia, upon the family member. Adolescent individuation and rebellion are typically perceived as a threat to the authority of the parents and risking the harmony of the family. This must be considered when suggesting assertive approaches to Asian clients.

A verse from Xiao Jing (The Classic of Filial Piety) depicts an important Chinese family honor value: "Your body with your hair and your skin is a gift from your parents. You must treasure this gift to be filial" (Xiao Jing, 1960). This teaching can be applied as a double-edged sword, on one hand it could encourage the anorexic child to recover, yet on the other hand it could encourage the parents to try to control the child even more than they already do. Individuation is discouraged for Chinese women. These women base their identity upon an idealized woman and mother that is socially construed. Throughout the various stages of life, Chinese women are expected to be submissive, subordinate, and subjugate to the will of the father, the husband, and the son (Ma, J., 2005). Asian adolescent girls and women acculturating to the United States are often torn between the individualistic Western society amidst which they now live, and the self-sacrificing and loyal cultural values of their heritage and family. This can leave Asian females feeling estranged from both cultures and caught in the middle in a state of cognitive dissonance (Ma, J., 2005).

Chinese adolescent females are concerned with maintaining the dignity and pride of the family. They are typically reluctant to seek outside help for eating disorders, because this would involve divulging private family matters to an outsider. Though Chinese parents are more willing to seek outside treatment for eating disorders if they perceive the health of their child to be threatened (Ma & Chan, 2004).

When treating an Asian individual or family for an eating disorder, it is important to recognize that the majority of literature regarding family therapy and eating disorders is written from a Western perspective. The insightful therapist can use the cognitive dissonance created in an Asian individual or family struggling to find a balance between eastern and western thought as an opportunity for the individual and family to explore values and beliefs; as well as reconsider how they relate to one another. The therapist can use this process to build up the family members' confidence and commitment to each other.

Understanding the family background of Chinese parents will empower both the therapist and eating disordered client to understand the parent's personal and social expectations in parenting. This can create important empathy on the part of the eating disordered individual and aid them in collaborating more effectively with their parents in recovery (Ma, J., 2005).

Additionally, when working with Chinese families, the family therapist must search out and acknowledge the subtle indicators of conflict amongst the family. Family conflicts must be patiently approached with observation of nonverbal cues used to indicate conflict (Chen, G., 2002).

African American Women

African American women prefer larger body shapes and report greater satisfaction with their bodies than Caucasian women (Ashley, Smith, Robinson, & Richardson, 1996; Miller, Gleaves, Hirsch, Green, Snow, & Corbett, 2000), and also reported fewer eating disorders than white women (Abrams, Allen, Gray, 1993; Rucker & Cash, 1992). Further, obese African-American women maintained a more positive body image than Caucasian women (Grogan, 1999). African American women who take pride in their cultural heritage are more likely to refer to the more liberal body ideal of their race when evaluating their own body. However, eating disorders have been found to be more prevalent in African American women who identified with a European American worldview. Dissatisfaction with body image was also pronounced in women who had not embraced their heritage and instead tended to view the dominant white culture as superior (Meshreki, L. & Hansen, C., 2004). O'Neill, S. (2003) published a compilation of data from eighteen studies examining the correlation between eating disorders and ethnicity amongst black and white women. White women were found to be more likely to develop an eating disorder overall. However, bulimia and binge-eating disorder behavior were found to be similarly prevalent in both African American and white women. Additionally, Petersons, Rojhani, Steinhan, and Larkin (2000) found that for African American college women, high socioeconomic status was correlated with eating disturbances.

Pacific Island Women

The American territory of Guam has a significant population of Chamorro females. These women report similar levels of body dissatisfaction and eating disorders as Caucasian women. This is attributed to the American economic and cultural influence upon Guam (Hattori, 2001; Hezel, 1987).

Traditional women from the Pacific Islands appreciate a rounded female shape. They view the curvaceous and robust woman as exuding health, power, and strength (Becker, 1995). Several studies report higher body mass index (BMI) levels among individuals from the Pacific Islands (Brewis, McGarvey, Jones, & Swineburn,1998; Craig, Halavatau, Comino, & Caterson, 1999; Metcalf, Scragg, Willoughby, Finau & Tipene-Leach, 2000). Interestingly, Samoans residing in Samoa and New Zealand preferred ideal body shapes smaller than their actual bodies, but did not view overweight bodies negatively (Brewis, et al. 1998). Fijian woman prefer a medium range body type for females. However, they are accepting of obese females, too. These women expressed contentment with their weight and body shape. Even if these women were obese and preferred a smaller frame, they were unlikely to be disappointed in their shape or try to diet. As the Pacific Islands become more influenced by Western culture, studies have shown that admiration of the thin female body image is becoming more prevalent (Craig, Swinburn, Matenga-Smith, Matangi, & Vaughn, 1996; Craig, Halavatau, Comino, & Caterson).

Native American Women

American Indian and Alaska Native adolescents are increasingly unhappy with their body weight and using unhealthy means to lose weight. In a study of 545 multicultural participants, American Indians exemplified the most eating disordered attitudes and behavior. A high level of bulimic behavior was identified amongst this group. Racism, low self-esteem, and pressure to look like the American ideal female may be the leading cause of developing eating disorders amongst Native Americans. To compound matters, frequently American Indians of both genders and all age groups are overweight (American Indian, 2005).

The extended family is the core family unit for most American Indians. Children may stay in various households of the extended family. This could be difficult for a western therapist to understand because typically American children are raised solely in the home of their parents, with occasional visits to grandparents and uncles and aunts. Whereas, it is not uncommon for American Indian children to stay at a distant cousin's home or even friends who are considered part of the extended family.

American Indians value sharing, this is in sharp contrast to the American value of accumulating goods. It would be important for the therapist to recognize that sharing is a cultural norm amongst Indians, and perhaps be more open to receiving small gifts from this client group.

Cooperation and the avoidance of discord are valued by Native American Indians. This would need to be considered by the therapist when addressing conflicts within families. Though Americans typically value confrontation and assertiveness, this direct approach might be harmful to an American Indian individual. Rather, amongst Indians, noninterference is valued. Respecting the rights of others is important. For example, a Native American Indian might be reticent to report spousal abuse of a neighbor or family member, because of this value. It would be important for the therapist to respect the underlying value system operating in the American Indian client's reluctance to step forward in such a situation.

Harmony with nature is desired by American Indians, rather than the American tendency to dominate the environment (Sue & Sue,

2003). This fundamental difference may influence the overall perspective of the American Indian, perhaps causing them to have a far more relaxed approach to addressing problems than the aggressive mentality of many Western mental health practitioners.

The time orientation of American Indians differs greatly from that of the dominant American culture. Future planning is not valued for Indians; rather living fully in the moment takes precedence (Sue & Sue, 2003). Punctuality is not highly valued by this group either, which is different than the norms of American culture. A therapist would need to be sensitive to this and not overreact to a late arrival of a client, misinterpreting it as passive aggression rather than a difference in cultural paradigms about time.

One generic counseling characteristic is to value emotional expression, and its perceived cathartic benefits. However, most American Indians and Alaskan Natives are understated in emotional expression (Sue & Sue, 2003). An overzealous Western therapist could cause the American Indian/Alaskan Native client to feel uncomfortable and forced to put on theatrics. It is important to respect the emotional expression norms of the culture that the practitioner is treating.

Another commonly valued generic counseling tool is in-depth discussions regarding deeply personal matters in the life of the client. However, privacy is valued by this group, and not revealing personal matters outside the extended family is the norm (Sue & Sue, 2003). Thus, opening up to a therapist and discussing issues would likely require a significant investment of time beforehand. Even then, it might be a far less intimate discussion than the therapist would like, because the American Indian/Native Alaskan client might not be willing to reveal too much. Disharmony is the commonly attributed cause of mental/emotional or physical illness amongst this group (Sue & Sue, 2003). Therefore, the common therapeutic approach of confrontation would likely be inappropriate for the American Indian/Native Alaskan client. Disregarding the cultural emphasis on disharmony and continuing to emphasize individualism and confrontation would be deeply unsettling to this client. Rather, recognizing the value of interdependent relationships amongst the extended family might be the first step. This group has the strength of many individuals to draw from to meet their needs. Therefore, they might be able to reconsider getting needs met by other individuals than the one that the therapist might have initially suggested confronting. Instead, they might work on accepting that flawed individual (as we all are flawed) and honoring what they do get from that relationship, and then moving on to others in their rich environment of extended family to meet their other needs.

Physiology

In addition to cultural factors, there likely is a significant genetic influence in the etiology of anorexia and bulimia. Several studies have demonstrated that an individual is seven to twelve times more likely to develop an eating disorder if it runs in the family. It is hypothesized that something goes awry in the neurotransmitter modulation in appetitive behaviors. This matter is complicated by the fact that the very dietary restrictions and abnormal behaviors inherent in anorexia and bulimia could cause monoamine or neuropeptide disturbances. That being said, abnormal serotonin (5-HT) is the neurotransmitter frequently blamed for contributing to eating disorders. Disturbance of serotonin activity, due to a gene that codes for an abnormal serotonin receptor, has been found in several studies of individuals with anorexia. Compared to a placebo control group, individuals taking antidepressants, specifically selective serotonin reuptake inhibitors (SSRI's), reduced their binge eating and vomiting. Additionally, SSRI's can reduce weight obsession and even encourage weight loss amongst eating disordered individuals. The SSRI's seem to aid the neurotransmitter system in modulating mood and impulse control. However, a severely emaciated anorexic is unlikely to see any improvement in her symptoms of anorexia from simply being treated with a selective serotonin reuptake inhibitor. This is due to the starving brain operating from a place of deficiency in serotonin to begin with. However, once the anorexic is recovering, eating a healthy diet, and has obtained a healthy weight, then the serotonin level is likely to naturally increase within the brain; selective serotonin reuptake inhibitors may then help the anorexic to avoid relapse (Kaye, W. & Strober, M., 1999).

When addressing physiology and medication with ethnically diverse populations, present the facts and allow the individual and family time to process this information through their own individual and cultural filters. They may need to pursue their own channels of advice and counsel before considering this option. The therapist should maintain a respectful appreciation of the individual and family's right to accept or reject Western medical practices.

Psychology

In addition to cultural influences and physiological predisposition, many eating disorder researchers have concluded that a disturbance in the self is the cause of anorexia and bulimia. These individuals are often dependent upon environmental cues for self-esteem rather than an inherent sense of worth. Self schemas are a complex array of memories that the individual draws upon to define the self. These schemas cover the gamut from skills and personality traits to physical characteristics. It has been suggested that eating disordered individuals suffer from more negative self schemas, thus resulting in depression and a desire to isolate. For example, this group is likely to have a fat self schema that haunts them and drives their eating disordered behaviors. Cognitive behavior therapy is frequently used in eating disorder treatment to reframe these self schemas (Stein, K. and Nyquist, L., 2001).

Treatment

The treatment of eating disorders amongst a multicultural population is challenging. For example, a multicultural limitation of rational emotive behavior therapy (the grandfather of cognitive behavior therapy) is that it emphasizes independence. Many cultures value interdependence and thus this theory can be disconcerting and threatening if applied insensitively to all cultures.

It has always seemed that Eastern and Western philosophy contradicted each other. The focus on control, conquering, and individuality of Western thought is incongruent with much of the Eastern thought that leans toward acceptance, working with nature, and interdependence with others. However, there is value to both schools of thought, and they can be successfully integrated when approached with sensitivity and caution. For example, in some cultures, folk healers represent the spiritual dimension of healing. Many of the great philosophers have sought to integrate the spiritual and logical when evaluating the human experience. Martin Buber, Christ, Carl Rogers, and others recognized the indivisibility of the spiritual and logical aspects of man. If approached mindfully, therapists, shaman, folk healers, and doctors have much in common. They all focus on healing the being. The being consists of physical, emotional, spiritual, and intellectual components. Thus, it is logical to conclude that addressing all aspects of the individual would lead to the greatest healing. Unfortunately, many problems can arise when working with multicultural spiritual practitioners as consultants. The training and education of the folk healer can be questionable, causing the therapist to lack trust in the suggestions of the spiritual advisor, no matter how sincere their desire to help. Also, the realm of uncredentialed spiritual healers can draw some unstable individuals that could unintentionally inflict harm upon a mutual client. The prudent therapist would respect the client's desire to gain spiritual insight, honor that, and yet maintain a professional distance from the spiritual advisor. The therapist would be wise to instruct clients to use both their intuition and intellect when evaluating potential spiritual advice and healing. Donald Meichenbaum designed cognitive behavior modification therapy. This theory is based upon cognitive restructuring which means to restructure one's self-dialogue and thus one's behavior. Clients must become aware of their scripted behavior patterns and what the underlying self-dialogue is, so that they can recognize what is motivating their behavior. Then change is possible. Meichenbaum emphasizes treating behavior problems such as impulsive and aggressive behavior by teaching clients to develop healthier coping skills. He outlined a specific treatment model of self-observation, creating a new internal dialogue and learning and implementing new skills. Meichenbaum developed a three-stage coping skills program entitled stress inoculation. This program consists of three techniques: (1) the conceptual phase: where the therapist and client work together to comprehend the stress-inducing issue and attempt to reframe the stressful event conceptually, (2) skills-acquisition and rehearsal phase: is about direct actions. Clients acquire and rehearse new self-dialogue techniques and stress management skills, (3) application and follow through phase: is emphasizing implementing the skills learned in therapy into the real world. Meichenbaum's cognitive behavior therapy is often ineffective for Middle-Eastern or Asian cultures. Disputing a motive or belief of a male in these societies is unacceptable. A therapist would need to be aware of this and modify their technique accordingly.

Two key psychological constructs, locus of control and locus of responsibility, as outlined by Kluckhohn and Strodtbeck's worldview model (Sue & Sue, 2003), can be useful in evaluating a client's level of acculturation. For example, a Japanese American client might present for treatment with a desire to fit in; thus rejecting her heritage and seeking to identify with the American culture. She may also view herself as a Japanese woman through the critical perception of an ethnocentric American rather than the culturally aware and sensitive woman that she has the potential to be. This client would benefit from encouragement to examine her beliefs about herself and her culture, and encouragement to question the paradigms that she has chosen for her worldview. The therapist would want to pose key questions regarding assimilation, such as: Why does she feel it is so important to fit in with the dominant culture? What value does her family place on their heritage? Additional important questions to be posed by the therapist regarding acculturation are: What does she like and dislike about the dominant culture and why? What benefits does she recognize in the dominant culture over her own heritage? What disadvantages? The therapist might also address her feelings of control and responsibility by posing questions, such as: How is she able to identify with the American cultural value of internal control? Did she feel that the Japanese culture failed to recognize the wisdom of the American emphasis on control? Or had she considered that perhaps an external locus of control might be a more accurate description of reality?

The capacity to accept oneself and take pride in oneself seems to be a cross-cultural need of all people. Feeling shame or embarrassment about one's heritage can lead to insecurity. The beauty of worldviews, paradigms, and other theories is that they can be changed. We, as growing human beings, can re-examine our assumptions and attitudes and reframe our perspectives.

An ideal therapist treating a multicultural population would embody Carl Rogers's (1967) core facilitative conditions of congruence, empathy and unconditional positive regard. Congruence would inspire trust in clients, as most cultures are likely to trust an individual capable of living at their highest level of integrity and demonstrating behavior, choices, and attitudes consistent with their internal value system. Empathy would be valuable because it would provide the client the opportunity to feel heard, understood, and accepted. Ideally, this client might feel that the therapist could see things from their perspective. Finally, unconditional positive regard would offer the client a safe and nurturing environment in which to explore themselves and deepen their self-acceptance.

The helping process stages consist of five areas: relationship building, assessment, goal setting, intervention and action, outcome evaluation and termination (Young, M., 2005). Initially, the rapport building of the therapist would be paramount to a new client of a different cultural background. The established quality of that relationship would be the foundation upon which the evolving stages of the relationship would rest. The therapist should be attentive and demonstrate that they understand the client's situation through reflective and advanced reflective skills. In the assessment stage, the therapist should be efficient in gathering pertinent data, and choose open-ended questions that delivered the maximum amount of needed tedious detail without making the client feel interrogated. It would be wise for the therapist to take notes, and later familiarize themselves with the client's data, so that they do not have to re-explain their story. The therapist should be sensitive to the client's need for encouragement and support; infusing the assessment stage with some of these nurturing qualities. The therapist should be enthusiastic and hopeful in the goal-setting stage. After the counselor has adequately ascertained the client's problems and pertinent background issues (Young, M. 2005), the therapist should provide assistance in setting realistic goals to change what the client has control over. In drawing up the treatment plan, specific behavioral changes should be detailed that would bring about the client's goals. During the intervention and action stage, the therapist and client should rely upon the strength of the counseling relationship, the personal importance of the goals to the client, and use therapeutic measures instigated by the therapist that are acceptable, not necessarily comfortable, for the client (Young, M. 2005). Finally, the therapist and client should engage in the outcome evaluation and termination stage, where together they would evaluate the progress made toward the client's goals and whether continuing treatment was needed.

References

Abood, D. A. & Chandler, S. B. (1997). Race and the role of weight, weight change, and body dissatisfaction in eating disorders. *American Journal of Health Behavior*, 21, 21–25.

Abrams, K. K., Allen, L., & Gray, J. J. (1993). Disordered eating attitudes and behaviors, psychological adjustment, and ethnic identity: A comparison of black and white female college students. *International Journal of Eating Disorders*, 14, 49–57.

American Indian and Alaska Native Girls. Eating disorder information sheet. Retrieved on March 13,2005 from:http://www.prevlink.org/clearing house/catalog/health_mental_health/eating_disorders/indian.pdf.

Ashley, C. D., Smith, J. F., Robinson, J. B., & Richardson, M. T. (1996). Disordered eating in female collegiate athletes and collegiate females in advanced program of study: A preliminary investigation. *International Journal of Sport Nutrition*, 6, 391–401.

Becker, A. T. (1995). *Body, self, and society: The view from Fiji*. Philadelphia: University of Pennsylvania Press.

Brewis, A. A., McGarvey, S. T., Jones, J., & Swinburn, B. A. (1998). Perceptions of body size in Pacific Islanders. *International Journal of Obesity*, 22, 185–89.

Chen, G. M. (2002). The impact of harmony on Chinese conflict management. In G. M. Chen & R. Ma (Eds.), *Chinese conflict management and resolution* (pp. 3–18). Westport, CT: Ablex.

Chiu, M.Y.L. (2002) Help-seeking of Chinese families in a Hong Kong new town. *Journal of Social Policy and Social Work*, 6, 221–40.

Craig, P., Halavatau, V., Comino, E., & Caterson, I. (1999). Perception of body size in the Tongan community: differences from and similarities to an Australian sample. *International Journal of Obesity Related Metabolic Disorders*, 23, 1288–94.

Craig, P., Swinburn, B. A., Matenga-Smith, T., Matangi, H., & Vaughn, G. (1996). Do Polynesians still believe that big is beautiful? Comparison of body size perceptions and preferences of Cook Island, Maori and Australians. *New Zealand Journal of Medicine*, 109, 200–203.

Crandall, Christian S. and Rebecca Martinez. 1996. Culture, Ideology, and Anti-Fat Attitudes. *Personality and Social Psychology Bulletin* 22: 1165–76.

Garner, D. M. (1991). Eating disorders inventory-2. Professional.

Hattori, A. P. (2001). Guam. In M. Ember, & C. Ember (Eds.), *Countries and their cultures* (Vol. 2). New York: Macmillan References.

Jung, J. and Lennon, S. Body Image, Appearance Self-Schema, and Media Images. *Family and Consumer Sciences Research Journal*, Vol. 32, No. 1, September 2003 27–51.

Kaye, W. and Strober, M. Serotonin: Implications for the Etiology & Treatment of Eating Disorders. *Eating Disorders Review*, May/June 1999, Vol. 10, No. 3.

Lai Bovenkerk, Y. (2001) An Investigation of the Experiences and Perspectives of Immigrant Chinese Canadian Mothers of Sons with Disabilities: Parent Involvement, Coping, and Related Beliefs and Values. PhD Thesis, University of British Columbia, Canada.

Muaki, T., Kambara, A., & Saski, Y. (1998). Body dissatisfaction, need for social approval, and eating disturbances among Japanese and American college women. *Sex Roles*, 39, 751–61.

Pandey, Shanta; Min Zhan; Collier-Tension, Shannon. Families' experience with welfare reform on reservations in Arizona. *Social Work Research*, June 2004, Vol. 28 Issue 2, 93.

Petersons, M., Rojhani, A., Steinhan, N., & Larkin, B. (2000). Effect of ethnicity on attitudes, feelings, and behaviors toward food. *Eating Disorders: The Journal of Treatment and Prevention*, 8, 207–19.

Stein, K. and Nyquist, L. Disturbance in the Self: A Source of Eating Disorders. *Eating Disorders Review*, January/February 2001, Vol. 12, No 1.

Sue, D. W. and Sue, D. (2003). *Counseling the culturally diverse: Theory and practice.*(4th ed.). New York: John Wiley & Sons, Inc.

Ma, Joyce L. C., Family Treatment for a Chinese Family With an Adolescent Suffering From Anorexia Nervosa: A Case Study. *The Family Journal*, January 2005, vol. 13, no. 1, pp. 19–26.

Meshreki, L. M.& Hansen, C. E. African American Men's Female Body Size Preferences Based on Racial Identity and Environment. *Journal of Black Psychology*, November 2004, vol. 30, no. 4, pp. 451–76.

XiaoJing: The Classic of Filial Piety. Retrieved on March 13, 2005 from: http://www.chinapage.com/confucius/xiaojing-be.html Young, M. (2005). *Learning the Art of Helping: Building Blocks and Techniques.* NJ: Pearson Merrill, Prentice Hall.

Chapter 22

Problems Frequently Co-Occurring with Eating Disorders

Chapter Contents

Section 22.1

Eating Disorders and Anxiety Disorders

Most people can find something they don't like about their body, and many take steps to eat more healthfully or start an exercise plan to improve their appearance.

Those with eating disorders develop habits that can cause a great deal of harm. They may fast or severely restrict their calories, exercise for hours on end each day, or take other actions to prevent any weight gain. Even though they are often underweight, they have an intense fear of becoming fat.

Usually appearing during adolescence or young adulthood, eating disorders can also develop during childhood or later in adulthood.

They are much more common among women and girls, but men and boys account for about 5 to 15 percent of those with anorexia or bulimia and about 35 percent of those with binge eating disorder.

Eating disorders commonly co-occur with anxiety disorders. For those who have an anxiety disorder, a co-occurring eating disorder may make their symptoms worse and recovery more difficult. It's essential to be treated for both disorders.

An eating disorder is present when a person experiences severe disturbances in eating behavior, such as extreme reduction of food intake or extreme overeating, or feelings of extreme distress or concern about body weight or shape. A person with an eating disorder may diet, exercise, or eats excessively, which can have life-threatening or even fatal consequences.

Anorexia Nervosa

People with the eating disorder called anorexia nervosa see themselves as overweight even though they are dangerously thin.

The process of eating becomes an obsession. Unusual eating habits develop, such as avoiding food and meals, picking out a few foods and eating these in small quantities, or carefully weighing and portioning food. They may repeatedly check their body weight or engage in other techniques to control their weight, such as intense and compulsive exercise, or purging by means of vomiting and abuse of laxatives, enemas, and diuretics.

Many people with anorexia also have coexisting psychiatric and physical illnesses, including depression, anxiety, obsessive behavior, substance abuse, cardiovascular and neurological complications, and impaired physical development.

Other symptoms may develop over time:

- Thinning of the bones
- Brittle hair and nails
- Dry and yellowish skin
- Growth of fine hair over body
- Mild anemia and muscle weakness and loss
- Severe constipation
- Low blood pressure, slowed breathing and pulse
- Drop in internal body temperature, causing a person to feel cold all the time
- Lethargy
- Infrequent or absent menstrual periods

Bulimia Nervosa

Bulimia nervosa is characterized by recurrent and frequent episodes of eating unusually large amounts of food and feeling a lack of control over the eating. This binge-eating is followed by purging (vomiting, excessive use of laxatives or diuretics), fasting, or excessive exercise.

People with bulimia usually weigh within a normal range, but like those who have anorexia, they fear gaining weight, wish to lose weight, and feel intensely dissatisfied with their bodies.

And like those with anorexia, people with bulimia often have coexisting psychological illnesses such as depression, anxiety, or substance abuse problems. Many physical conditions also result from their behavior, including electrolyte imbalances, gastrointestinal problems, and oral and tooth-related problems.

Other symptoms:

- chronically inflamed and sore throat;
- swollen glands in the neck and below the jaw;

177

- worn tooth enamel and increasingly sensitive and decaying teeth as a result of exposure to stomach acids;

- gastroesophageal reflux disorder (GERD);

- intestinal distress and irritation from laxative abuse;

- kidney problems from diuretic abuse;

- severe dehydration from purging of fluids.

Binge Eating Disorder and Eating Disorder Not Otherwise Specified (EDNOS)

Another category is "eating disorder not otherwise specified," or EDNOS, which includes several variations of eating disorders. Most of these disorders are similar to anorexia or bulimia but with slightly different characteristics. Binge eating disorder is one type of EDNOS.

People with binge-eating disorder experience frequent episodes of out-of-control eating. But they do not purge their bodies of excess calories, and many people with this disorder are overweight or obese. They experience feelings of guilt, shame, or distress, often leading to another cycle of binge eating.

Obese people with binge eating disorder often have other psychological illnesses, too, including anxiety, depression, and personality disorders. In addition, obesity is associated with cardiovascular disease and hypertension.

Anxiety or Eating Disorder: Which Comes First?

A 2004 study found that two-thirds of people with eating disorders suffer from an anxiety disorder at some point in their lives and that around 42 percent had developed an anxiety disorder during childhood, well before the onset of their eating disorder. Other studies also confirm that an anxiety disorder usually precedes the onset of an eating disorder, but panic disorder often follows.

Obsessive-compulsive disorder (OCD) is the most common anxiety disorder to co-occur with an eating disorder. Those who have both disorders often develop compulsive rituals connected to food, such as weighing every bit of food or cutting it into tiny pieces, or even binge eating.

The odds of developing bulimia are greater for women with posttraumatic stress disorder (PTSD) and social anxiety disorder is also commonly found among people with an eating disorder.

Treatment

Anxiety and eating disorders may be treated at the same time and in the same manner. Even so, recovery from one disorder does not ensure recovery from another, so it is necessary to seek help for both.

A well-established, highly effective, and lasting treatment is cognitive-behavioral therapy, or CBT, which focuses on identifying, understanding, and changing thinking and behavior patterns. Benefits are usually seen in twelve to sixteen weeks, depending on the individual.

Taking medications under a doctor's supervision and joining a support group are also sound treatment options.

Treatment for eating disorders also includes nutritional management and nutritional counseling. Those who experience severe symptoms may require hospitalization to help restore them to a safe and healthy weight.

Section 22.2

Eating Disorders and Attention Deficit Hyperactivity Disorder

"Adolescent Girls with ADHD Are at Increased Risk for Eating Disorders, Study Shows," © 2008 The Rector and Visitors of the University of Virginia. Reprinted with permission.

Girls with attention deficit hyperactivity disorder (ADHD) stand a substantially greater risk of developing eating disorders in adolescence than girls without ADHD, a new study has found.

"Adolescent girls with ADHD frequently develop body-image dissatisfaction and may go through repeating cycles of binge eating and purging behaviors that are common in bulimia nervosa," said University of Virginia psychologist Amori Yee Mikami, who led the study.

The findings appear in the February 2008 issue of the *Journal of Abnormal Psychology*.

ADHD is a disorder that affects about 5 percent of school-age children, and three times more boys than girls. Symptoms include a short attention span, poor organization, excessive talking, disruptive and aggressive behavior, restlessness, and irritability. Many children with ADHD suffer through a range of problems, from poor grades to poor relations with parents and teachers, and more than half have serious problems making friends.

Because the disorder is far more common in boys, researchers are still learning its long-term effects on girls.

"Our finding suggests that girls may develop a broader range of problems in adolescence than their male counterparts," Mikami said. "They may be at risk for eating problems, which are a female-relevant domain of impairment. We know that eating disorders occur ten times more often in girls than boys."

Additionally, Mikami noted that because ADHD is more common in boys, many girls with the disorder may go undiagnosed and untreated.

"Girls with ADHD may be more at risk of developing eating problems as adolescents because they already have impulsive behaviors that can set them apart from their peers," Mikami said. "As they get older, their impulsivity may make it difficult for them to maintain healthy eating and a healthy weight, resulting in self-consciousness about their body image and the binging and purging symptoms."

The study was conducted with an ethnically diverse sample of 228 girls in the San Francisco Bay area; 140 who had been diagnosed with ADHD and 88 matched comparison girls without ADHD. They were first assessed between the ages of six and twelve and again five years later.

Girls with the "combined type" of ADHD (those with both inattention and hyperactivity/impulsivity) were most likely to have adolescent bulimia nervosa symptoms, relative to girls with the "inattentive type" of ADHD (those with inattention only) and girls without ADHD. Girls with both types of ADHD were more likely to be overweight, to have experienced harsh/critical parenting in childhood, and to have been peer-rejected than girls without ADHD. Mikami said she believes these factors could contribute to the bulimia nervosa symptoms.

"An additional concern is that stimulant medications used to treat ADHD have a side effect of appetite suppression, creating a risk that overweight girls could abuse these medicines to encourage weight loss, though we have not yet investigated that possibility," Mikami said.

She warned parents and teachers to be aware that adolescent girls with ADHD may develop an array of female-relevant symptoms beyond the standard ADHD symptoms, to include eating disorders, depression, and anxiety.

Section 22.3

Eating Disorders and Depression

Having an eating disorder is not a lifestyle choice, a "diet gone wrong" nor an attempt to get attention. A person with an eating disorder has a mental illness.

Eating disorders are serious, potentially fatal conditions and most people with eating disorders need psychological treatment and/or physical health treatment (e.g., nutritional advice) to promote recovery.

Many people who have an eating disorder will also experience depression and/or anxiety at some point in their lives.

This section looks at the links between eating disorders and other mental health problems, such as depression and anxiety disorders. It also looks at where to get help, treatment options, and what family and friends can do to support people with eating disorders.

What Are Eating Disorders?

Eating disorders involve an unhealthy preoccupation with eating, exercise, and body weight/shape. Distorted thoughts and emotions about body image and self-worth can lead to marked changes in eating and exercise behaviors—these may include excessive dieting, fasting, overexercising, using medications (e.g., slimming pills, diuretics, laxatives), vomiting, or binge eating.

Eating disorders vary in characteristics and causes, but can generally be linked to negative feelings and low self-esteem. An unhealthy relationship with food is often an attempt to deal with underlying mental health problems.

Eating disorders are common and increasing. In Australia, one in four people knows someone who has experienced an eating disorder. About two to three in every one hundred Australian females has anorexia or bulimia nervosa, and around four in one hundred Australians have symptoms of binge eating disorder. It is not uncommon for a person to progress from one eating disorder to another.

Eating disorders can affect people from any age group, gender, or socioeconomic and cultural background.

Warning Signs of an Eating Disorder

Anyone experiencing several of the following warning signs should seek help straight away.

Table 22.1. Features of Eating Disorders

Anorexia nervosa	Distorted body image and obsessive fear of gaining weight
	Extremely limited food intake and increased levels of exercise
	Can lead to a dangerously low body weight, malnutrition, and starvation
Bulimia nervosa	Often starts with dieting to lose weight
	Binge-eating followed by vomiting, fasting, or overexercising
	Binge/purge/exercise cycle can become increasingly compulsive and uncontrollable over time
Binge eating disorder	Eating of excessive amounts of food, often when not hungry, as a distraction from other problems
	No purging, but feelings of intense guilt, shame, and self-hatred after binges
	May involve sporadic fasts and repetitive diets
Eating disorders not otherwise specified (EDNOS)	EDNOS is a term used when a person shows signs of disordered eating, but does not meet all the criteria of a specific eating disorder. For example, a person could show all of the psychological signs of anorexia and be losing weight, but still be menstruating and not yet be underweight for their height. There are a number of types of EDNOS, though many may not be recognized or diagnosed by a doctor.

Behavioral Signs

- Dieting or overeating excessively
- Eating very quickly or very slowly
- Eating only certain types and amounts of food
- Avoiding social situations that involve food
- "Playing" with food rather than eating it
- Going to the bathroom straight after meals
- Wearing loose-fitting clothes to hide weight loss

- Preparing and cooking meals for others, but not actually eating

- Engaging in repetitive or obsessive behaviors relating to body shape and weight (e.g., weighing)

- Exercising excessively, feeling compelled to perform a certain number of repetitions of exercises or experiencing distress if unable to exercise

Physical Signs

- Weight loss or weight fluctuations

- Sensitivity to the cold or feeling cold most of the time, even in warm temperatures

- Changes in or loss of menstrual patterns

- Swelling around the cheeks or jaw, calluses on knuckles, or damage to teeth due to vomiting

- Fainting

Emotional or Psychological Symptoms

- Thinking and talking a lot about body image, body weight, and food

- Expressing extreme dissatisfaction with body or having a distorted body image

- Becoming irritable or withdrawing from family and friends

- Being sensitive to comments about food, exercise, weight, or body shape

- Feeling depressed or anxious

- Having difficulty concentrating

- Having problems with relationships

- Having suicidal thoughts or behavior

Eating disorders can result in a wide range of physical health problems, including severe malnutrition, or brain, heart, or kidney problems, which may lead to loss of consciousness or death. People with untreated anorexia and/or bulimia can die as a result of these illnesses.

What Are the Links between Eating Disorders and Depression?

People with eating disorders are twice as likely to experience depression when compared to people in the wider community. One study found that close to 50 percent of adolescents with eating disorders had high levels of depression and anxiety, especially those with bulimia.[2]

However, it is unclear whether depression is a risk factor for an eating disorder, or occurs as a result of an eating disorder. Depression can make people more likely to feel negatively about their bodies and themselves—this may put them at risk of developing an eating disorder. Eating disorders may also make people more at risk of developing depression, particularly if they experience rapid weight loss or starvation.

The two conditions also share many risk factors:

- Biological factors
- Genetic factors, e.g., a family history of mental health problems
- Social factors, e.g., media emphasis on a "thin ideal" of beauty
- Psychological factors, e.g., low self-esteem, ineffective coping strategies, and poor relationships.

Taking Action Against Eating Disorders

All eating disorders are treatable. Because they are mental illnesses, most people experiencing them benefit from professional help. The sooner they get help, the easier it is to overcome the problem and the more likely they are to make a full recovery. A delay in seeking treatment can lead to serious long-term consequences for the person's physical and mental health.

Helping Yourself

The first step: If you suspect you may have an eating disorder, the first step is to acknowledge that something isn't quite right and that you have to do something about it.

Reaching out: Once you have acknowledged you have a problem, it's good to seek help from others. Trying to tackle an eating disorder alone is very difficult as the underlying psychological issues are often complicated. You could start by talking to someone you know well and trust, before seeking professional help. Telling someone for the first time can be daunting, but can also bring a great sense of relief as you are no longer carrying your concerns alone.

Getting professional help: A good place to start is a health professional with specialist knowledge about eating disorders, such as a general practitioner, psychiatrist, psychologist, or dietitian. These health professionals can give an initial assessment of your physical state and diagnose the nature and severity of the eating disorder. A doctor can also outline treatment options and provide referrals for further treatment, according to your personal circumstances and current physical state.

Helping Someone Else

Getting someone with an eating disorder to acknowledge his or her problem can be difficult. People who experience eating disorders often go to great lengths to hide their illness due to feelings of shame or not wanting to give up their behavior, or because it's their way of coping with an issue.

Encouraging someone to seek professional help, and supporting them during the process, can be the most important thing that a family member, friend, or partner can do. But ultimately, the responsibility for accepting help and getting better lies with the person themselves.

Your aim should be to provide support for the person so that he or she feels safe and secure enough to seek treatment or to find someone else he or she can trust to talk to openly.

Offering Your Support [3]

What Is Helpful?

- Learn as much as you can about eating disorders before approaching the person.

- Stay calm, and try to be nonjudgmental, respectful, and kind.

- Discuss your concerns with the person in an open and honest way. Try to use "I" statements that are not accusing, such as "I am worried about you," rather than "you" statements such as "You are making me worried."

- Give the person plenty of time to discuss his or her feelings and reassure the person that it's safe to be open and honest.

- Suggest that he or she may benefit from seeking professional help.

- Offer to assist the person in getting the help he or she needs, but be careful not to overwhelm the person with information and suggestions.

Table 22.2. Common Myths about Eating Disorders

The Myth	The Facts
Eating disorders only affect females.	Anorexia and bulimia nervosa are more common in females, but both males and females experience these disorders. Males and females experience binge eating disorder more equally. Females with eating disorders are more likely to focus on weight loss, while males are equally likely to focus on increasing muscle mass or weight loss.
Eating disorders occur in only young people.	Eating disorders can be found in people as young as seven and as old as seventy. Most eating disorders start in adolescence—but if untreated, they can last long into adulthood. They can also develop for the first time or only become apparent in adult life.
Eating disorders are an attempt to get attention.	The causes of eating disorders are complex and often involve individual, biological, familial and sociocultural factors. The behaviors associated with eating disorders may sometimes be interpreted as "attention seeking," however they are a sign that the person is struggling with issues and needs help. People with eating disorders often prefer to avoid drawing attention to themselves.
Eating disorders are about appearance.	Eating disorders are psychological illnesses and have little to do with food, eating, appearance, or beauty. Eating disorders are usually related to emotional issues such as control and low self-esteem.
People with eating disorders are always thin.	A person with an eating disorder can be underweight, within a healthy weight range, or overweight.

What Is Unhelpful?

- Don't avoid talking to the person because you fear it might make him or her angry or upset, or make the problem worse.

- Don't approach the person in situations that may lead him or her to become sensitive or defensive (e.g., when either of you is feeling angry, emotional, tired, or frustrated).

- Don't be critical of the person.

- Don't give simple solutions to overcoming the person's problems, like saying "All you have to do is eat."

- Don't make generalizations such as "never" and "always" (e.g., "You're always moody" or "You never do anything but exercise").

- Don't say or imply that what the person is doing is "stupid" or "self-destructive."

- Don't take negative reactions personally or show disappointment or anger.

- Don't make promises to the person that you cannot keep.

- Don't try to solve the person's problems for him or her.

Treatment Options

Professional treatment for eating disorders involves managing physical health (including nutritional advice) and promoting mental health. In addition, drug treatment, support groups, and some alternative therapies may be useful.

Physical health management aims to monitor, restore, and maintain a person's nutritional balance (avoid starving or overeating) and also treat the longer-term physical problems that result from unhealthy eating patterns. The treatment usually involves seeing a doctor and/or a dietitian, developing a plan for healthy eating, and having regular check-ups.

Some people need more intense and structured care in a hospital. Being admitted to a hospital for treatment of weight loss occurs only if the individual is very malnourished.

Psychological treatment begins to address eating patterns and related thoughts, feelings, and behaviors by helping people find new ways of thinking about and handling issues such as self-esteem, control, perfectionism and family problems. This can include individual and family therapy and psycho-education (information on psychological issues). These psychological therapies are also used to treat depression and anxiety:

- **Cognitive Behavior Therapy (CBT):** Often people with eating disorders and/or depression have negative ways of seeing situations and themselves. Cognitive behavior therapy is one of the most researched psychological therapies and has a lot of evidence to support its effectiveness in treating people for depression and anxiety disorders. CBT teaches people to think realistically about common difficulties, helping them to change their thought patterns and the way they react to certain situations. Behavioral therapy approaches have been shown to be very helpful for many anxiety disorders.

- **Interpersonal Therapy (IPT):** Interpersonal therapy (IPT) has also been researched and found to be effective for treatment of depression. It helps people find new ways to get along with others and to resolve losses, changes, and conflict in relationships.

Antidepressant medication can play a role when people become severely depressed or when other treatments are ineffective in the treatment of depression. Deciding which antidepressants are best for a person can be complex. There is a range of factors that should be discussed with a doctor before starting antidepressants.

Antidepressant medication can take fourteen to twenty-one days before beginning to work effectively. The prescribing health professional should discuss differences in effects and possible side-effects of medications. Stopping medication should only be done gradually, on a doctor's recommendation and under supervision.

Most people taking medication will benefit from psychological therapies as well, as this will reduce the likelihood of relapse once the medication is ceased.

The Therapeutic Goods Administration (Australia's regulatory agency for medical drugs) and manufacturers of antidepressants do not recommend antidepressant use for depression in young people under the age of eighteen.

Facts about Depression and Anxiety Disorders

Depression

- Depression is more than just a low mood—it's a serious illness. People with depression find it hard to function every day and may be reluctant to participate in activities they once enjoyed. Depression has serious effects on physical and mental health. It is very common for people with an eating disorder to experience a level of depression at some time or another.

- One in five females and one in eight males will experience depression in their lifetime.[4]

Anxiety Disorders

- Everyone feels anxious from time to time, but for some people, anxious feelings are overwhelming and cannot be brought under control easily. An anxiety disorder is different from feeling stressed—it's a serious condition that makes it hard for the person to cope from day to day.

- Nearly one in seven people will experience some type of anxiety disorder in any one year (around one in six women and one in ten men) and one in four people will experience an anxiety disorder at some stage of their lives.[4]

Things to Remember

- Eating disorders often go hand in hand with one or more other mental illnesses, such as depression or anxiety disorders, due to the associated negative feelings and low self-esteem that are present with both conditions.

- Eating disorders can be difficult to detect. This is because the person may actively conceal their eating or exercise behaviors, deny that they have a problem, or find it difficult to ask for help from family members and friends.

- The sooner a person with an eating disorder gets help, the better. Recovery from an eating disorder and depression or anxiety requires appropriate support from family members, friends, the community, and health professionals.

- Helping a family member or friend with an eating disorder involves providing support in a nonjudgmental and respectful way. The most important step is to encourage the person to seek professional help and offer to assist him or her to find the help they need.

Sources

This section was adapted from the following sources:

1. Victorian Centre of Excellence in Eating Disorders & Eating Disorders Foundation of Victoria (2004) An Eating Disorders Resource for Schools. A Manual to Promote Early Intervention and Prevention of Eating Disorders in Schools.

2. Patton GC, Coffey C & Sawyer SM (2003) "The outcome of adolescent eating disorders: findings from the Victorian Adolescent Health Cohort Study." *European Child & Adolescent Psychiatry* 12: I/25–29.

3. Adapted from the Mental Health First Aid Training and Research Program (2008). Eating disorders: first aid guidelines for assisting adults. Melbourne: Orygen Youth Health Research Centre, University of Melbourne. Available at www .mhfa.com.au.

4. Australian Bureau of Statistics (2008) 2007 National Survey
    of Mental Health and Wellbeing: Summary of Results (4326.0),
    Canberra, ABS.

Eating Disorders Foundation of Victoria (www.eatingdisorders.org).

Russell S, Fuscaldo G and Ealey W (2008). Eating Disorders with Comorbid Depression and Anxiety: A Mapping Project of Eating Disorder
Organisations in Australia. Beyondblue Limited: Melbourne

Russell S, Fuscaldo G and Ealey W (2008). Eating Disorders with
Comorbid Depression and Anxiety: Literature Review. Beyondblue
Limited: Melbourne

Section 22.4

Eating Disorders and Diabetes

"Diabetes and Eating Disorders," © Diabetes Australia. Reprinted with
permission. Diabetes Australia is the peak consumer body representing all
people affected by diabetes and those at risk. We provide comprehensive
information about diabetes awareness, prevention, and management. Additional information is available at www.diabetesaustralia.com.au or the
Diabetes Infoline 1300 136 588. The full text of this document is available
online at http://diabetesaustralia.com.au/Documents/Eating%20Disorders
%20Booklet.pdf; accessed October 2010.

Eating disorders are a considerable issue for many people living
with diabetes. This information resource has been developed for people
with type 1 diabetes, their family and friends to explain the different
types of eating disorders and why people with type 1 diabetes may
have a higher risk of developing an eating disorder.

What Is an Eating Disorder?

There are many different types of eating disorders.
Anorexia nervosa involves:

• severe restriction of food intake;

• loss of body weight to an unhealthy level;

- loss of menstrual periods; and

- an intense fear of getting fat and losing control of eating.

Bulimia nervosa involves:

- eating binges with large amounts of food, usually secretly; and

- attempts to compensate for these binges to avoid weight gain through unhealthy measures such as misuse of laxatives, fluid or diet pills, self-induced vomiting, excessive exercise and periods of strict dieting.

Binge eating disorder involves periods of binge eating but without the compensatory behavior which bulimia nervosa involves such as vomiting or excessive exercise.

There is a wide range of disordered eating patterns.

Not all people with an eating disorder or disordered eating have a clear-cut diagnosis. For example, some people can have both anorexia and bulimia at the same time, or one of the conditions might develop into the other at a later date. Other people may be severely restricting their food intake without fulfilling all of the other criteria for a diagnosis of anorexia nervosa but this is still an eating disorder. All of these conditions are serious and need assistance and attention.

Why Do People Develop an Eating Disorder?

Eating disorders are serious and complex health issues relating to eating behaviors, body image, body shape, and weight. They are more common among young women and adolescent girls but can also affect males. People of all ages and from all backgrounds can experience eating disorders.

Many factors are known to affect the development of eating disorders, for example:

- physical changes during adolescence;

- pressure to achieve and succeed;

- major life changes such as ending a relationship;

- abuse, trauma, or a fear of the responsibility of adulthood;

- personality characteristics such as perfectionism, low self-esteem, high achievers and people who have a strong need to seek approval and please others; and

- family situations where an emphasis is placed on physical appearance, body weight, and shape and expectations of children are high.

Type 1 Diabetes and Eating Disorders

Managing type 1 diabetes is a complex balancing act between different management techniques and support from a diabetes healthcare team. Your diabetes healthcare team is you, working with your doctor, diabetes educator, dietitian, podiatrist, and eye specialist to ensure you live well.

A healthy eating plan is a central part of managing type 1 diabetes, alongside insulin injections or a pump and a program of physical activity. This means that a person with diabetes will have to focus on their food intake, over a long period of time and sometimes since early childhood, which can sometimes lead to a problematic relationship with food and eating.

I Have Type 1 Diabetes. Am I at Greater Risk of an Eating Disorder?

Anyone living with type 1 diabetes may be at risk of an eating disorder but adolescents and young adult women are most at risk.

As well as individual, family, and social stresses that can contribute to eating disorders there are additional factors for people with diabetes.

Some parts of the management and living with type 1 diabetes that may increase the risk of developing an eating disorder are:

- the dietary counseling and advice involved in diabetes healthcare can sometimes focus too much on restricting food intake;

- feelings of depression, guilt, and/or anxiety can be increased by some aspects of diabetes, such as the constant monitoring of blood glucose levels and worry about the long-term complications of diabetes;

- hypos (low blood glucose levels) need to be treated by eating extra sugar and carbohydrate and this extra food can sometimes cause weight gain. As some people find hypos unavoidable if they are to have tighter blood glucose control, this situation can become very complicated. New diabetes management techniques such as insulin pumps and new insulins are, however, being shown to allow tighter control without so many extra hypos; and

- weight loss is a common symptom of undiagnosed diabetes and others may comment favorably about this weight loss during the period around when type 1 diabetes is first diagnosed, and there may be some disappointment when the diabetes diagnosis and treatment means that good health is restored and normal weight returns.

Are Eating Disorders Worse for a Person with Diabetes?

Eating disorders can create extra risks for a person with diabetes. They can make managing diabetes more complicated and may lead to a range of short- and/or long-term health problems associated with diabetes:

- Weight loss can occur with continued high blood glucose levels, however the risk of long-term complications also increases significantly.

- Missing or decreasing insulin doses so that glucose and calories are lost through the urine will lead to high blood glucose levels and may cause diabetic ketoacidosis (DKA), a potentially life-threatening condition.

- Severe hypos can occur if food is restricted or purged (vomited), especially if this is done secretly, so it can be very difficult to take the appropriate insulin doses in these situations.

Could I Have an Eating Disorder?

Dieting is the single most common risk factor for the onset of an eating disorder, especially in young women.

There are many warning signs of an eating disorder. It is important to seek help if you suspect that you or someone you know may have an eating disorder.

The warning signs of an eating disorder can include:

- unhealthy and excessive preoccupation with body appearance, weight, and food;

- periods of dieting and overeating;

- avoidance of social situations involving food;

- increased mood changes, irritability, social withdrawal;

- change in clothing style or wearing baggy clothes to hide weight loss;

- frequent excuses not to eat or wanting to eat alone;

- playing with food. i.e., cutting food in small pieces;

- excessive exercise;

- faintness, dizziness, fatigue, weakness;

- anxiety, depression, mood swings;

- trips to the bathroom after meals;
- vomiting;
- feelings of being out of control with food;
- impaired concentration, alertness, comprehension; and
- evidence of binge eating.

Some more warning signs of an eating disorder in a person who has diabetes can include:

- extreme fluctuations in blood glucose levels;
- frequent high or low blood glucose levels and/or diabetic ketoacidosis (DKA), possibly resulting in hospital admission;
- consistent extremely high HbA1c (a blood test which measures the overall blood glucose levels over the last two to three months);
- missing insulin doses, or changing doses significantly or frequently; and
- weight loss without beginning a healthy eating plan or exercise program.

Who Can I Speak to for Help?

If you think you may have an eating disorder, it is important to seek help and treatment from a team of health professionals that understand both type 1 diabetes and eating disorders. You may find it challenging at first to find someone to help you who has experience in both areas but there are many places to start.

The health professionals that may be able to help you include an endocrinologist or a family doctor, diabetes educator, dietitian, social worker, or psychologist.

Many hospitals provide services through an eating disorders clinic. Your doctor can refer you to a clinic or you can phone your nearest major hospital directly and ask how you can attend an eating disorders clinic.

You may feel that you are able to manage your eating disorder but inevitably this situation will be out of your control and seeking professional help is the best way to start to address the problem.

If you are studying at school, your school counselor or welfare officer will be able to refer you to people who may help. It is important to remember that although counselors are not experts in diabetes and eating disorders, they may be a useful first point of contact for finding help. You can ask them to help you find someone experienced in diabetes and eating disorders.

What Can I Do to Help My Child, Partner, or Friend Who Has Type 1 Diabetes and May Have an Eating Disorder?

If someone you know with type 1 diabetes is showing signs of an eating disorder, you are encouraged to help them. Early intervention is important. Firstly, suggest the person seeks professional help as explained above.

Section 22.5

Eating Disorders and Self-Harm

"Eating Disorders and Self-Harm: A Chaotic Intersection," by Randy A. Sansone, M.D., John L. Levant, Ph.D., and Lori A. Sansone, M.D., reprinted from *Eating Disorders Review*, May/June 2003, Volume 14, Number 3. © 2003 Gürze Books. Reprinted with permission. Reviewed by David A. Cooke, M.D., FACP, October 2010.

There is clear empirical evidence that a subgroup of individuals with eating disorders (ED) engage in self-harm behavior (SHB). Individually these disorders are difficult to treat; in combination they represent a chaotic intersection. SHB ranges from various non-lethal forms of self-injury to genuine suicide attempts. Some examples of non-lethal self-injury include hitting, burning, scratching, or cutting oneself; pulling out one's hair and eyelashes; purposefully precipitating harmful "accidents," and participating in physically abusive relationships.

SHB may also manifest as overt eating disorder symptoms, such as abusing laxatives, inducing vomiting, or exercising excessively with the expressed or primary intent to experience pain or cause self-injury. Therefore, when assessing ED symptoms, it is essential to determine the intent or function of the symptoms (i.e., food, body, and weight issues vs. purposeful self-harm).

The Prevalence of SHB among Eating Disorders Patients

The prevalence of non-lethal self-injury among ED patients is approximately 25 percent, regardless of the type of eating disorder or the treatment setting (*Eating Disorders* 2002; 10:205). As for suicide attempts, the prevalence rates appear to vary, depending on the ED diagnostic subgroup and study setting. The prevalence of suicide attempts is lowest among outpatients with anorexia nervosa (16 percent). Prevalence rates are higher for bulimic individuals treated as outpatients (23 percent) and inpatients (39 percent). The highest rates of suicide attempts are reported among bulimic individuals who have comorbid alcohol abuse (54 percent) (*Eating Disorders* 2002; 10:205).

Causes of SHB among Those with ED

The precise etiology of self-harm behavior among those with ED is unknown, but it is suspected to be complex, with many underlying causes. It is also known to vary between individuals. About 25 percent of self-harming individuals with ED appear to meet the criteria for borderline personality disorder (BPD).

Variables that contribute to BPD include temperament, traumatic triggering events, family-of-origin dysfunction (e.g., inconsistent treatment by a caretaker, a negative family environment, or "biparental failure"), and various biological abnormalities, including possible aberrations in serotonin levels. Because BPD is frequently associated with a history of abuse during childhood (e.g., sexual, physical, and emotional abuse and witnessing violence), it is difficult to ascertain if associated biological findings are the causes of and/or outcomes of early developmental trauma. However, early violation of body boundaries appears to foster dissociative defenses in young victims, as well as a separation of body self and psychological self ("You can hurt my body, but not me"). These processes appear to subsequently lower the threshold for SHB in adulthood.

Multi-Impulsive Bulimia

A related construct, multi-impulsive bulimia, also involves impulsive SHB (e.g., suicide attempts), in addition to other forms of impulsivity such as substance abuse and sexual promiscuity. Compared with BPD, considerably less is known about multi-impulsive bulimia in terms of etiology. It may be that this syndrome is actually made up of a subset of individuals with BPD.

Assessment

When assessing an individual with suspected SHB and an eating disorder, it is crucial to explore in depth not only ED symptoms, but also the presence of concomitant SHB. These may include: (1) past suicide attempts; (2) repetitive, ongoing, non-lethal self-harm behavior; and (3) ED symptoms that do not appear to be related to concerns about food, body, and/or weight. An example of the latter could include self-injury equivalents such as inducing vomiting without food in one's stomach.

Although proven thresholds for various symptoms have not been established, an ongoing pattern of SHB is the conceptual benchmark. Several instruments to help detect and measure self-harm are now available to clinicians, including the Self-Harm Inventory (*J Clin Psychol* 1998; 54:973), the Self-Injury Survey (1994; Providence, RI), and the Impulsive and Self-Harm Questionnaire (Dissert Abstr Int 1997; 58:4469).

Treatment Strategies

There is no consistent, empirically proven treatment strategy for SHB in those with ED. However, a variety of interventions, used in assorted combinations, appear to offer promise.

Psychotherapy

Many psychotherapeutic techniques for SHB have been described for years in the literature on borderline personality disorder. Here are some of the approaches:

- Cognitive restructuring (eliciting and restructuring faulty cognitions that promote SHB)

- Dynamic approaches (e.g., uncovering the deeper dynamic themes around SHB, such as self-punishment or eliciting caring responses from others, and bringing these themes into the patient's conscious awareness)

- Sublimation (defined as rechanneling SHB into more socially acceptable alternatives, such as drawing or writing out self-destructive urges in detail)

- Interpersonal restructuring (using a consistent verbal phraseology at the time of a crisis that restructures the meaning and function of self-harm behavior in an interpersonal relationship)

- Family intervention (i.e., uncovering and translating what the patient may be trying to communicate through SHB)

- Various forms of contracting (i.e., encouraging personal control, establishing limits around the treatment)

- Group therapy

Again, none of these approaches alone is effective, whereas combinations appear to promote some degree of stabilization in most patients.

Dialectical behavior therapy is a formal approach that includes a combination of techniques, including individual and group intervention, cognitive and dynamic therapy, and psychoeducation. Like other forms of combination treatment, this systematized approach holds promise for the treatment of these complex patients.

Psychotropic Medication

Three clinical issues are relevant when considering whether to use psychotropic medications in this population: (1) the meaningful reduction of SHB; (2) selection of medications that are reasonably weight-neutral; and (3) avoidance of medications that are dangerous in overdose.

Most prescribing clinicians initially choose treatment with a weight-neutral selective serotonergic reuptake inhibitor (SSRI). As caveats, both sertraline (Zoloft®) and fluoxetine (Prozac®) appear to be relatively weight-neutral, whereas paroxetine (Paxil®) is frequently associated with weight gain. In addition, citalopram (Celexa®) overdose is associated with cardiac conduction changes that may foreshadow an arrhythmia, which can be lethal.

When there is no meaningful response with an SSRI, a second medication may be added. We typically choose an anticonvulsant. Gabapentin (Neurontin®; 100–600 mg per day) is seemingly weight-neutral at lower doses, and is safe in overdose. Topiramate (Topamax®) is associated with weight loss, and may be particularly helpful among those with binge eating disorder. Safety in overdose with topiramate is not well studied, but reports indicate no adverse effects.

Low-dose, atypical antipsychotic drugs may also be used as an augmentation strategy, either with the SSRI alone, or with the combination of an SSRI and anticonvulsant. Ziprasidone (Geodon®) is weight-neutral at all doses (e.g., 20 mg once or twice daily) and low-dose risperidone (Risperdal®; e.g., 0.25–0.5 mg per day) also appears to be reasonably weight-neutral. In contrast, olanzapine (Zyprexa®), quetiapine (Seroquel®), and clozapine (Clozaril®) are noted for producing weight gain in susceptible patients. These latter three atypical antipsychotics may also cause metabolic abnormalities such as elevated serum glucose, cholesterol, and triglyceride levels.

Finally, several studies indicate that eicosapentaenoic acid (EPA), an omega-3 fatty acid found in fish oil, may reduce depressive and aggressive symptoms as well as suicidal ideation (*Am J Psychiatry* 2003; 160:167; *Am J Psychiatry* 2002; 159:477). In the empirical literature, the suggested dosage of EPA has been 1,000 mg/day, although this explicit formulation is not seemingly available over the counter (e.g., a 432- mg softgel capsule is available). EPA appears to be weight-neutral and safe, even in overdoses.

Given the preceding pharmacologic suggestions, medications appear to offer modest yet meaningful reductions in SHB (an estimated 30 percent reduction in symptoms). As is the case with any trauma-based syndrome, including post-traumatic stress disorder, full remission is unlikely with the use of medications alone. The outcome data for the combination of psychotherapy strategies and medications varies, of course, from moderate remissions to refractory courses.

Conclusions

Patients with SHB constitute a substantial minority of individuals with eating disorders. While our understanding of the causes for SHB in this population remain somewhat elusive, it is likely that this phenomenon has many causes. Assessment of all ED patients should include clinical inquiry into the presence of SHB. In addition, formal measures of SHB are available.

Treatment approaches need to be individualized, and consist of a combination of psychotherapeutic strategies and medications. A reduction in SHB is a reasonable expectation, but a full and sustained remission is less likely to occur in the short term. Whether full remission occurs with longer follow-up periods is unknown. Clearly, these patients remain complex enigmas in our clinical realms.

Suggested Reading

Wonderlich S, Myers T, Norton M, et al. Self-harm and bulimia nervosa: A complex connection. *Eating Disord* 2002; 10:257.

Sansone RA, Levitt JL. Self-harm behaviors among those with eating disorders: An overview. *Eating Disord* 2002; 10:205.

Sansone RA, Sansone LA. Assessment tools for self-harm behavior among those with eating disorders. *Eating Disord* 2002; 10:193.

Sansone RA, Levitt JL, Sansone LA. Self-harm behavior and eating disorders. *J Prof Counselor* 2004; 18:55–69.

Levitt JL, Sansone RA, Cohn LS. *Self-Harm Behavior and Eating Disorders*. New York: Brunner-Routledge, 2004.

Section 22.6

Eating Disorders and Sexual Abuse

"Sexual Abuse and Eating Disorders," by Mary Anne Cohen, CSW. Mary Anne Cohen is director of the New York Center for Eating Disorders. This article is adapted from her book, *French Toast for Breakfast: Declaring Peace with Emotional Eating* (Gurze Books, 1995). Reviewed by David A. Cooke, M.D., FACP, October 2010.

In my eating disorder practice, 40 to 60 percent of the men and women who come to therapy for an eating problem have been sexually or physically abused. "It was my father's best friend." "It was my father." "It was my brother." "It was my mother's boyfriend." "It was my mother." "And so I starved myself." "And so I binged and purged." "And so I got fat." "And so I started using laxatives."

What is the connection between sexual abuse and developing an eating disorder? The answer is guilt, shame, anesthesia, self-punishment, soothing, comfort, protection, and rage.

Sexual abuse can have many different effects on the eating habits and body image of survivors. Sexual abuse violates the boundaries of the self so dramatically that inner sensations of hunger, fatigue, or sexuality become difficult to identify. People who have been sexually abused may turn to food to relieve a wide range of different states of tension that have nothing to do with hunger. It is their confusion and uncertainty about their inner perceptions that leads them to focus on the food.

Many survivors of sexual abuse often work to become very fat or very thin in an attempt to render themselves unattractive. In this way, they try to de-sexualize themselves. Other survivors obsessively diet, starve, or purge to make their bodies "perfect." A perfect body is their attempt to feel more powerful, invulnerable, and in control, so as not to re-experience the powerlessness they felt as children. Indeed, some large men and women, who are survivors of sexual abuse, are afraid to lose weight because it will render them feeling smaller and child-like. This, in turn, may bring back painful memories that are difficult to cope with.

A patient described how she gained thirty pounds at the age of eight. Her mother accused her of eating too many raviolis at the school cafeteria. She was scared to tell her mother that her uncle was sexually molesting her. Another patient had been abused by her alcoholic father starting at age seven. As a teenager, she binged and made herself throw up before going out with her boyfriend because she felt dirty, anxious, and guilty about her sexual feelings.

Sexual abuse and emotional eating both have one element in common. It is secrecy. Many eating disorder patients feel guilty about the sexual abuse in their childhoods, believing they could have prevented it but chose not to because of some defect in themselves. So they push their secret underground, and then distract and anesthetize themselves by emotional eating.

Children do not tell about their abuse for a variety of reasons. Sometimes they don't realize that anything wrong was happening at the time, or they don't want to believe anything is wrong. Sometimes a child is dependent on the abuser, so he or she may not want to risk upsetting the security of the status quo. Sometimes children keep the abuse secret for fear they will not be believed. And sometimes they keep the abuse secret because they are threatened or are bribed to keep silent.

Sexual abuse can come in many shades of nuance beyond overt touching. One father repeatedly bragged to his daughter about the size of his sexual organs and how he needed special large underwear to accommodate them. Another patient reported how her father and brother would forcefully hold her down and tickle her all over until she became hysterical and was gasping for breath.

People with eating problems often suffer from symptoms of post-traumatic stress disorder without realizing that its origins lie in sexual abuse. Post-traumatic stress may be characterized by depression, feeling chronically "dead" inside, having recurrent anxiety or nightmares, or feeling constantly and painfully vigilant to one's surroundings. Victims of post-traumatic stress disorder may begin to engage in self-destructive behavior such as entering into repetitive abusive relationships, losing themselves to drugs, alcohol, promiscuity, and even self-mutilation. Self-mutilation refers to inflicting bodily harm on themselves, such as cutting, burning, or even excess body piercing.

Of course, none of these symptoms is absolute confirmation of abuse, but they are strong indicators of past sexual trauma. Connecting these symptoms to an actual event of sexual abuse can be a validating experience because the symptoms of inner turmoil begin to make sense.

What can you do to heal from sexual abuse? The first step is to recount your experience to someone you trust, someone who can witness the full brunt of your pain and rage. Since the experience of sexual abuse is about being out of control, you need to be in a protected setting where your feelings can re-emerge and let loose. Releasing pain and guilt is not an intellectual experience, but something that comes from deep within the heart. This can be a difficult step because exposing your emotions can feel like a repetition of the original trauma.

Although there is more media coverage than ever before about the prevalence of sexual abuse, this does not relieve the shame that many people feel about it. If you have been a victim of incest, facing the abuse means facing not only the shame that you come from the kind of family where abuse is perpetrated, but also that no one in your family protected you. Additionally, men who have been sexually abused as children, either by a male or by their mother, have distinct shame issues related to feelings of passivity and weakness.

Sometimes eating disorder patients feel enormous guilt for having enjoyed the sexual contact with their abuser. Binge eating, purging, or starving then becomes their ongoing self-induced punishment. When we scratch the surface of the lives of these children, though, we discover that sexual abuse may have been the only real affection or caring they received. A child who is lonely or starved for affection may revel in the attention, even if it is abuse. But the truth is that children are never the seducers—they are always the victims. The only thing a child is guilty of is the innocent wish to be loved.

Confronting your shame, releasing your pain, and experiencing rage and guilt are part of the process of reclaiming your inner self as well as your sexual self. The need to detour your feelings through destructive eating will subside when you are able to grieve for the little child who was betrayed.

Lately much has been written about "false memory syndrome," in which a person "remembers" sexual abuse that never occurred. This, indeed, can happen in certain vulnerable people. Therefore, it is crucial that you not work with a therapist who "leads" you to a false memory of the experience. Memories of the abuse, if present, should evolve over the course of therapy rather than being planted in your head for you to "try on for size." If you suspect that something may have happened to you, trust your perception and let your inner "knowing" be your guide.

Section 22.7

Eating Disorders and Substance Abuse

Food for Thought: Substance Abuse and Eating Disorders—the first comprehensive examination of the link between substance abuse and eating disorders—reveals that up to one-half of individuals with eating disorders abuse alcohol or illicit drugs, compared to 9 percent of the general population. Conversely, up to 35 percent of alcohol or illicit drug abusers have eating disorders compared to 3 percent of the general population. The seventy-three-page report by the National Center on Addiction and Substance Abuse (CASA) at Columbia University was released on December 18, 2003, by CASA president and former U.S. secretary of health, education and welfare, Joseph A. Califano Jr.

"For many young women, eating disorders like anorexia and bulimia are joined at the hip with smoking, binge drinking, and illicit drug use," said Califano. "This lethal link between substance abuse and eating disorders sends a signal to parents, teachers, and health professionals—where you see the smoke of eating disorders, look for the fire of substance abuse and vice versa."

The exhaustive report finds anorexia nervosa and bulimia nervosa as the eating disorders most commonly linked to substance abuse and for the first time identifies the shared risk factors and shared characteristics of both afflictions.

Substance Abuse and Eating Disorders

Shared risk factors:

- occur in times of transition or stress;
- common brain chemistry;
- common family history;

- low self-esteem, depression, anxiety, impulsivity;
- history of sexual or physical abuse;
- unhealthy parental behaviors and low monitoring of children's activities;
- unhealthy peer norms and social pressures;
- susceptibility to messages from advertising and entertainment media.

Shared characteristics:

- obsessive preoccupation, craving, compulsive behavior, secretiveness, rituals;
- experience mood altering effects, social isolation;
- linked to other psychiatric disorders, suicide;
- difficult to treat, life threatening;
- chronic diseases with high relapse rates;
- require intensive therapy.

The report lists caffeine, tobacco, alcohol, diuretics, laxatives, emetics, amphetamines, cocaine, and heroin as substances used to suppress appetite, increase metabolism, purge unwanted calories, and self-medicate negative emotions.

The report found that because health professionals often overlook the link between substance abuse and eating disorders, treatment options are virtually nonexistent for these co-occurring conditions.

"The public health community, parents, and policy makers must educate our children about healthy body images from a very young age, and treatment and prevention programs must address the common co-occurrence of substance abuse and eating disorders," stated Susan Foster, vice president and director of policy research and analysis at CASA, who spearheaded the project.

"Advertisers put children at greater risk of developing an eating disorder through the portrayal of unrealistic body images," noted Mr. Califano. "The average American woman is 5'4" tall and weighs approximately 140 pounds, but the average model that purportedly epitomizes our standard of beauty is 5'11" tall and weighs 117 pounds." The report found that women's magazines contain more than ten times more ads and articles related to weight loss than men's magazines, which is the same gender ratio reported for eating disorders.

The report finds that while only 15 percent of girls are overweight, 40 percent of girls in grades one through five and 62 percent of teenage girls are trying to lose weight. These girls are especially vulnerable to eating disorders and related substance abuse problems.

Other notable findings include:

- Middle school girls (ten- to fourteen-year-olds) who diet more than once a week are nearly four times likelier to become smokers.

- Girls with eating disorder symptoms are almost four times likelier to use inhalants and cocaine.

- 12.6 percent of female high school students take diet pills, powders, or liquids to control their weight without a doctor's advice.

- Bulimic women who are alcohol dependent report a higher rate of suicide attempts, anxiety, personality and conduct disorders, and other drug dependence than bulimic women who are not alcohol dependent.

- Hispanic girls are slightly more likely than Caucasian girls and significantly more likely than African American girls to report having fasted for twenty-four hours or more and having vomited or taken laxatives to lose weight.

- As many as one million men and boys suffer from an eating disorder; gay and bisexual males are at increased risk of such disorders.

Part Three

Causes of Eating Disorders

Chapter 23

Identifying and Understanding the Causes of Eating Disorders

Chapter Contents

Section 23.1

What Causes Eating Disorders?

Excerpted from "Eating Disorders," © 2010 A.D.A.M., Inc.
Reprinted with permission.

There is known no single cause for eating disorders. Although concerns about weight and body shape play a role in all eating disorders, the actual cause of these disorders appears to involve many factors, including those that are genetic and neurobiologic, cultural and social, and behavioral and psychologic.

Genetic Factors

Anorexia is eight times more common in people who have relatives with the disorder. Studies of twins show they have a tendency to share specific eating disorders (anorexia nervosa, bulimia nervosa, and obesity). Researchers have identified specific chromosomes that may be associated with bulimia and anorexia.

Biologic Factors

The body's hypothalamic-pituitary-adrenal axis (HPA) may be important in eating disorders. This complex system originates in the following regions in the brain:

- **Hypothalamus:** The hypothalamus is a small structure that plays a role in controlling our behavior, such as eating, sexual behavior and sleeping, and regulates body temperature, hunger and thirst, and secretion of hormones.

- **Pituitary gland:** The pituitary gland is involved in controlling thyroid functions, the adrenal glands, growth, and sexual maturation.

- **Amygdala:** This small almond-shaped structure lies deep in the brain and is associated with regulation and control of major emotional activities, including anxiety, depression, aggression, and affection.

The HPA system releases certain neurotransmitters (chemical messengers) that regulate stress, mood, and appetite. Abnormalities in the activities of three of them, serotonin, norepinephrine, and dopamine, may play a particularly important role in eating disorders. Serotonin is involved with well-being, anxiety, and appetite (among other traits), and norepinephrine is a stress hormone. Dopamine is involved in reward-seeking behavior. Imbalances with serotonin and dopamine may explain in part why people with anorexia do not experience a sense of pleasure from food and other typical comforts.

Cultural Pressures

The media plays a role in promoting unrealistic expectations for body image and a distorted cultural drive for thinness. At the same time, cheap and high-caloric foods are aggressively marketed. Such messages are contradictory and confusing.

Section 23.2

Altered Sense of Taste in Women with Anorexia Gives Clues to Causes of Eating Disorders

Although anorexia nervosa is categorized as an eating disorder, it is not known whether there are alterations of the portions of the brain that regulate appetite. Now, a new study finds that women with anorexia have distinct differences in the insula—the specific part of the brain that is important for recognizing taste—according to a new study by University of Pittsburgh and University of California, San Diego researchers currently online in advance of publication in the journal *Neuropsychopharmacology*.

The study also implies that there may be differences in the processing of information related to self-awareness in recovering anorexics compared to those without the illness—findings that may lead to a better understanding of the cause of this serious and sometimes fatal mental disorder.

In the study led by Angela Wagner, M.D., University of Pittsburgh School of Medicine, and Walter H. Kaye, M.D., of the University of Pittsburgh and the University of California, San Diego (UCSD) Schools of Medicine, the brain activity of thirty-two women was measured using functional magnetic resonance imaging (fMRI.) The research team looked at images of the brains of sixteen women who had recovered from anorexia nervosa—some of whom had been treated at the Center for Overcoming Problem Eating at Western Psychiatric Institute and Clinic of the University of Pittsburgh Medical Center—and sixteen control subjects. They measured their brains' reactions to pleasant taste (sucrose) and neutral taste (distilled water). The results of the fMRI study are the first evidence that individuals with anorexia process taste in a different way than those without the eating disorder.

In response to both the sucrose and water, imaging results showed that women who had recovered from anorexia had significantly reduced response in the insula and related brain regions when compared to the control group. These areas of the brain recognize taste and judge how rewarding that taste is to the person. In addition, while the controls showed a strong relationship between how they judged the pleasantness of the taste and the activity of the insula, this relationship was not seen in those who had recovered from anorexia.

According to Kaye, it is possible that individuals with anorexia have difficulty recognizing taste, or responding to the pleasure associated with food. Because this region of the brain also contributes to emotional regulation, it may be that food is aversive, rather than rewarding. This could shed light on why individuals with anorexia avoid normally "pleasurable" foods, fail to appropriately respond to hunger, and are able to lose so much weight.

"We know that the insula and the connected regions are thought to play an important role in interoceptive information, which determines how the individual senses the physiological condition of the entire body," said Kaye. "Interoception has long been thought to be critical for self-awareness because it provides the link between thinking and mood, and the current body state."

This lack of interoceptive awareness may contribute to other symptoms of anorexia nervosa such as distorted body image, lack of recognition of the symptoms of malnutrition, and diminished motivation to change, according to Kaye.

Anorexia nervosa is a serious and potentially lethal illness, which may result in death in 10 percent of cases. It is characterized by the relentless pursuit of thinness, emaciation, and the obsessive fear of gaining weight. Anorexia commonly begins during adolescence, but strikes throughout the lifespan, and is nine times more common in females than in males. These characteristics support the possibility that biological processes contribute to developing this disorder.

Many individuals with anorexia nervosa have difficulty obtaining treatment because it is not considered a biological illness. Toward this end, Kaye is working with the National Eating Disorders Association (NEDA) to promote new public understanding and improve treatment of eating disorders.

Section 23.3

Genetics and Anorexia

A new study led by University of North Carolina at Chapel Hill (UNC) researchers estimates that 56 percent of the liability for developing anorexia nervosa is determined by genetics.

In addition, the study found that the personality trait of "neuroticism" (a tendency to be anxious and depressed) earlier in life is a significant factor associated with development of the eating disorder later.

Anorexia nervosa is a psychiatric illness characterized by an individual's refusal to maintain a minimally acceptable body weight, intense fear of weight gain, and a distorted body image. It occurs primarily among females in adolescence and young adulthood and is associated with the highest mortality rate of any mental disorder.

This study is the first published in the medical literature to estimate how much liability for developing anorexia nervosa is due to genetics, and the first to find a statistically significant association between the prospective risk factor of neuroticism and later development of anorexia, said Dr. Cynthia M. Bulik, lead author of the study, published in the March 2006 issue of the *Archives of General Psychiatry*.

"What this study shows is that anorexia nervosa is moderately heritable and may be predicted by the presence of early neuroticism, which reflects proneness to depression and anxiety," Bulik said. "Fifty-six percent heritability—that's a fairly large contribution of genes. The remaining liability is due to environmental factors."

Bulik is the William R. and Jeanne H. Jordan distinguished professor of eating disorders in UNC's School of Medicine and director of the UNC Eating Disorders Program at UNC Hospitals. She also is a professor of nutrition, a department housed in the schools of public health and medicine, and holds the only endowed professorship in eating disorders nationwide.

The reason she and her co-authors reached these conclusions where previous studies could not, Bulik said, is that their study was based on data obtained from screening a very large sample of twins. Their sample, from the Swedish Twin Registry, consisted of 31,406 individuals born between 1935 and 1958. None of the previous studies had samples nearly as large, Bulik said.

Working with colleagues at the Karolinska Institute in Stockholm, Bulik's team screened members of the sample for a range of disorders, including anorexia nervosa, using diagnostic criteria from the American Psychiatric Association's *Diagnostic and Statistical Manual of Mental Disorders—Fourth Edition*. Information from sample members collected in 1972–73 was used to examine prospective risk factors.

About half of the members of the sample were monozygotic, or identical, twin pairs, who are genetically identical. The other half were dizygotic, or fraternal, twins, who are no more similar genetically than siblings who are not twins.

"In this big population, we compared the group of monozygotic twins with the group of dizygotic twins and asked the question, 'How often do both twins in a twin pair have the disorder?' If you find that both members of monozygotic twin pairs have the disorder more frequently than both members of dizygotic twin pairs, that suggests there's a genetic component to the disorder," Bulik said.

That's what the researchers found, she added.

"It was more common for both members of identical twin pairs to have it than for both members of fraternal twin pairs."

A statistical analysis of the data they collected from the twins in the sample estimated that genetics accounted for 56 percent of the liability for developing anorexia within that population.

Since the Swedish Twin Registry contained data on sample members dating back to 1972–73, Bulik's team also was able to determine the factors or features that these people had earlier in life that predicted they were going to develop anorexia nervosa later.

"What we found was that neuroticism, measured in 1973, was the strongest predictor of the development of anorexia nervosa later in life," Bulik said. Other prospective risk factors that were examined, including a low body mass index and excessive exercise levels, were not found to be predictive.

One of the next steps, Bulik said, is to put these two pieces of information together to figure out exactly what is inherited. "We suggest that there are some basic biological differences between people with anorexia nervosa and everybody else," Bulik said. "When most of us get hungry, or starved, we get more anxious. But these people's bodies respond differently. They say that food deprivation makes them feel more calm and more in control, which is one reason they keep doing it."

Section 23.4

Impaired Brain Activity Underlies Impulsive Behaviors in Bulimia

Excerpted from "Impaired Brain Activity Underlies Impulsive Behaviors in Women with Bulimia," National Institute of Mental Health, July 15, 2009.

Women with bulimia nervosa (BN), when compared with healthy women, showed different patterns of brain activity while doing a task that required self-regulation. This abnormality may underlie binge eating and other impulsive behaviors that occur with the eating disorder, according to an article published in the January 2009 issue of the *Archives of General Psychiatry*.

Background

Rachel Marsh, Ph.D., Columbia University, and colleagues assessed self-regulatory brain processes in women with BN without using disorder-specific cues, such as pictures of food.

In this study, twenty women with BN and twenty healthy controls viewed a series of arrows presented on a computer screen. Their task was to identify the direction in which the arrows were pointing while the researchers observed their brain activity using functional magnetic resonance imaging (fMRI).

People generally complete such tasks easily when the direction of the arrow matches the side of the screen it is on—an arrow on the left side pointing to the left—but respond more slowly and with more errors when the two do not match. In such cases, healthy adults activate self-regulatory processes in the brain to prevent automatic responses and to focus greater attention on resolving the conflicting information.

Results of the Study

Women with BN tended to be more impulsive during the task, responding faster and making more mistakes when presented with conflicting information, compared with healthy controls.

Patterns in brain activity also differed between the two groups. Even when they answered correctly to conflicting information, women with BN generally did not show as much activity in brain areas involved in self-regulation as healthy controls did. Women with the most severe cases of the disorder showed the least amount of self-regulatory brain activity and made the most errors on the task.

Significance

Altered patterns of brain activity may underlie impaired self-regulation and impulse control problems in women with BN. These findings increase the understanding of causes of binge eating and other impulsive behaviors associated with BN and may help researchers to develop better-targeted treatments.

Chapter 24

Body Image and Eating Disorders

Chapter Contents

Section 24.1

Facts about Body Image and Eating Disorders

What Is Body Image? Body Image Facts

Body image refers to the way we perceive our own bodies and the way we assume other people perceive us. "Body image involves our perception, imagination, emotions, and physical sensations of and about our bodies. It's not static, but ever-changing; sensitive to changes in mood, environment, and physical experience. It is not based on fact. It is psychological in nature, and much more influenced by self-esteem than by actual physical attractiveness as judged by others. It is not inborn, but learned. This learning occurs in the family and among peers, but these only reinforce what is learned and expected culturally." [Lightstone, 1999]

Some general facts about body image:

- The average size of the idealized woman (as portrayed by models), has stabilized at 13 to 19 percent below healthy weight. [Garner et al., 1980]

- The thin ideal is unachievable for most women and is likely to lead to feelings of self-devaluation, dysphoria (depression), and helplessness. [Rodin et al., 1984]

- Eighty-nine percent of women in a study of 3,452 women wanted to lose weight. [Garner, 1997]

- Constant dieting and the relentless pursuit of thinness has become a normative (thought to be normal) behavior among women in Western society. [Rodin et al., 1984]

- Thinness has not only come to represent attractiveness, but also has come to symbolize success, self-control, and higher socioeconomic status. [Forehand, 2001]

- The weight-loss industry brings in at least $55.4 billion in revenue per year. [Marketdata Enterprises, 2007]

- A disturbed body image is a significant component of eating disorders and plays an important role in the development and continuation of eating disorders. [Stice, 2002]

Body Image and Dieting

When women and girls experience poor body image, they often turn to dieting as a solution. There are numerous studies that cite the psychological connection between poor body image and dieting, and some studies are being published that detail the physical effects of dieting. In order to understand dieting and weight loss, it is important to have a good grasp of the possible mindset or intentions around it as well as the types of behaviors involved.

For a summary of the effects of dieting on eating disorders, see the article "Does Dieting Increase the Risk for Obesity and Eating Disorders?" in the 2006 edition of the *Journal of the American Dietetic Association*. [Spear, 2006]

Dieting During Adolescence

- Dieting is a common practice among adolescents, especially girls.

- In a survey of adolescents in grades nine through twelve (approximately ages fourteen to eighteen), more than 59 percent of females and 29 percent of males were trying to lose weight. Over 18 percent of girls and 8 percent of boys had gone without food for twenty-four hours or more to lose weight in the last thirty days. Of the girls, 11.3 percent had used diet pills and 8.4 percent had vomited or taken laxatives to lose weight. [Centers for Disease Control, 2004]

- 56.2 percent of teenagers ate less food, fewer calories, or foods low in fat to lose weight or keep from gaining weight; 65.7 percent exercised to lose weight. [Centers for Disease Control, 2004]

- Adolescent girls who engaged in extreme weight-loss behaviors (vomiting and using laxatives or diet pills) were significantly less likely to eat fruits and vegetables compared with nondieters and dieters using more healthful approaches. [Centers for Disease Control, 2004]

- Dieting may compromise healthy growth and cause nutrient deficiencies. Adolescent girls most often diet to improve their appearance, and although this behavior is widespread, teenagers continue to be more overweight than ever before. [Calderon et al., 2004]

219

Relationship between Dieting and Eating Disorders

- Eating disorders are eighteen times more likely to develop in adolescent girls who dieted at a severe level than in those who did not diet. [Patton et al., 1999]

- In one study, an eating disorder was five times more likely to develop in teens who dieted at a moderate level than teenagers who did not diet. [Patton et al., 1999]

- Two-thirds of new cases of eating disorders arise in female adolescents who have dieted moderately. Eating disorders are largely predicted by higher rates of early dieting. [Patton et al., 1999]

- The fact that someone is dieting increases the risk that she or he will overeat or binge to counteract the effects of calorie deprivation. Dieting encourages a shift from a reliance on physiological reasons for eating (feelings of hunger) to psychological control over eating behaviors (a person's feeling that he or she shouldn't eat so much, for example). Lowered body satisfaction, appearance satisfaction, and pressure to be thin all increase with an increase in binge eating. [Stice et al., 2002]

- Dieting is the most important predictor of new eating disorders. Differences in the incidence of eating disorders between sexes were largely accounted for by the high rates of early dieting in the female subjects. [Patton et al., 1999]

Body Image and Mental Health (Including Impact on Psychology, Shame, Depression, Self-Worth, Attitudes, Self-Esteem)

In February 2007, the American Psychological Association (APA) released a report, *Report of the APA Task Force on the Sexualization of Girls*, examining and summarizing the best psychological theory, research, and clinical experience addressing the sexualization of girls via the media and other cultural messages [APA, 2007]. This superb report connects the dots between girls' psychological health, their behaviors, and media influences. You'll find many references to those findings below.

When women and girls feel bad about their bodies, they often feel bad about themselves. This outcome is what the field of eating disorders treatment is trying to capture when pointing out the seriousness of poor body image. Yet weight-loss products focus on instilling feelings of body hatred in consumers:

- The thin ideal is unachievable for most women and is likely to lead to feelings of self-devaluation, dysphoria (depression), and helplessness. [Rodin et al., 1984]

- Studies also show that self-objectification is associated with negative mental-health outcomes in adolescent girls. In early adolescence, girls who had a more objectified relationship with their bodies were more likely to experience depression and had lower self-esteem. [Ward, 2002]

- Among African-American and white adolescent girls, self-objectification is a significant predictor of depression, body shame, and disordered eating, even when controlling for race, grade in school, and body-mass index. [Ward and Rivadeneyra, 1999]

- One study exposed undergraduate women to forty full-page photographs from *Cosmopolitan*, *Vogue*, and *Glamour* magazines. Young women exposed to images of idealized models indicated more eating-disorder symptoms than women in the control group, as well as more negative mood states and lower self-esteem. [Zurbriggen and Morgan, 2006]

Attitudes

Girls and young women who more frequently consume or engage with mainstream media content also support the sexual stereotypes that paint women as sexual objects. [Ward, 2002; Ward and Rivadeneyra, 1999; Zurbriggen and Morgan, 2006]

Media exposure has been found to constrain young women's conceptions of femininity by putting appearance and physical attractiveness at the center of women's values:

- Frequent viewing of reality TV programming among young women is associated with a stronger belief in the importance of appearance. [Tolman et al., 2006]

- When they were asked to rate the importance of particular qualities for women, white and African-American high school students who consumed more mainstream media attributed greater importance to sexiness and beauty than did students who consumed less media. [Ward, 2004; Ward and Averitt, 2005]

Self-Esteem

In psychology, self-esteem (also called self-worth, self-confidence, and self-respect) reflects a person's overall self-appraisal of their worth.

According to the *Report of the APA Task Force on the Sexualization of Girls* (2007), low self-esteem is associated with health-compromising behaviors in adolescence, such as substance use, early sexual activity, eating problems, and suicidal ideation. Surprisingly, there is little longitudinal research addressing this issue. Just at the time when girls begin to develop their identities, they are more likely to suffer losses in self-esteem:

- In the eighth grade, girls who objectify their bodies more have much lower self-esteem. For this reason, diminishing self-esteem arising in early adolescence may make girls particularly vulnerable to cultural messages that promise them popularity, effectiveness, and social acceptance through the right "sexy" look. On the other hand, the drop in self-esteem may be a result of how responsive they are to these cultural messages. [McGeer and Williams, 2000]

- In one study, white and African-American girls (ages ten to seventeen years) threw a softball as hard as they could against a distant gymnasium wall. The researchers found that the extent to which girls viewed their bodies as objects and were concerned about their bodies' appearance predicted poorer motor performance on the softball throw. Self-objectification, it appears, limits the form and effectiveness of girls' physical movements. [Van den Berg et al., 2007]

- Perhaps the most insidious consequence of self-objectification is that it breaks down one's thinking process. Ongoing attention to physical appearance leaves fewer resources available for other mental and physical activities.

- White college students who were alone in a dressing room were asked to try on and evaluate either a swimsuit or a sweater. While they waited for ten minutes wearing the garment, they completed a math test. The young women in swimsuits performed significantly worse on the math problems than did those wearing sweaters. No differences were found for young men. In other words, thinking about the body and comparing it to sexualized cultural ideals disrupted mental capacity in young women. [Fredrickson et. al., 1998]

  - This impairment also occurs among African-American, Latina, and Asian-American young women. [Hebl et al., 2004].

  - This impairment extends beyond mathematics to other cognitive domains, including logical reasoning and spatial skills. [Gapinski et al., 2003]

- Low self-esteem is often associated with health-compromising behaviors in adolescence such as substance use, early sexual activity, eating problems, and thoughts that may lead to suicide. Surprisingly, there is little longitudinal research addressing this issue. [APA, 2007]

- One longitudinal study examines the predictive association between self-esteem in young New Zealanders ages nine to thirteen years and a variety of health-compromising behaviors at age fifteen. Low levels of self-esteem significantly predicted adolescent reports of problem eating, suicidal ideation, and multiple health-compromising behaviors. [McGeer and Williams, 2000]

Section 24.2

Fostering Healthy Body Image

"Healthy Body Image and Weight in Your Pre-Teen or Teen," by Wendy Oliver-Pyatt, M.D. © 2010 Eating Disorder Hope (www.eatingdisorderhope.com). Reprinted with permission.

Puberty is a tumultuous time in a child's life: the first giant step into the unknown world of adulthood, with its excitement and fears. And no area of puberty and adolescence is more fraught with both promise and worry than a child's changing body image.

Suddenly, after growing slowly and steadily for years, a child approaching puberty rapidly begins to shoot up and round out. In addition, sexual characteristics make their appearance, as hormones trigger breast development, pubic hair growth, and a host of other changes including that hallmark of the teenage years: radical mood swings.

To help your teenager through this exhilarating but also frightening time, it's important to begin by understanding normal pubertal changes.

As children's bodies undergo these changes, they also develop a new image of their own sexuality and attractiveness. In addition, as they add weight and round out, their casual relationship with food and eating becomes more complex.

Children who navigate these changes successfully can mature into confident, healthy individuals who value their own bodies and are in control of their eating. Those who fall prey to societal pressures or destructive dieting during their teen years, however, are targets for eating disorders or lifelong obesity. That's why parents need play an active role in understanding their children's changing bodies and feelings during puberty and adolescence, and promoting a positive body image and a healthy relationship with food and eating.

Why Puberty Changes Can Trigger Body Issues

The onset of normal puberty changes often leads to insecurity and negative body image in formerly confident, self-assured children. Consider these three typical examples:

- Fourteen-year-old Katie weighed 110 a year earlier before her periods started, but quickly shot up to 145. She became terrified about getting fat and weighed herself every day, because her P.E. teacher said she was getting "a little too hefty" for the gymnastics activities she loved.

- Latisha, a nine-year-old, was a happy child who loved life and made friends easily. She was sturdy and athletic like her dad, and already nearly as tall as her mom. When she started at a new school in the fall, the other kids started calling her "Jumbo" and "Whale." She began to feel insecure, and when she came home from school she would ask her mom worriedly, "Why am I so big?"

- Thirteen-year-old Miguel was a whiz at computers and a genius at video games. But the boys at his school didn't care about his brain; all they noticed was that he was fifteen pounds heavier than most of them. At lunch, they called him the Pillsbury Dough Boy, and poked him in the belly. The girls laughed, and Miguel wanted to crawl in a hole and die.

Just like their children, parents too may react to normal pubertal changes with concern, thus "pathologizing" these changes. For example, the parents of the children described above reacted in the typical way: by putting them on diets. All three sets of parents followed diet plans recommended by their children's doctors. Latisha's mother also hired a personal trainer and purchased low-calorie frozen dinners for her, and Miguel's mom paid him $5 for each pound he lost. Katie's stepmom spent hours in the kitchen trying to create low-fat, low-calorie versions of Katie's favorite foods.

One year later, Katie was in the early stages of bulimia. Latisha was self-conscious and was starting to sneak food into her room, and Miguel continued to gain weight with each passing month and ate compulsively while playing video games.

What happened to these children? The answer to this question involves two modern-day culprits: fat phobia, and the harmful dieting that it generates. Understanding the toxic effects of both fat phobia and dieting can help you give your child the tools she needs to traverse normal development safely while maintaining a healthy self-esteem and relationship with her body.

The Toxic Effects of "Fat Phobia" and Dieting on Normal Human Development

Spend an afternoon watching your child's favorite shows, or looking through fashion magazines for teens. Do you see anyone who looks like your child? Probably not, because the "ideal body" of today's TV star or fashion model is generally a product of dangerous starvation diets and plastic surgery.

Statistically, only three in every one hundred women has a fashion-model figure—meaning that ninety-seven in one hundred girls think their bodies are "abnormal" compared to the artificial ideal promoted by the media. This dissatisfaction rises as children enter their teen years and become more interested in looks and aware of their own appearance.

In other cultures, a child's first steps into manhood or womanhood are celebrated. For instance, women in some African tribes receive special tattoos when they reach puberty and begin developing womanly curves, and Judaism honors both boys and girls who reach the age of fourteen with a special ceremony. But for most American girls (and a growing number of boys), there is no celebration or ceremony. Instead, there's a growing realization that their bodies are growing thicker, plumper, or curvier in a culture that despises a healthy body as "fat," "weak," and "gross."

As a result, more than half of thirteen-year-old girls, and more than three-quarters of seventeen-year old girls, are unhappy with their bodies. By the time they hit college, nearly all will be dieting and more than 10 percent will have life-threatening eating disorders. Boys, too, are now becoming victims of the unrealistic images they see in the media. As a result, eating disorders now affect around 3 percent of boys, and at least one-third of male teens engage in extreme dieting or binge eating.

Ironically, the media's promotion of dangerous thinness as an ideal leads millions of children to begin dangerous dieting when they aren't actually overweight—an ordeal they frequently undertake with the blessing of parents and doctors who focus on weight tables instead of factoring in children's genes and development. For instance, consider the three children I described at the beginning of this section:

- The first girl, Katie, was actually at an appropriate and healthy weight for her height and age. She just "felt" big because she wasn't as slim as a fashion model, and because she was being pressured by a coach to maintain an unnaturally childlike figure. By accepting the idea that her weight was a problem, and aiding her efforts to go below her natural weight, her parents played a strong role in pushing her into an eating disorder.

- The second child, Latisha, inherited her father's genes, and is biologically designed to be taller and somewhat larger than her more slender peers and her mother. Moreover, her body was preparing to reach puberty at ten years of age, which is a common phenomenon for African American girls (who often begin menstruating a year or so earlier than other girls). But because she was bigger than her mother, both her parents and her doctor bought into the idea that she was "fat." She also started to feel ashamed about her size—and when her parents fostered her anxiety about her body by supporting her dieting, it reinforced her sense of shame about her body and who she is.

- As for Miguel, he was initially only a few pounds overweight—most likely the result of his transition from childhood to adolescence, as well as his lack of physical activity. His parents' decision to put him on a diet and pay him to lose weight backfired by driving him to "retaliatory grazing."

If dieting actually worked, or at least did no harm, then it wouldn't really matter if these children had spent a few weeks counting calories or carbs—even though they didn't need to. But in reality, a child's first diet is often the initial step toward a dangerous eating disorder or obesity. In fact, parents need to be aware that dieting often creates lifetime food, body image, and weight problems.

Here's how the vicious cycle works. Fewer than 5 percent of dieters successfully keep off the pounds they lose, and more than one-third of them gain back more weight than they lost. That's because dieting triggers excessive hunger and causes our bodies to store fat more efficiently.

As a result, the child who initially diets to get rid of a few pounds of "baby fat" is likely to gain weight instead, causing feelings of shame and distress—feelings that in turn can lead to secretive eating and bingeing. That's the first step in a cycle of failed diets, out-of-control eating, and weight gain—a cycle that often lasts a lifetime. Worse yet, failed diets lead many children to ever-more-restrictive diets, eventually culminating in full-blown bulimia or anorexia. More than one in three dieters progresses to extreme dieting, and a quarter of those people will develop eating disorders.

In addition to setting children up for obesity or eating disorders, dieting is dangerous in other ways. For example, 45 percent of skeletal mass develops during the teen years, and strict dieting can dramatically reduce bone mass. Dieting also impairs thinking and memory and mood, making it more difficult for children to succeed at school and enjoy their lives. In addition, extreme dieting can damage the kidneys, heart, and immune system.

In short, dieting creates weight problems and eating disorders in children who aren't overweight to begin with, and it doesn't help children who are overweight to lose their excess pounds.

Dealing with "Fat Phobia," Weight Concerns, and Human Development in a Productive Way

To raise children who are free from weight problems, or to help children who actually are overweight, parents need to focus on two objectives—neither of which involves dieting. The first is to counter the toxic effects of the "culture of thinness" by teaching their children (whether they have weight issues or not) to have realistic ideas about their own bodies, and to offer knowledge and reassurance about human development. The second is to create lifestyle changes that foster a relaxed relationship with food, free of bingeing, restricting, and emotional eating.

The most important step in this process is to immunize your child against unhealthy cultural messages. For instance, share stories about models and actors with eating disorders so your child will understand the ugly truth behind the size-zero fairytale. Also, keep an eye out for good role models—for instance, many of the contestants on *American Idol*—who aren't unnaturally slender and who have confidence in their own beauty. In addition, see if you can steer your child toward programming where he'll see real-life people in all shapes and sizes who lead successful and interesting lives.

The next step is to address your own fears and misconceptions about weight—both your own weight and your child's. Start by examining your own relationship with food and your body. A child who grows up hearing, "Ugh, I look disgusting in this dress—I can't go to the party" or "I hate myself for eating that cake!" learns to think of food as an enemy and his or her own body as an object of shame or disgust. A child who grows up watching a parent's unsuccessful diets and witnessing the resulting anxiety over weight gain will feel a lack of control over her own eating and weight. Avoid these issues by expressing positive thoughts about your own body and about your relationship with food— and, even more important, by avoiding fad dieting—and you'll pass healthy attitudes on to your child.

Also, examine how you feel about your child's size and weight. This is especially important if you have a strong case of "fat phobia" yourself, or if your child is larger than you (particularly if you have a daughter). Often, today's children are taller and heavier than their parents. If you have a mental picture of your child as a "little you," it's important to realize that it's just fine if she's three inches taller or twenty pounds heavier than you by the time she's a teen. Also, if you've battled weight issues all of your life, it's important not to start your child on the same path by panicking when she gains a few pounds in puberty. Expecting a child to be a size 6 like you when her body's blueprint dictates otherwise is a prescription for eating disorders.

It's also crucial to be aware of the normal pattern of weight and height gain in children as they near or pass the turning point of puberty. Here are some guidelines, although children's weight and height will vary according to their genes and environment:

- It's normal for a child to gain thirty to forty pounds between the ages of eleven and fourteen. It is normal for your child to gain twenty pounds (or more) in a year.

- In girls, puberty-related weight gain generally appears first as a layer of fat all over the body and then gradually appears more around the breasts, thighs, and hips. Thus, some girls will appear "fat" for a time before their curves appear. Others, however, will develop a curvaceous body well before their peers—and still others will remain very thin and un-curvy. Girls in any of these groups need assurance that they are perfectly normal. Boys, too, may go through a "baby fat" stage before growing into their weight gain, and need to know that this is healthy and normal.

- Boys tend to be shorter than girls until they reach puberty. At that stage, both girls and boys often "shoot up." This means that your child may be much shorter or taller than her classmates, and she needs to know that this is normal. It's also normal for a child's feet or arms to grow quickly (hence the cliché about "gangly" teens). Boys may also develop a temporary swelling of the breast, and need reassurance that this is normal.

Children proceed through puberty in different ways according to their own genetic blueprint. Help children recognize and prepare for this by discussing the facts about differences in body size and shape that are inherent in all living creatures.

When Should I Talk to My Child about His or Her Development?

When you see your child's body starting to change, talk about what's happening! Don't wait until your child starts to receive misinformation from others. When you and your child recognize these changes as normal and healthy—even as exciting—you can set the stage for emotional and physical health. In particular, make sure your child knows that weight gain is a normal, healthy part of becoming a young woman or man. (Are children embarrassed when you bring up these topics? Yes. But they'll appreciate the information, because you'll be addressing their own unspoken fears and concerns.)

In addition, take active steps to teach your children healthy ideas about food and eating. Here are effective strategies for giving children the gift of a healthy relationship with food and their bodies:

- Never portray any food as an enemy. Help your child to develop a natural, healthy relationship with food and eating. Educate your child about the health benefits of high-nutrition foods, but don't place junk food completely off-limits. We crave what we can't have, so a child who occasionally eats a cupcake or candy bar is much less likely to become overweight than a child who thinks that all tempting foods are taboo and thus obsesses about them.

- Treat all family members equally with regard to food. Never single out a child based on his or her weight. Do not make different rules for different family members (e.g., Johnny can have all the dessert he wants, but Sarah really should eat fruit instead).

- Teach your child to recognize hunger and satiation. Ask a young child things like, "How does your tummy feel right now? Is it hungry?" After a meal, ask, "Is your tummy really full?" Also, don't make your child clean her plate—a habit that trains people to overeat. Instead, let her decide when she's eaten enough. A good rule of thumb: You decide what, when, and where your child eats, while your child decides whether or not to eat, and how much to eat. Trying to control how much your child eats will backfire!

- Encourage "mindful eating." Often, both kids and adults eat on autopilot. One way to increase your child's awareness of her own hunger and how much she's eating is to serve snacks in bowls rather than letting family members grab an entire bag of chips or box of cookies. This helps a child recognize when she's full, instead of zoning out and eating the entire box or bag of food. Also, encourage your children to eat in the kitchen or the dining room. Another good rule of thumb: your entire family should make it a habit to avoid eating while watching television.

- Beware of pressures from coaches. Kids involved in sports often experience pressure to lose weight, especially in activities like gymnastics, ballet, track, and wrestling. This puts your child at greatly heightened risk for an eating disorder. If you sense that a coach or instructor is pressuring your child to diet, meet with the coach and explain that this is unacceptable to you.

- If your child truly is overweight, and you're quite sure that it's not a temporary weight gain due to puberty or an emotional upset such as a divorce or death in the family, realize that "quick fixes" don't work. Instead, make gradual and positive life changes (not just for your child affected by weight gain, but for your entire family) that will pay off over time. Here are the most important steps you can take to promote a healthy and adaptive relationship with food and body image, through normal development and for a lifetime.

- Increase your child's activity. If your child isn't routinely physically active, plan regular family activities that involve movement; for instance, put up a basketball hoop or go on family bike rides. (But don't present these activities as a way for your child to lose weight. Instead, offer them as something fun to do.) Also, reduce the amount of time your family spends watching TV—one of the biggest culprits in weight gain. Put away the video games for the weekend, too.

- Avoid tasteless, artificial diet foods. Instead, teach your child to enjoy and appreciate natural, well prepared, and tasty foods— whether they're low in calories or carbohydrates or not. Your child will respond with satiety and stop eating on her own, when given the opportunity to eat delicious and nourishing foods in a setting which promotes mindfulness.

- Find a knowledgeable pediatrician. If your current pediatrician pushes a diet for your child, seek out a doctor who understands the impact of dieting and food restriction. Also, be sure this doctor rules out physical problems that can contribute to weight gain, such as sleep apnea (a surprisingly common problem in children) and thyroid conditions.

- Teach your child that his weight and his body size and shape aren't the most important things about him. Involve your child in esteem-building activities that make him feel competent and proud of his abilities. (For example, foster an artistic talent by signing your child up for sculpture classes, or encourage his musical abilities by buying him a guitar.) Getting a teenager involved with a volunteer organization such as Special Olympics can also increase her activity level while helping her realize that there are more important things in life than how much a person weighs. It may seem strange, but taking your child's mind off her weight is one of the best ways to help her become fit!

- Love your child unconditionally. Never bribe your child to lose weight, or say "You'd look so pretty in that dress if you lost a few pounds," or say, "Look how good Kathy looks now that she's thinner—you could do the same thing." Let your child know that you love her just as she is now—absolutely and unconditionally. Don't make critical comments about her current weight, and don't lavish her with praise and presents if she loses weight. A child who realizes that her parents' love doesn't hinge on her weight is far less likely to sneak food and eat secretly—a major contributor to obesity and emotional problems.

- Buy clothes that your child enjoys wearing, and that fit well. It's important that your child have access to attractive, well-fitting clothing that matches who she is. Make sure she has an adequate supply of clothes that fit. Try L.L. Bean and Land's End for plus sizes. Don't expose your child to a shopping trip to a store that doesn't supply the clothing she needs. Remember that your developing child will be growing quickly, and you may need to invest more in clothing than you expected during developmental changes.

None of these fixes will work overnight—but unlike dieting, they almost always will work in the long run. More importantly, they will give your child self-confidence and the secure feeling that she's loved and valued—no matter what the scale says, and no matter how different she looks from the anorexic model on the cover of this month's *Vogue*. That sense of self-esteem will do more to make her happy in life, and more to give her control over her weight and her health, than any diet could ever do.

Chapter 25

Environmental Factors in Eating Disorder Development

Chapter Contents

Section 25.1

Sociocultural and Psychological Factors in Eating Disorders

Excerpted from "Eating Disorder Causes" by Nancy A. Rudd, Liz Davis, and Penny Winkle. © 2010 The Ohio State University Body Image Health Task Force. Reprinted with permission. For additional information, visit http://ehe.osu.edu/cs/bitf/.

Sociocultural

Cultural pressure is said to contribute to unattainable images of beauty that create pressure for meeting impossible standards.

Sociocultural factors get significant attention, especially in the media. Eating disorders tend to be more common in industrialized countries; however, this is changing as less developed parts of the world have access to new technology and become Westernized.

Generally, cultural factors are thought to stress standards and ideals of beauty and thinness that are difficult, if not impossible, to attain. These images of beauty have been said to be aimed mainly at women and act to oppress them by demanding conformity to transitory standards that come and go with time.

Anorexics are sensitive to society's influence and subsequent approval and disapproval. As a result they attempt to attain the ideal societal perception that thin is superior and become obsessed with weight and body image. It is thought that self-worth is therefore equated with a slim appearance and vulnerability to eating disorders increases.

Western culture is blamed for being obsessed with the human body and a lean and lithe appearance. Beauty is sold as the key to happiness and the ultimate goal. Such images of beauty are delivered in a daily barrage in numerous women's magazines, on television, film, and other forms of mass media. However, as powerful as these influences may be, sociocultural factors should not be considered to be the only cause of eating disorders, but one ingredient in a complicated formula.

Psychological

Psychological factors help explain some of the features of eating disorders that sociocultural factors fail to address. A number of psychological factors have been suggested as being relevant in the development of eating disorders. In discussing the issue, it is important to remember the integral relationship between psychological and familial factors. The individual is part of the family system and develops within it. Thus, both individual and family psychology has been implicated and theories of causation tend to be related to this interaction. Eating disorders are typically considered to be related to problems during upbringing, family dysfunction, low self-esteem, overcontrolling parents (particularly mothers and distant fathers), and sexual abuse. The family is strained and experiences difficulties long before the patient moves to receive treatment. There has usually been a struggle with the eating-disordered child over eating and conflicts around food over some period of time before treatment.

Individuals suffering from eating disorders are typically described as having low self-esteem and experiences of feeling inadequate. They often report fearing sexual maturation, have trouble coping with stress, and tend to behave with a non-assertive manner. They are conflict avoidant and rarely resolve conflicts with others in a mature way. There are usually problems for the adolescent with separating from the family and normal individuation. These are thought to be problematic because of disturbances in communication, role structure, affect modulation, and boundary diffusion. These families have been described as enmeshed, overprotective, and as co-opting the anorexic daughter in destructive alliances with one parent or another (triangulation). It is postulated that the family has difficulty coping with stress, that the parents have an unacknowledged problem in their relationship, and that the daughter is enlisted to balance an otherwise unhealthy situation. Parents have even been described as affectionate, intrusive, but also neglectful and controlling. The anorexic daughter is more submissive than are teens without eating disorders.

In conclusion, it is important to consider all factors in the etiology of eating disorders. It has roots in the biological, psychological, and sociocultural. All these complex factors interact and are interrelated. It is important to consider individual differences in assessing an individual with a possible eating disorder.

Section 25.2

Eating Disorders as Adaptive Functions

Excerpted from *The Eating Disorder Sourcebook, Third Edition* by Carolyn Costin, MA, MED, MFCC. © 2007 The McGraw-Hill Companies, Inc. Reprinted with permission.

A struggling will, an insecure feeling, and despair may manifest themselves in problems with the care and feeding of the body but are fundamentally a problem with the care and feeding of the soul. In her aptly titled book *The Obsession: Reflections on the Tyranny of Slenderness*, Kim Chernin has written, "The body holds meaning . . . when we probe beneath the surface of our obsession with weight, we will find that a woman obsessed with her body is also obsessed with the limitations of her emotional life. Through her concern with her body she is expressing a serious concern about the state of her soul." What are the emotional limitations commonly seen in individuals with eating disorders? What is the state of their souls?

Common States of Being for the Eating Disordered Individual

How and why a particular person uses starving, bingeing, or purging as a way to cope is an individual issue but it is easy to understand how a person in one or more of the following emotional states will naturally seek comfort for, alleviation of, or distraction from his or her feelings:

- Low self-esteem

- Diminished self-worth

- Belief in the thinness myth

- Need for distraction

- Dichotomous (black or white) thinking

- Feelings of emptiness

- Quest for perfection

236

- Desire to be special/unique
- Need to be in control
- Need for power
- Desire for respect and admiration
- Difficulty expressing feelings
- Need for escape or a safe place to go
- Lack of coping skills
- Lack of trust in self and others
- Terrified of not measuring up

Not everyone who is exposed to the culture's idealization of thinness and goes on a diet develops an eating disorder. Some may even have the genetic predisposition—in other words, the gun is loaded—and be in a trigger-pulling environment, but no disorder. Why? These are people who, for whatever reason, are strong enough, together enough, stable enough, resilient enough, or protected enough to be inoculated against developing an eating disorder. Some might develop subclinical eating disorders and escape serious consequences or even recognition. Others might develop an anxiety disorder or a phobia but not have eating problems. Others go unscathed.

For the most part, people who develop eating disorders have some psychological vulnerability or sensitivity; or there is an event, trauma, or family dysfunction in their lives that occurs at the right time, or is of the right duration or severity, to set them up for being the one person out of all their dieting friends who goes from diet to disorder. If, as the research shows, people can recover from this illness, what do they recover from? What have we treated when people get better? So far, not their genes and not (unfortunately) the culture. What unique features or events in a person's life (aside from dieting) contribute to eating disorder susceptibility that can be dealt with to help him or her heal? My answer to this question relies in large part on my experience of treating eating disorder clients and their families for almost thirty years. I am not a researcher, but I have gathered countless hours of data on this subject and have collaborated with my colleagues and my clients, who have indeed been my best teachers.

Disordered Eating Behaviors: Serving a Purpose

Even if they started out as dieting techniques, eating disorder symptoms end up serving some kind of purpose that goes well beyond weight loss as a goal. Certain people begin to use disordered eating behaviors as substitutes for psychological functions that have not been developed: "If I don't purge, I'm anxious and distracted. After I purge, I can calm down and get things done," or "Not eating makes me feel safe and in control."

In trying to understand the meaning behind someone's behavior, it is helpful to think of the behavior as serving a function or "doing a job." Once the function is discovered, it becomes easier to understand why it is so difficult to give the behavior up and what might have to be done to replace it with something else. Paradoxically then, an eating disorder, for all of the problems it creates, is an effort to cope, communicate, defend against, and even solve other problems. This concept is critical in understanding and treating these disorders. For some, starving may be in part an attempt to establish a sense of power or control, self-worth, strength, and containment. Bingeing may be used to numb pain because of a developmental deficit in the ability to express grief or sadness or self-soothe. Purging may become an acceptable physiological and psychological release of anger or anxiety if the expression of one's feelings in childhood was not fostered or was met with neglect, criticism, or abuse.

Whether consciously or not, when people cannot cope in a healthy way, they often develop adaptive measures, the purpose of which is to make them feel whole, safe, secure, and in control. Some individuals use food, weight loss, and eating rituals to cope with other problems and to either avoid or meet emotional needs.

The following is a list of adaptive functions that eating disorder behaviors commonly serve:

- Comfort, soothing, nurturance
- Numbing, sedation, distraction
- Attention, a cry for help
- Discharge of tension, anger, rebellion
- Predictability, structure, identity
- Self-punishment or punishment of "the body"
- Self-cleansing or self-purification
- Protection or safety (through creation of a small or large body)
- Avoidance of intimacy
- Proof for self-blame instead of blaming others (for example, abusers)

As an eating disorder therapist, I help my clients discover the adaptive function(s) their eating disorder symptoms serve and what their specific manifestation of behaviors means. The behaviors often express inner conflict and can be paradoxical:

- **An expression of and defense against early childhood needs and feelings:** It's too scary to need anything, I try not to even need food.

- **An expression of self-destructive and self-affirming attitudes:** I will be the thinnest girl at my school, even if it kills me.

- **An assertion of self and a punishment of self:** I insist on eating whatever and whenever I want, even though being fat is making me miserable. . . . I deserve it.

The Eating Disorder Self

Eating disorder symptoms are the behavioral component of a separate, split-off self, or what I have come to call the "eating disorder self." This self has a special set of needs, behaviors, feelings, and perceptions, all of which are dissociated from the individual's core or "healthy self." The eating disorder self functions to express, mitigate, or in some way meet underlying needs and make up for the developmental deficits.

To get beyond this, the adaptive functions that the eating and weight-related behaviors serve must be "put out of a job" and replaced with healthier alternatives. To accomplish this, the eating disorder self must be recognized and understood in terms of why it exists. In addition, the person's healthy self has to be strengthened in order to take over the job. Eventually healing takes place when the two selves are integrated and no longer functioning as separate entities.

Treatment involves helping clients get in touch with their unconscious, unresolved needs and providing or helping to provide in the present what was missing in the past.

Eating Disorder Behaviors and Attachment

Research data and literature on attachment and eating disorders suggest that eating disorder symptoms may be substitutes for a secure attachment to help the patient overcome a real or perceived sense of inadequacy, insecurity, or fear. Data suggest that the frequency and intensity of anxious attachment in eating disordered individuals is greater than in control subjects. It seems that those with eating disorders are capable individuals who can use their intelligence and skill to manage major life issues but are highly sensitive and overreact to life's daily stresses and complexities.

In a summary of their research on eating disorders and attachment, Ainsworth and Roth (1989) reported that the development of a sense of secure attachment and the ability to respond to situations with self-reliance may have been derailed in some way for all kinds of eating disordered individuals, resulting in self-blame, anger, and rejection as well as denial of these emotions. These people feel inadequate and essentially unworthy even in the face of many accomplishments. They are unable to validate themselves internally and look for external means to do so, making them more susceptible to an exaggerated focus on appearance.

Uncovering and repairing any attachment issues can be an integral part of recovery.

Section 25.3

Bullying and the Link to Eating Disorders

Bullying is nothing new. It is a dark side of human nature, and often people view this behavior as something that comes with the territory—whether at school or in the workplace. But the far reaching tentacles of bullying are something that may not be immediately apparent. What if bullying is also responsible for triggering eating disorders in many individuals?

Recent studies suggest bullying behaviors have caused people to develop eating disorders. The girl teased about her weight in the gym class, or the woman humiliated by her boss, are much more prone to develop anorexia nervosa or a related illness.

Research shows prejudice and bullying behaviors toward overweight children begin as early as nursery school. Preschoolers are less likely to play with or befriend "the fat kids." Building Understanding Love & Learning for Youth (B.U.L.L.Y.) reports one of every four children is bullied, and one child is bullied every seven minutes. Bullying behaviors among children occur on many levels, including physical, verbal, nonverbal, and even online cyber-bullying.

Verbal bullying includes teasing, while nonverbal bullying includes intimidation through gestures. Cyber-bullying can include name calling through email. Many bullied victims cope with pain in ways which endanger their health. Children teased about weight and body shape are likely to develop low self-esteem, depression, negative body image, and an eating disorder.

Emotional states, especially social anxiety and shame, can trigger an eating disorder. Social anxiety is when one feels vulnerable to the negative criticism of others. Shame brings on feelings of hopelessness and inferiority. Such feelings are associated with poor body image.

The National Youth Violence Prevention Resource Center reports both males and females are bullied because of appearance. Male bullies will likely use aggression toward their target. Female bullies will use indirect forms of aggression, such as rumor and exclusion.

Swedish scholar Carolina Lunde recently conducted a study to understand the link between peer influence and body image. Participants were between ages ten and fourteen. Lunde found bullied and teased children were especially critical of their own looks. According to Lunde, girls were teased more about appearance than boys. Girls were also less comfortable with their appearance and body image.

Another study conducted in 2004 at the United Kingdom Centre for Eating Disorders looked at adolescent girls suffering from anorexia nervosa and their experiences with bullies and peer pressure. Participants were between ages fourteen and eighteen. All participants claimed bullying, cliques, and stereotyping led to their eating disorders. One young woman suggested if a student is disliked, he or she will likely be teased about weight. Also, participants claimed particular body types were associated with high social status.

Bullying is also found in adults. According to a 2007 survey conducted by the Workplace Bullying Institute, close to 40 percent of workers were subjected to workplace bullying.

Workplace bullying is classified as inappropriate and repeated behaviors directed toward one or more employees. The target is left humiliated, offended, and intimidated. Workplace bullying tactics include rumors, rolling eyes, name calling, and waving fists. Bullied victims are more likely to make mistakes on the job. Workplace bullying negatively impacts the economy by decreasing productivity and increasing turnover. The victim's health is also at stake. Victims may blame themselves, causing low self-esteem. Feelings of stress and trauma can lead to depression, nausea, ulcers, eating disorders, and suicidal thoughts. Other health problems from bullying include headaches, high blood pressure, and post-traumatic stress disorder.

Bullies ingrain negative labels into the heads of their victims. It is unfortunate that bullying is a major part of society from preschool years through adulthood. No matter how old the victim is, self-esteem and health are ultimately jeopardized.

This is why we must do our part to ensure that the problem of bullying does not flourish unchallenged. We can reaffirm to ourselves with the National Association of Anorexia Nervosa and Associated Disorders' (ANAD's) pledge: I will accept myself as I am. I will accept others as they are, and I will not tolerate physical or mental abuse.

Take action by:

- Talking to parents, teachers, counselors, school principals.

- Explaining to the child or adolescent it is not their fault. Express concern and ask them to talk to you about what is going on.

- If you feel no one is helping, ask the principal about school policy on bullying. If there is not a policy, ask that one be created and enforced.

For workplace bullying, specific actions include:

- Let the bully and others know in no uncertain terms that you will not be harassed or intimidated by that person by refusing to be victimized. Let others know of the problem; don't keep it to yourself.

- Keep a diary detailing the nature of the bullying (e.g. dates, times, places, what was said or done and who was present).

- Report the unacceptable behavior to a supervisor, manager or the human resources department of your employer.

- To help give you the skills to fight back, you may need to take assertive skills training.

Section 25.4

Boundary Invasion as a Cause of Eating Disorders

Where does an eating disorder come from? Countless parents and eating disorder patients ask me this question in person, on the phone, in emails from around the United States and different parts of the world. The tone of the question is bewilderment, anguish, and deep sincerity. Where do eating disorders come from? Why can't I (or my loved one) stop the behavior and eat normally?

As I listen to the unique stories of individuals and family members plagued by an eating disorder, one common theme I hear relates to boundary invasion. People with eating disorders, at some vulnerable time in their lives, experienced relentless, continuous, thorough, and inescapable boundary invasion. The eating disorder developed as a way to escape, protest, and, tragically, duplicate that boundary invasion.

Blatant and severe boundary invasions involve extreme behavior such as physical assault, sexual assault, and sexual molestation. A body of research now exists that explores the consequences of severe invasions and includes the work in the areas of post-traumatic stress disorder (PTSD) and dissociation identity disorder (DID). You can use your search engines to find some quality websites that provide excellent information on these conditions.

More subtle invasions can also wreak havoc on the mind and spirit of a developing person. Such a person, if she is creative, bright, and determined to survive the assaults on her identity, can develop an eating disorder. The function of the eating disorder is to block out pain and resist invasion. Unfortunately, the eating disorder also stops psychological development as it numbs emotions and awareness plus creates a disorder that mimics the hurt the person seeks to escape.

These noncriminal violations are powerful forces that can create an environment in which a young powerless person may need to develop an eating disorder in order to maintain her sanity and, sometimes, her actual survival.

When a young person has no privacy and no right to say, "No," it means she has no boundary between herself and others. No privacy means she can be invaded at any time in any way. When her diary is read, when her possessions are borrowed or taken without permission, when her efforts in school or sports or the arts are overwhelmed by someone else's ideas, goals, or personality, when her choices are disregarded or treated with disdain, when she has little or no choice in terms of clothes, foods, friends her boundaries are being violated.

Lack of boundaries means that no clear and agreed upon understanding exists in the young person or her caretakers about consequences of behavior. Essentials can be ripped away. Luxuries can appear for no reason. Emotions acted out in kindness or cruelty, material objects, abuse, and gifts have no understood criteria for coming and going.

Boundaries are invaded when a young person has no responsibilities of her own and no recognized consequences for her actions. If she can have anything she asks for with no effort on her part she learns nothing about personal effort, limits, consequences, or what enough means. If someone picks up her clothes, does her laundry, fixes her car, pays her bills, lets her borrow money or objects without expecting them to be returned, the young person experiences no boundaries and no limits. She lives in a confusing chaotic world that doesn't respect her boundaries or the boundaries of others.

She doesn't have an opportunity to recognize and develop her own identity boundaries. If she learns that she doesn't have to keep promises, if she doesn't appreciate and reciprocate the generosity of others then she doesn't learn how to be in effective and warm relationships. She learns that she has no limits in her behavior and desires. She learns this when her caretakers don't keep their promises, and/or don't have empathy and compassion for her experiences.

Gratifying a child's every whim is not a loving act nor is it spoiling a child through overindulgence. Such treatment is actually neglect. The child's identity, taste, capacity to grow, learn, and function, her potential to be competent and responsible are neglected. Worse, this neglect may be based on the caretakers' assertion that the child is incompetent and could not now or ever assume responsibility for her self-care. Worse yet, out of their own insecurities and personal weaknesses, caretakers may need to feel powerful and in control. They may feel threatened by a rising competent person in their midst.

When a powerless person is flooded with the agenda of others, even if well meaning, it's as if a steamroller is bearing down on her psyche.

She may learn to please, manipulate, compete, or control in order to cope and survive, but she is unable to learn to be fully present as her genuine self. She may also learn to escape the pain of being steamrolled by entering into eating disorder behaviors.

Boundaries are also invaded when a child is given too much responsibility, especially if the tasks require acceptance of deceit and family secrets. If a person with a mental disorder is given authority in a family and the child must defer to that person's illogical and emotional reasoning or outburst as if this were normal, the child either develops a distorted view of the world or develops an eating disorder to block out the assault on her own mind. If she is criticized, insulted, told she is crazy, stupid, clumsy, incompetent, or sick for experiencing and expressing her honest response, she will either be severely damaged or develop an eating disorder to help protect herself.

Here are some examples of excessive responsibility that become intolerable psychic assaults:

- She knows about a sexual affair of one parent and knows the other parent is ignorant of the affair.

- She knows about a crime or act of cruelty or deceit that she must keep secret or be branded disloyal.

- She is expected to witness crimes, acts of cruelty and neglect within her family (against people or animals) without protest or experience the pain of ridicule, punishment, or rejection.

- She lives with and must accept the behavior and authority of a caretaker who behaves irrationally, i.e., screams, throws objects; dissembles appliances, computers, cars; takes charge of mail or money and doesn't follow through; must be the driver even though careless or tends toward road rage behavior; hallucinates.

The psyche of a young and powerless person in such situations can create an eating disorder to block her from pain and these identity assaults. With the aid of the eating disorder the person places her heart and mind in cold storage until the day she is safe enough or strong enough to come out of hiding.

The tragedy is that she never learns the concept of enough. Furthermore, eating disorders have a tenacious hold on people because the disorder is deeply linked to survival issues. Even if she frees herself of the actual boundary-invading environment or even if the authority figures change, she still lives the tragedy through the duplication of the invasive experiences in the disorder itself. After all, eating disorders can invade a person's life, making normal activities difficult or impossible. Work, school, family, and social responsibilities can be impossible to honor when a person is in the grip of an eating disorder.

From within that grip the person criticizes herself so harshly that she is paralyzed and cannot take independent action in the world. She chooses abusive relationships because they are familiar to her. She is kidnapped for no reason she understands by the compulsive urge to binge or purge or hide through isolation. She cannot express her true feelings out of fear of punishment or abandonment and lives via a false self. A sense of despair is ever present.

Recovery work involves far more than the end of eating disorder behavior related to food. Through work with trustworthy and responsible treatment professionals the individual undergoes an internal restructuring. She moves through developmental stages she missed while her heart and mind were in cold storage. She learns to cope with what seems to be a new and different world as her psyche matures. She learns how to nourish her body, heart, and mind so she can be healthy and strong. From a position of health and strength she learns to recognize danger and make self-caring decisions. She learns that she can take responsibility for choices she makes to build a life for herself that is worth living.

Boundary invasions forced her to go into survival mode. It may be that during the survival mode she unknowingly developed a kind of psychic strength and courage that equips her to journey through the arduous path to recovery. Once she finds and commits to her recovery path and works with the professional who understands her journey she can use strength and courage and move to a healthy life where she can take care of her true self.

Chapter 26

The Media and Eating Disorders

Chapter Contents

Section 26.1

Media Influence and Eating Disorders

"Media/Advertising," © 1998 Deborah J. Kuehnel, LCSW. Reprinted with permission. For additional information, visit www.addictions.net. Editor's note added by David A. Cooke, MD, FACP, 2010.

Society pays a significant amount of attention to body image and physical attractiveness, youthfulness, sexuality, and appearance. The covers of magazines display pictures of men and women alike, whose images are offered as near perfection in society's consensus. These photographs are often additionally computer-enhanced and taken in near perfect circumstances. The average man or woman could not possibly compete with these images. Perhaps the models themselves cannot live up to these expectations. Eating disorders are not foreign illnesses to the modeling industry. What is unfortunate but interesting is the fluidity of society and the alterations imposed due to its changeableness. The impact of these changes can be enormous to those who strive for that perfection. It guarantees they may never quite be able to reach those goals and almost ensures a sense of failure, shame, and guilt (Grub, Sellers, & Waligroski, 1993; Stice, Schupak-Neuberg, Shaw, & Stein, 1994; Wiseman, Gray, Mosimann, & Ahrens, 1992).

One of the strongest messengers of sociocultural pressures may well be the mass media (Stice, Schupak-Neuberg, Shaw, & Stein, 1994). Irving (1990) discovered a direct relation between media exposure and eating disorder symptomatology over the last several decades. The increase in eating disorders through the years has coincided with a decrease in women's ideal body weight as portrayed in the media (Wiseman, Gray, Mosimann, & Ahrens, 1992).

Paralleling the rise in eating disorders was an increase in the number of articles and advertisements promoting weight-loss diets in women's magazines (Anderson & DiDomenico, 1992). Anderson and DiDomenico (1992) established that women's magazines contained 10.5 times more advertisements and articles promoting weight loss than men's magazines, the same sex ratio reported by Anderson (1990) for eating disorders. Irving (1990) exposed women to slides of thin, average, and heavy models, which resulted in lower self-esteem and decreased weight satisfaction for these women. A similar experiment utilizing pictures of models from women's magazines found that exposure to thin models, rather than average-sized models, produced increased depression, stress, guilt, shame, insecurity, and body dissatisfaction (Stice et al, 1994).

These associations support the assertion that exposure to the media-portrayed thin ideal is related to eating pathology and suggests that women may directly model disordered eating behavior presented in the media (e.g., fasting or purging) (Stice et al, 1994). Leon, Fulderson, Perry, and Cudeck (1993) established strong associations between body dissatisfaction and eating disorders. The internalization of the media's thin ideal produces heightened body dissatisfaction, which leads to the engagement in disordered eating behavior. Additionally, the focus on dieting in the media may promote dietary restraint, which appears to increase the risk for binge eating (Polivy, 1996; Stice et al., 1994).

Body dissatisfaction is a widespread and common phenomenon among women in general (Andrews, 1997). One of the most central aspects of shame pertains to individual concerns about how one is regarded by others and self-conscious feelings about the body have been consistently noted in the shame literature (e.g., Gilbert, 1989; Mollon, 1984). There is evidence that bulimia is related to general public self-consciousness (Striegel-Moore, Silberstein, & Rodin, 1993). Bodily shame aspects include self-consciousness and embarrassment about general appearance and about exposing specific body parts, concealment of different body parts, and feelings of disgust about oneself concerning others' comments about appearance and body parts (Andrews, 1997). Stice and Shaw (1994) demonstrated that greater ideal-body stereotype internalization predicted increased body dissatisfaction, which was related to heightened eating disorder symptoms. Consistent with these findings, Leon (1993) also drew a path from body dissatisfaction to eating pathology. Stice and Shaw (1994) indicated a strong positive relation between internalization of the thin-ideal and disordered eating. Specifically, it may be that exposure to ideal-body images results in negative affects including shame, guilt, depression, and stress, as well as a lack of confidence which also shows a strong relation to eating pathology (Stice et al., 1994). Further body dissatisfaction leads to restrained eating, which has been linked to the onset of binge eating and bulimia (Wiseman et al, 1992).

Although most women are exposed to the media portrayed thin-ideal images, only a small proportion develop eating disorders. It may be that women with perfectionistic tendencies are more inclined to feel dissatisfied with their bodies when they compare themselves to those images presented in the media. Coping skills may also moderate the relation between negative affect, binge eating, and restricting, as women with better coping skills would likely ameliorate negative affect in more adaptive ways (e.g., seeking social support) (Stice & Shaw, 1994; Stice et al, 1994).

Notes from the Health Reference Series *Medical Advisor*

Unrealistic male body portrayals have also become an issue in recent years. Increasingly, "ideal" male bodies in popular media have very high muscle mass and degrees of muscle definition. This is quite pronounced in comic books, animated children's programs, and action figure toys (Pope et al., 1999). It is especially striking if modern characters are compared to those in similar media from several decades ago; characters such as Superman, Batman, and Spiderman are now portrayed as far more muscular than in the 1940's, 1950's, and 1960's. The widespread use of anabolic steroids among professional sports further promotes an unrealistically lean and muscular body ideal. A new disorder, coined "muscle dysmorphia," is being increasingly seen in men, and it has been suggested that media portrayals are contributing factors (Mosley, 2008). Individuals with this disorder share many features seen in eating disorders, including distorted body image and an obsession with exercise to increase muscle mass and lose fat. The prevalence and cause of this disorder is less well characterized than eating disorders, but it may well represent a new variation on an old theme.

Section 26.2

Pro–Eating Disorder Websites

"Web of Controversy: Investigating Pro–Eating Disorder Sites,"
by Jessica Setnick, MS, RD/L. *Today's Dietician.* © 2007 Great Valley
Publishing Co. Reprinted with permission.

The internet isn't the world's safest playground—and web pages that seemingly promote, even glorify, thinness may be real cause for concern.

Critics have labeled them "accomplices to suicide" and founders have heralded them as "supportive havens."[1] Behind all the media hoopla, what do you need to know about so-called pro–eating disorder websites to best serve your clients?

A Look at Content

The truth is that few of these sites contain original content. Many are small, personal websites or weblogs with content lifted from other related sites. Much of the content can be found elsewhere on the internet, including weight-loss-related websites that do not associate themselves with pro–eating disorder sites.

Many of the websites feature photos of underweight or emaciated women, dubbed thinspiration. A minority are personal photos of individuals photographing themselves in a mirror; the vast majority are paparazzi shots of celebrities, photos taken during fashion shows, and models in advertisements—all of which are readily available in major magazines.

The singularity of focus is what makes the pro–eating disorder websites so unique. Instead of four or five pages of emaciated, elongated, computer-manipulated models spaced out in a magazine among editorial content, these sites stockpile these images exclusively. To curious observers, rather than having a temptation to emulate these images, more likely their reaction may be surprise at how absolutely commonplace they are. In other words, the majority of these images are by no means underground, subversive, or secret. They are merely purloined from the many media images we encounter on a daily basis without even trying.

There is one style of thinspiration that is unique to pro–eating disorder websites: photos portraying underweight individuals, always girls or women, participating in questionable behaviors, such as kneeling over a toilet, exercising, or showing off their skeletons. The more disturbing websites include captions such as "I love your bones," indicating that such appearances are desirable.

Many websites include language insisting that their goal is to "offer support," a "safe haven," or a "nonjudgmental" forum for those with eating disorders. It is unclear whether these statements are merely a standard disclaimer to cover a more devious and dangerous purpose or whether those who develop the sites are merely as confused about eating disorders as those they claim to serve.

For example, The House of ED, whose home page motto is Latin for "What nourished me, destroyed me," provides on one page The Diet Coke Diet:

- Breakfast: 12–20 oz. Diet Coke
- Snack: 12 oz. Diet Cherry Coke
- Lunch: 12–24 oz. Diet Vanilla Coke
- Snack: 12 oz. Diet Coke with Lemon
- Dinner: 24–36 oz. Diet Coke with Lime
- Snack: 12 oz. Diet Caffeine [sic] Free Coke

And on another page, there is substantial information on first aid and seeking help for self-injury.

Some self-described anorexia tips are much like what you would find on a reputable weight loss site—for example, detailed directions on how to eat small portions, keep a food diary, use clothes to monitor weight loss instead of the scale, and avoid refined foods. Some sites include a body mass index calculator, restaurant guides, suggestions for how to get through a weight loss plateau, and distractions to keep you busy when tempted to eat. Out of context, none of these would be surprising to a dietetics professional; in fact, many use these same tools on a daily basis with clients.

"Think of all the positive changes you can experience by losing weight." This quote is not, as you might suspect, from a pro–eating disorder website but in fact from the weight loss page on about.com. A quick review of standard weight loss websites finds few specify that before attempting weight loss, one should ensure that weight loss is recommended. In other words, a normal weight or underweight person who nevertheless wants to lose weight could find a large portion of the information on pro–eating disorder websites without ever finding a pro–eating disorder website.

Viewers Beware

So what is unique about pro–eating disorder websites? Along with flippant, directionless, but possibly influential blurbs such as "EDNOS, the smart choice," a small but important minority of the information on some pro–eating disorder websites is clearly harmful if followed.

"An Anorexic Mind" is a web article compiling dozens of pro-anorexia "tips" from various websites. Although the author introduces "An Anorexic Mind" as a mocking commentary on anorexia, to an impressionable reader contemplating weight loss at any cost, it is a detailed, helpful, and instructive guide. Consider the following excerpts:

- "Be sure to [expletive deleted] your relationship with food from the start. You want to make yourself as neurotic as possible about food, eating, kitchens, cutlery, refrigerators, restaurants, and . . . start hating the source of foods."

- "Associate food with disgusting things. . . . Draw pictures of juicy red apples somehow morphing into giant dead rotting pigs."

- "Create a list of suitable punishments either for thinking of food or for caving in and eating food itself . . . include ridiculous amounts of exercise, purging, self-mutilation, isolation, basic denial of necessary comforts such as blankets on a cold night or shelter when it is raining, or simply menial, disgusting tasks such as cleaning the bathroom. Remember, you need discipline."

- "Believe in the power of dieting as though it were a religion."

In addition to the philosophical tips, "An Anorexic Mind" includes lists of thinspirational books and music, as well as tips to burn calories, deny hunger, and hide unhealthy behaviors. Nowhere does it list the dangers of anorexia, which we all know to be damage to every major organ system in the body, permanent bone loss, and eventual death.

And herein lies the major concern with pro–eating disorder websites: With a few exceptions, they fail to address the negative consequences of eating disorders, much less the actual dangers to life and limb. If negative health effects are mentioned at all, they are minimized or factually misrepresented. One site insists that ketosis is a desirable metabolic state, menstrual irregularities do not have serious effects, and although "lethal heart rhythms" is listed as a complication of bulimia, somehow "there are few major health problems" for a "bulimic of normal weight."

Implying that eating disorders are a handy and safe method for weight loss is clearly incorrect and irresponsible and could prevent someone who is already in danger from seeking medical care and treatment.

Hide and Seek

The websites themselves are well hidden, in part due to a crackdown by free web hosts at the request of the National Eating Disorders Association (NEDA) on the grounds that they violate the terms of service by being harmful to minors. (See NEDA's stance on pro–eating disorders websites below.) Some sites have moved to private hosting, and some have moved to solely bulletin board status. Others appear to have disbanded but may have morphed into another format or site. The names of the websites cannot be merely typed into a browser. In most cases, they must be linked to from another site, as the full site name is usually long and/or coded. If you are interested in perusing these sites, typing "pro ana" into your search engine is far less helpful than typing "pro ana" into the search engine at xanga.com, for example. Likewise, typing "thinspiration" into a standard search engine will provide less pro–eating disorder imagery than typing "thinspiration" into youtube.com.

Although some media reports have suggested that pro–eating disorder sites have legions of loyal fans and are responsible for hundreds of new eating disorder cases, there is no evidence of that on the pro–eating disorder websites themselves. There is no bragging about success at "converting" new followers and no accounting of new members seduced. To the contrary, many sites appear to be one-woman creations, even those (e.g., Anorexia Nation) whose names imply a voluminous following.

The Power to Influence?

Because the mechanism(s) of eating disorder development are currently not well understood, it is difficult to determine the impact of anything on the incidence or prevalence of eating disorders, including pro–eating disorder websites.

We do know that for most people with eating disorders, a desire for weight loss preceded the development of the disease, and many patients with eating disorders implicate a diet or other weight loss attempt as the immediate pre-disorder trigger. There are many cases in which involuntary weight loss triggered an eating disorder; however, it appears that in the majority of these cases, weight loss was considered desirable, even if it was not voluntarily attempted. Long before pro–eating disorder websites existed, mainstream weight loss media—diet books, diet programs, diet websites, and so on—have been implicated as triggers by patients with eating disorders. It is weight loss itself that triggers the eating disorder, regardless of the mechanism of action or education.

Even the pro–eating disorder websites themselves seem to be ambivalent about the role they play in the development of eating disorders. Some pro–eating disorder websites insist in their content that they aren't doing anything wrong, as no website can cause anorexia. Other sites include a disclaimer or warning on the home page indicating that images within may be "triggering" to some viewers.

Anorexics Unite attempts to cover all the bases in its homepage "Mission Statement":

> Anorexics Unite is a Pro–Anorexic website. We are not responsible for the underage viewing of this website or any injuries that may come of viewing this site. If you are of the many who are faint-of-heart, please turn back now. You will find many possibly disturbing images and material throughout this website. If you are recovering from an eating disorder or planning on recovering, or don't have an eating disorder, turn back now. We do not "teach" anyone to become eating disordered. You cannot "learn" an eating disorder. It is a disease acquired [sic] over time. I would also like to add that a website cannot "brainwash" you into becoming eating disordered. Thank you for understanding.

The House of ED provides the following "Disclaimer":

> If you do not have an eating disorder or are in recovery, do not view this website because it may cause you to relapse or obtain an eating disorder. The owner of this site does not promote eating disorders but simply provides a safe haven for those already affected by it. Enter at your own risk.

For someone who is intrigued or interested, it seems unlikely that such a disclaimer would discourage him or her from proceeding. On the other hand, someone with an eating disorder who is truly attempting to recover may appreciate the warning that triggering material is waiting inside. It is too bad the equally triggering highway billboards and fashion magazines don't provide the same courtesy.

The fallacy behind the hype that pro–eating disorder websites cause eating disorders is that one simply cannot choose to develop an eating disorder. Anorexia, bulimia, and other eating disorders are physiologic brain disorders of multifactorial origin. The exact mechanisms that cause them remain unclear, but we do know that one cannot choose to have an eating disorder, much the same way one cannot choose to have cancer. Many people undertake diets; arguably only a portion develop eating disorders. One pro–eating disorder website offers this comparison: "A man can shave his head and look bald, but he is still not bald." Some people force themselves to throw up once or twice, and then walk away without developing bulimia.

On the other hand, no one knows what makes an individual susceptible to eating disorder development, so potentially everyone is at risk. The House of ED, site of violent contradictions that it is, states that every person in a developed country could reasonably be considered in danger of developing an eating disorder. In other words, it is impossible to predict the level of impact, if any, that a pro–eating disorder website (or any other media literature or image) will have on an individual's eating disorder propensity.

An adult who is comfortable with his or her weight but is curious about the pro–eating disorder movement might not be influenced by a pro-anorexia or pro-bulimia website. However, an impressionable teen who is interested in "fitting in" by losing weight may find the information fascinating and inspirational. In other words, the effect of a pro–eating disorder website is likely a result of the user's mindset prior to viewing the site. This leads to the conclusion that if the site viewer comes to the pro–eating disorder site predisposed or susceptible to an eating disorder, the information on the site may contribute to the further development of the disease.

Only one study to date has assessed the influence of pro–eating disorder sites on patients with eating disorders, and none has analyzed their potential influence on creating eating disorders. In the one available study, "Surfing for Thinness: A Pilot Study of Pro–Eating Disorder Usage in Adolescents with Eating Disorders," patients who frequented pro–eating disorder websites required longer treatment and more hospital admissions.[2] Future research might assess the impact of pro–eating disorder websites on internet users without eating disorders, study the long-term effects of participating in a pro–eating disorder online community vs. an eating disorder recovery group, and provide more information on the influence of these sites.

How Can Dietetics Professionals Help?

Dietetics professionals visiting pro–eating disorder websites will experience them much differently than affected individuals; therefore, the impact on and meaning of these websites to each client is infinitely more important than the professional's view. As with all subjective portions of assessment, hearing from the client will guide the treatment plan and course of action rather than standard guidelines regarding hours of internet usage per day, etc.

In the meantime, dietetics professionals working in behavioral health, eating disorders, weight management, and adolescent medicine may consider adding questions regarding internet usage to their general assessment of clients. Although no evidence-based guidelines currently exist, common sense investigation of how much time is spent on the internet, which type of sites are visited, and what the client considers the role of the professional team vs. the internet community may be helpful in determining a course of action. Possible interventions may include parental supervision of adolescent internet usage to prevent any viewing of pro–eating disorder sites, voluntary limits on time spent or type of sites viewed, and/or required discussion of internet content during nutrition counseling or psychotherapy sessions.

In an ideal world, an individual attempting to recover from an eating disorder would not view pro–eating disorder websites or any other triggering media, but this can be accomplished only in a full-time treatment center. Ultimately, internal coping skills must be developed to provide protection from visual and other external triggers that influence eating disorder recovery and relapse. Media literacy is already accepted as one essential skill, since complete abstinence from all potential triggers is nearly impossible outside of treatment. With regard to pro–eating disorder websites, media literacy may include education regarding the computer manipulation of images; dissection of nutrition myths and misconceptions promoted on a website; exploration of the mindset of someone trying to justify his or her eating disorder by recruiting "followers"; and how weight-obsessed pro–eating disorder websites reflect or distort the weight-obsessed general culture.

It remains to be seen how pro–eating disorder sites will impact the eating disorders landscape and the prevalence of eating disorders in general. It seems possible that once the bulk of the information is out there, interest will be lost, and the websites will fade. On the other hand, with stated goals that "someday the pro-anorexic lifestyle will be accepted in society," we may be confronting these websites and their repercussions for many years to come.

References

1. "Mixed Messages: Proponents say they offer 'support,' but a Stanford University study finds that patients who visited

pro–anorexia Web sites were sicker longer." Newsweek online at MSNBC.com.

2. Wilson JL, Peebles R, Hardy KK, et al. "Surfing for thinness: A pilot study of pro–eating disorder Web site usage in adolescents with eating disorders." *Pediatrics*. 2006;118(6):1635–43.

The National Eating Disorders Association's Stance

"The National Eating Disorders Association actively speaks out against pro-anorexia and pro-bulimia websites. These sites provide no useful information on treatment but instead encourage and falsely support those who, sadly, are ill but do not seek help. These sites could have a severe negative impact on the health of those who consult them and encourage a 'cult' type destructive support system that discourages people from the treatment they so desperately need. Anorexia nervosa is a potentially lethal disease and has the highest mortality rate of any mental illness. Bulimia is also a very dangerous illness with serious long-term health consequences. Eating disorders cannot be taken lightly.

"Our emphasis is on steering people toward treatment and health. We offer educational materials for all ages, and a toll-free helpline (800-931-2237) with referrals to treatment professionals. Each February during National Eating Disorders Awareness Week, we support hundreds of events created by volunteers around the country. Our annual conference every autumn brings together treatment providers and families of those with eating disorders, informing and inspiring thousands of conference attendees with the latest knowledge and new personal connections.

"A goal of the National Eating Disorders Association is to raise awareness of eating disorders as serious, life-threatening illnesses—which are treatable. Most of those who enter treatment recover. Please visit us at www.NationalEatingDisorders.org."

Part Four

Medical Complications
of Eating Disorders

Chapter 27

Overview of Medical Complications of Eating Disorders

There are frequently seen with those suffering from eating disorders or who have had a history of an eating disorder a vast array of physiological complications and health risks. No two individuals are the same. Their bodies may respond and react differently to the abuse which they succumb to under eating disorder behaviors. Very rarely can someone who "dabbles" in eating disorders (no matter which, anorexia, bulimia, or compulsive overeating) simply walk away from the behavior alone. Additionally, it is not uncommon to experience a switching of behaviors from one to the other or to additional self-destructive behaviors like self-injurious behavior, compulsive spending, gambling, substance abuse, and stealing behavior, to state a few.

As a therapist I have to be very in tune with the possible complications, more now than ever since insurance companies are not very helpful in providing the right levels of care an individual may need. For the most part to date insurance companies are dictating treatment and eating disorders are illnesses they decline adequate treatment for very frequently. Individuals suffering from eating disorders and their family members need help in understanding the serious ramifications of these destructive behaviors on the body, soul, and mind of the individual.

"Physiological Complications," © 2002 Deborah J. Kuehnel, LCSW. Reprinted with permission. For additional information, visit www.addictions.net. Reviewed and updated by David A. Cooke, M.D., FACP, September 2010.

Electrolyte Imbalances

Minerals make up the electrolyte system. They are essential for the balanced chemistry of the body and its ability to function correctly. They ensure healthy nerve and muscle impulses, kidneys and heart, blood sugar levels, and the delivery of oxygen to the cells of the body. When this system is disrupted the results can be devastating, including heart attacks and stokes. You will see electrolyte imbalances especially with behaviors associated with purging (vomiting, abuses of diuretics and laxatives), as well as in drowning the body by binging on large quantities of fluids such as water, milk, or soda.

Dehydration

This is caused by the depletion (frequently seen with purging behaviors) or lack of intake of fluids into the body. Restricting, vomiting, laxative and diuretic abuse, and extended exercise without appropriate hydration are the primary causes. Symptoms include: Possible dark circles under eyes, a "drawn" look to the face itself, dizziness, weakness, and darkening of urine. In extreme cases it can lead to kidney failure, heart failure, and death.

Malnutrition

Can be caused by significant undereating and in some cases overeating to the point of flooding the body and its systems. It can also be seen with binging and purging behavior especially when the individual is purging following everything eaten. The body requires fuel (food) as its primary energy source and when deprived of that it can result in respiratory infections, kidney failure, blindness, heart attack, and death.

Hyponatremia

A flooding of the system with water. (Drinking more than eight eight-ounce glasses of water a day.) One client I worked with drank five gallons of water per day. Often seen with those who binge on fluids. This is a very serious condition which requires immediate medical attention. Due to the influx of water the body cannot balance its sodium level adequately and this can cause fluid in the lungs, the brain to swell, nausea, vomiting, severe confusion, and even death. It can also appear as a drug overdose to medical personal because of an enormous amount of strength an individual may experience in conjunction with some psychotic and delusional orientations.

Muscle Atrophy

A wasting away of muscle tissue and a decrease in muscle mass due to the body feeding off of itself. Usually accompanies restricting.

Lanugo

An unusual soft downy hair on the face, back, or arms. This is caused by the body's protective mechanism in malnutrition to help keep the individual warm. It is a result of hormonal imbalances. It may take an extended period of time for this to go away after the individual begins eating appropriately due to the body's need to protect itself.

Edema

This is a swelling of the soft tissues as a result of excess water accumulation and retention. Pitting edema is the type of swelling which when you apply pressure to the swollen area an indentation is left. It is most common in the legs, feet, and fingers of all three eating disorders. For bulimics and anorexics it can also be present in the abdominal area. Can be caused by laxative and diuretic abuse.

Re-Feeding Edema

A very serious condition which requires medical supervision. It usually occurs during the time the individual who has been depriving themselves of sustenance and begins to eat again. Generally one of the causes of this edema is the lack of protein in the system. Patients or clients who resume normal eating should be monitored for this because it is a natural reaction of the body to the reintroduction of food.

Impaired Neuromuscular Functioning

Inability to be able to move in a normal fashion. Due to vitamin and mineral deficiencies.

Temporary Paralysis

An extreme weakness of the muscles which may disable the individual to move at all. Frequently caused by low levels of potassium but also by the degeneration of nerve cells in the spinal cord or in the brain which have been deprived of essential nutrients. After onset they may occur more frequently and more severely and may lead to permanent muscle weakness and possible death.

Esophageal Reflux

This is a regurgitation of partially digested items in the stomach, mixed with acid and enzymes. This can lead to damage in the esophagus, stomach, and larynx. This can be a precancerous state to the esophagus and voice box and requires medical attention and medication often. Often seen in bulimics who purge through vomiting, reflux can become so bad that food cannot be kept down at all and purging becomes involuntary for the individual.

Barrett Esophagus

A condition associated with cancer of the esophagus and caused by reflux. It brings about a change in the cells of the esophagus.

Mallory-Weiss Tears

Mallory-Weiss tears are rips in the lining in the esophagus caused by forceful vomiting. They may occur during purging, and typically lead to vomiting blood. Some of these tears can be life-threatening.

Digestive Difficulties

There can be two issues in this area. One is a deficiency in digestive enzymes, which leads to the body's inability to properly digest food and absorb nutrients. This may lead to malabsorption problems, malnutrition, and electrolyte imbalances. Additionally, when one purges one risks a change in the signals from the stomach to the brain resulting in slowed digestion because the body has become accustomed to purging behavior. For bulimics this can be disturbing because the small intestine does not send its signal to the brain to tell the individual that they are full at the appropriate time. Additionally, the individual tends to feel full for a longer period of time, which is very uncomfortable for the individual trying to recover from an eating disorder.

Pancreatitis

Digestive enzymes attack the pancreas. This can be very painful. It can be caused by the repeated stomach trauma of vomiting, alcohol consumption, or the excessive use of laxatives or diet pills.

Peptic Ulcers

Caused by increased stomach acids, high consumption of caffeine as seen in some forms of diet pills, or alcohol consumption.

Cramps, Bloating, Constipation, Diarrhea, Incontinence

Increased or decreased bowel activity. Many patients are treated for irritable bowel syndrome. Laxative abuse can damage nerves in the intestine, which can lead to severe and permanent constipation.

Weakness and Fatigue

Caused by insufficient nutrients or malnutrition, electrolyte imbalances, vitamin and mineral deficiencies, increased depression, insomnia, and heart problems.

Swelling in Face

Particularly noticeable where the glands lie connecting the upper and lower jaws. Often follows purging by vomiting.

Bloodshot-Appearing Eyes or Tiny Blood Vessels Torn on the Face

A direct result of violent purging by vomiting behavior.

Gastrointestinal Bleeding

A bleeding which occurs in the digestive tract which primarily is seen through elimination or blood in the stool.

Gastric Rupture

A sudden perforation or rupture in the stomach.

Hair Loss, Dry Skin, Brittle Lusterless Hair, Brittle Nails

Vitamin deficiencies.

Seizures

Due to dehydration there is an increased risk to anorectic and bulimic individuals of seizures (which are surges of electricity within the brain). In these individuals lesions on the brain may develop as a result of long-term malnutrition, in which a lack of the oxygen-carrying cells the brain requires to function adequately causes chemical imbalances.

Low Blood Pressure, Hypotension

A condition brought about by malnutrition, dehydration, and a lowering of the body temperature. Can cause heart arrhythmias, shock, or myocardial infarction.

Orthostatic Hypotension

This is seen as a sudden drop in blood pressure when changing positions from sitting or laying down to the standing position. The individual may experience a momentary inability to see, dizziness, blurred vision, passing out, heart pounding, and headaches.

High Blood Pressure, Hypertension

Seen primarily in compulsive overeaters, the blood pressure elevates beyond 140 over 90. It causes abnormal thickening of the heart muscle, resulting in heart attacks. Additionally, it may cause strokes, either fatal or brain damaging, and kidney failure.

Hypoglycemia

A disturbance in blood sugar resulting in low blood sugar especially seen in anorectic or bulimic patients. Sweating and shakiness are symptomatic and can indicate problems with the liver or kidneys, which can lead to neurological and mental deterioration. Dietary attention is important.

Diabetes

A high blood sugar as a result of an inadequate production of insulin. Often seen in malnourished individuals as well as compulsive overeaters. For some this condition may be treated with dietary changes. Some patients who develop diabetes which requires medical attention and medication during the eating disorder are able as they recover more fully to be rid of the symptoms of diabetes, but need to be watched medically for a recurrence. Some warning signs are frequent urination and inability to quench thirst, nervousness, weakness, trembling, weak rapid pulse, seizures, and possible appearance of intoxication.

Ketoacidosis

A state which involves high levels of acids which build up in the blood caused by the body burning fat rather than sugar and carbohydrates to get energy. The shift from utilizing carbohydrates as energy to fat results in the formation of ketoacids. Kidneys are overwhelmed by the continuous production of ketone bodies, resulting in profound acidosis. Common causes are alcohol abuse, starvation, excessive purging, dehydration, and hyperglycemia. Untreated diabetes can cause ketoacidosis (also known as DKA).

Kidney Infections and Potential Kidney Failure

The function of the kidneys is to purify the poisons from the body, regulate acid concentration, and maintain water balance. The risk of difficulties with the kidneys increases with dehydration, infection, low blood pressure, and vitamin deficiencies. Untreated diabetes causes significant strain on the kidneys and can lead to kidney failure.

Amenorrhea

Loss of menstrual cycle because the hormone estrogen secreted by the ovaries ceases to be produced. This can lead to osteoporosis and osteopenia.

Osteopenia

A below normal bone mass, which may lead to osteoporosis. This may result from nutrient and vitamin deficiency, as well as menstrual disturbances that may accompany eating disorders.

Osteoporosis

A thinning of the bones with a reduction in bone mass, which leaves bones vulnerable to fractures. Like osteopenia, this may result from nutrient and vitamin deficiency, as well as menstrual disturbances that may accompany eating disorders.

A bone density test is helpful in evaluating damage caused from eating disorder behaviors of restriction, binging, and purging.

Temporomandibular Joint (TMJ) Syndrome

A form of degenerative arthritis within the temperomandibular joint in the jaw. This is often seen in bulimic patients who purge through vomiting, causing unnecessary strain on the joint. There is often pain in the joint area, with difficulty chewing as a result, and headaches.

Dental Problems

Stomach acids and enzymes from vomiting can cause erosion of tooth enamel especially seen on the insides of the teeth where the tongue meets the teeth. This erosion ultimately leads to severe decay and lays the groundwork for gum disease. Vitamin D and calcium deficiencies and hormonal imbalances can lead to decalcification of the teeth.

Heart Attack, Cardiac Arrest, Dysrhythmia, Angina (Chest Pain), and Irregular Heartbeat

Sudden heart attacks can cause permanent damage to the heart or death. A cardiac arrest is sudden death. Electrolyte imbalances such as potassium deficiency, extreme orthostatic hypotension, low blood pressure, slow heart rates, malnutrition, hormonal imbalances, high blood pressure, high cholesterol, and accumulations of fat deposits around the heart muscle can all be contributing factors which involve complications with the heart. All eating disorders have the potential for serious complications with the heart and even death.

Liver Disturbances and Failure

The liver is a very important organ of the body. It works to eliminate waste from cells and works in conjunction with your digestive system. Some patients attempt suicide through the use of acetaminophen, which causes in some cases extreme liver damage and can ultimately lead to death. Also the abuse of ipecac syrup also causes damage to the liver and it cannot be eliminated from the body. Severe malnutrition can also cause liver disease.

Infertility

This is a condition which leaves an individual unable to have children. In eating disorders it may be caused by the lack of menstrual cycle and other hormonal imbalances. Malnutrition and various vitamin deficiencies can also make it impossible to carry a child to full term. Additionally the lack of proper nutrition during pregnancy can lead to the birth of a baby with birth defects.

Problems during Pregnancy

Due to malnutrition, dehydration, vitamin and hormone deficiencies, pregnancies while actively involved in eating disorder behavior put the unborn child at high risk of chronic illness, still birth, and death.

Death

Ultimately eating disorders, which are very self-destructive in nature and can be viewed as slow attempts at suicide behavior, can lead to heart attacks, strokes, internal bleeding, gastric rupture, perforated ulcers, liver failure, kidney failure, pancreatitis, and suicide. Eating disorders have the highest fatality rate of all psychiatric disorders, with risk estimated at 5 to 20 percent.

Chapter 28

Medical Symptoms and Complications Associated with Anorexia

Any child who undereats is at risk for the conditions we will describe. The longer the undereating goes on, the more likely it is that it will turn into full-blown anorexia nervosa. We use the term "anorexic" here, recognizing that bulimics and binge eaters can also experience the same medical complications and symptoms from bouts of undereating.

Anorexia nervosa, in severe cases, can affect almost all the major organ systems. In this chapter, we will discuss the symptoms of anorexia, which we have organized by different functions and areas of the body.

Growth

In children, the effects of anorexia are particularly devastating because the child has not yet finished growing and maturing. Height, for instance, can be compromised in anorexic children. While most children are expected to be as tall or taller than their parents, children whose anorexia has become chronic will likely be shorter than would have been predicted without the illness.

Sexual Development

Anorexia can also delay sexual development. Anorexic girls may stop getting their menstrual periods, a change that gives rise to mixed

Excerpted from *The Parent's Guide to Eating Disorders*, by Marcia Herrin, EdD, MPH, RD, and Nancy Matsumoto (Gürze Books: Carlsbad, CA, 2007), © 2007 Gürze Books. Reprinted with permission.

feelings in most girls. At first, they are glad not to have to bother with a monthly cycle. They may have heard that athletic girls are likely not to have periods, so their condition seems even somewhat desirable. On this point, you can inform your child that doctors today believe that loss of menstrual periods among athletes is almost always the result of undereating, not overexercise, although it is true they need to eat more to meet their caloric needs.

Girls may also admire the way anorexia delays the development of hips and breasts, physical features they associate with being fat. Girls whose anorexia predates menarche (the beginning of menstruation), on the other hand, will usually not realize that their starvation has delayed its onset. By substantially delaying puberty and permanently interfering with height and breast development, anorexia at this young age has an even more detrimental effect on health and development than does anorexia in adolescents. One reason that children are thought to be at an increased medical risk from anorexia is that they naturally have smaller fat stores than do adolescents and so lose vital tissues more quickly with weight loss.

Boys and young men with anorexia may also experience delayed sexual development. The primary symptom of this is decreased levels of serum testosterone, a condition that can be determined by blood tests.

Gastrointestinal Symptoms

Anorexics may experience a variety of gastrointestinal symptoms, all of which are believed to be caused by malnutrition and underuse of the gastrointestinal tract. Chronic undereating actually causes the musculature of the small and large intestine, which churns and digests food, to atrophy. The anorexic may experience stomachaches and bloating as food sits in the stomach longer than usual. The constipation anorexics often suffer from is frequently confused with fullness, a feeling they use to rationalize not eating.

This delayed emptying of the stomach and the bloating that accompanies it can lead to yet another uncomfortable symptom, reflux. Slightly different from the "acid reflux" caused by eating too much spicy food that many over-the-counter medications claim to eliminate, this type of reflux causes food to rise up into the esophagus or sometimes even into the mouth, and can increase the likelihood of developing bulimia.

All of these problems normally reverse relatively quickly with weight gain.

Low Blood Pressure, Dizziness, Hypothermia, and Poor Concentration

Anorexics also often experience dizziness and low blood pressure, which can lead to fainting spells. Although Olivia's coach noticed she was thinner, he didn't suspect a problem until Olivia fainted two weeks in a row at soccer practice. Parents should be alert to complaints by their children of feeling faint; this is not a common occurrence in healthy children, but can be an early symptom of an eating disorder.

Fainting spells can show up even before the child has lost a significant amount of weight, and can be dangerous. Maggie, an accomplished young horsewoman, was lucky she was not seriously hurt when undereating led her to lose consciousness while atop her jumping horse. Maggie had a hard time believing that just skipping breakfast and lunch could result in passing out. She had only lost a few pounds that month and was still technically within a normal weight range.

Another frequently seen symptom, loss of too much of the body's essential fat stores, causes hypothermia, or low body temperature, which in turn will cause the anorexic child to feel cold when everyone else is comfortable, and require layers and layers of clothing to feel warm. The anorexic's surprisingly cold hands are another tip-off to a developing eating disorder. Other common symptoms are lethargy, apathy, and poor concentration. For reasons that are not well understood, most anorexics are able to concentrate on academic schoolwork, but may have difficulty following a simple conversation.

Natalie's parents were falsely reassured about some of the symptoms they were seeing because Natalie continued to get straight A's even as she struggled to remember what plans she had made for after-school transportation or to engage in a casual chat. Although she had clearly become more absentminded, it was hard for her parents to point to any clear sign of illness since all the changes were so gradual and subtle.

Adaptations to Starvation: Hair, Nails, Skin, and Muscle Changes

The anorexic's body adapts to starvation by focusing on maintaining the most essential major organ functions, while withholding nourishment from more superficial parts of the body, such as hair and nails. Brittle nails and extreme dryness of the skin caused by lack of protein and fat in the diet are common signs of anorexia, as well as loss of scalp, body, and even pubic hair.

Sarah's response to the realization that the thinning of her beautiful, flaxen hair was due to her weight loss was to break down into wrenching sobs. As superficial as it may seem, the loss of hair is often the only symptom anorexics worry about. I have seen a number of patients who were motivated to change their eating-disordered behavior solely for the sake of saving or restoring their hair. Because anorexics will often worry more about such minor symptoms than the more life-threatening aspects of the disorder, I often tell parents to explore what it is about the disorder that scares their child most, and to help them understand that improving their eating will help solve that problem.

With more extreme weight loss, patients may develop lanugo, a fine, downy body hair on their back, arms, and legs (and sometimes faces and necks) that is characteristic of the human fetus while it is still in the womb. On the bodies of anorexics, lanugo is thought to be a primitive attempt by the body to maintain body temperature, as this type of hair takes fewer calories to produce than normal hair. Anorexics may also experience bone pain when exercising, and despite the fact that they are exercising, muscle wasting. Muscle loss is particularly noticeable in the arms and legs, a change that at first thrills many anorexics.

Cardiac Symptoms

Although the following information may be frightening to you as parents, it is important to remember that the body is capable of making a remarkable recovery once food intake is improved and eating-disordered behaviors are discontinued. Because cardiac symptoms are among the most serious complications associated with eating disorders, however, it is important to be able to recognize them if and when they occur in your child. Early signs that anorexia may be affecting the heart are fatigue, lightheadedness (feeling dizzy upon standing or sitting up from a sitting or prone position), or cold, bluish, splotchy hands and feet. More serious symptoms, which warrant calling your doctor immediately, include slowed or irregular heartbeat, shortness of breath, chest pain, leg pain, and rapid breathing.

Heart palpitations (the subjective awareness of one's own irregular heartbeat) and chest pains are often experienced at night in bed, causing anorexics to fear they may be dying. Often these symptoms go hand-in-hand with bradycardia (slow heart rate indicated by a slow pulse) and low blood pressure. Although bradycardia is quickly resolved by adequate nutrition, unless it is rectified it can, in the most serious cases, put the anorexic at risk for congestive heart failure. An electrocardiogram (EKG) can confirm slowed heart rate and/or arrhythmias. Because the malnutrition of anorexia can reduce the size of the heart to a dangerous degree, chest x-rays are used to detect changes in heart size.

Some patients, keenly aware of their slow heart rate, become obsessed with measuring it. Heather was sure, as she counted heartbeats per minute as she lay in bed at night, that her heart had stopped between beats. Amy, noticing the same phenomenon, became hysterical and had her parents call an ambulance to take her to the emergency room.

Victoria told me that as scary as some of these physical signs are, she found them oddly reassuring. In her case, constantly feeling cold, having a slowed heart rate, and even brittle nails and hair all meant she could not be eating too much.

In rare cases, anorexics experience edema, or fluid retention, in their abdomen or legs, especially when they have entered a period of weight gain after sudden refeeding or have stopped abusing laxatives or diuretics. Edema is an early sign that the heart is not functioning well enough to handle the increases in fluid that naturally result when weight is gained or laxatives and diuretics are discontinued. If your child does experience such edema, close monitoring by your doctor can ensure that your child is not in acute danger. Again, while this symptom and others we describe are potentially dangerous, good, close medical supervision and a wholehearted effort to reverse the disorder is the approach that will get your child out of medical danger most quickly and safely.

As the anorexic body wastes away, so does the heart. Some researchers have noted that even a week or two of severe dieting can lead to substantial loss of heart muscle.

One example of a rare cardiac complication associated with severe anorexia is mitral valve prolapse. This type of heart-valve prolapse occurs because although the malnourished heart muscle shrinks, the valves inside the heart chamber do not. The result is a set of misshapen valves that do not close properly. The faulty valves cause blood to leak back into the heart chamber, which in turn causes palpitations and chest pain. Although mitral valve prolapse is a potentially fatal condition, it appears to be reversible with weight gain.

In the most extreme cases of anorexia, the cumulative effects of long-term starvation (an irregular heartbeat, edema, bradycardia, to name a few possible contributing factors) can cause sudden heart failure. Malnutrition has caused the heart to shrink, resulting in decreased cardiac output and low blood pressure. Finally, the heart simply gives out.

Most often, this type of sudden death occurs while the anorexic is asleep. Such is the insidious nature of anorexia; a disease in which slow starvation can coexist with such a surprising degree of functional well-being that sometimes an autopsy will show no obvious heart problems. The thought of chronic anorexia leading to sudden death is an extremely frightening one, but this tragedy does occasionally happen. Those most at risk are severe anorexics who have suffered a long period of extreme emaciation. By intervening early, you can be assured that you are protecting your child from this, the most devastating consequence of an eating disorder.

Bone Problems

Osteopenia (reduced bone density) and later, osteoporosis (extremely serious bone loss), are among the most common and serious medical complications of anorexia. Osteopenia occurs early in anorexia and makes it unlikely that an adolescent will be able to accumulate normal amounts of bone mass. As the anorexic girl or boy matures, the risk that the low bone mass of osteopenia will progress to osteoporosis increases.

Anorexic women as young as in their late teens have been diagnosed with osteoporosis. Their bone loss is the direct result of both hormonal changes and malnutrition. Extreme weight loss renders the anorexic's emaciated body unable to produce the female hormone estrogen, which normally keeps the body's bones strong and healthy. A sure sign of dangerously low estrogen is the loss of menses. Nutritionally, extreme weight loss diets are usually low in protein and calcium, among other nutrients. As a rule, these deficiencies also contribute to bone loss, although some anorexics manage to consume adequate amounts of protein and calcium and still have serious bone loss. Another crucial nutrient is dietary fat. Too little fat affects the body's ability to make estrogen and absorb vitamin D, without both of which calcium absorption is seriously compromised. The result of these anorexia-driven changes is brittle bones that can fracture or break easily.

Unremitting weight loss is associated with continued decreases in bone density. The good news is that once an adolescent anorexic reaches a healthy weight, bone density improves, and the body builds even more bone with the return of menses. Yet most patients never fully restore their bone mass and are more likely than the average person to face bone problems in the future.

It is important to remember that simply getting periods back is not always enough to begin rebuilding bone; full weight restoration must occur before that happens. We stress this point because some medical doctors still mistakenly believe that getting periods back is enough to protect bones. It is not uncommon for some girls to resume menses at a lower-than-healthy weight. (For older teens healthy weight is defined as having a body mass index [BMI] of 20; for younger girls a BMI that is on a normal growth curve is considered to be healthy.) These anorexics may continue losing bone until they reach a healthy weight. Recent research, in fact, points to body weight as the most important determinant of bone density.

Some girls believe they are beginning to rebuild bone after being prescribed replacement hormones (estrogen, progesterone, or oral contraceptives). In fact, however, often they are not. Researchers are still trying to tease out why this is so, but it is likely that to be fully effective, hormones must interact with a constellation of nutrients (calcium and phosphorous are just a few of those).

Unfortunately, the underweight anorexic often cannot supply enough of these nutrients to spark the complex interactions necessary for bone formation. Adolescent anorexia is particularly devastating because adolescence is a time when children should be building bone to last a lifetime, not losing it. Ninety percent of a person's bone mass is accrued by the time he or she turns twenty. For this reason, any disruption in hormone levels should be taken seriously.

Researchers have also found that anorexic adolescent patients lose more bone than adults with anorexia. Anorexics of any age are at risk for bone fractures. Usually, fractures will occur as the person ages or engages in high-impact exercises such as running on hard pavement.

Testing Bone Density

A bone density test commonly known as a "DEXA" (dual-energy x-ray absorptiometry) is the state-of-the art method for measuring bone mineral density. For anorexic adolescents whose disorder is a longstanding problem, and includes amenorrhea for six months or more, having your doctor order a DEXA (also known as a densitometry) can sometimes be helpful in breaking through the anorexic's denial that her eating behaviors are having an effect on her health.

After two years of maintaining a below-normal weight, first-year graduate student Selena finally agreed to have a DEXA. Her results came back comparing her bones to those of someone four times her age. "But I feel fine!" was her first response. Over the course of time, she was able to motivate herself to gain some much-needed weight by focusing on doing everything she could to protect her bones from more damage.

As with Selena, bone density tests are compared to a statistical norm, and do not measure actual bone loss unless they are repeated periodically. Only by doing a baseline test and then repeating it six months or a year later will you be able to tell if your child's bone density has improved or deteriorated.

Because it can take six months to a year of amenorrhea and restricted eating before any measurable bone loss occurs, DEXAs are not usually advised unless the anorexic has a long-term eating disorder. Many experts recommend a bone density test on anorexics whose amenorrhea lasts longer than six months.

For anorexics who fit this description, the test can be quite helpful and is offered by most major hospitals at a cost of $250 to $450. The test is relatively safe; the exposure to radiation is one-tenth of that of a chest x-ray.

Recovering Bone Density

Most experts believe that once it is lost, bone density cannot be improved without weight gain. Even with weight gain, only partial recovery of bone density is likely. As we have mentioned, supplemental hormones are not particularly effective in helping the anorexic rebuild bone, probably because the anorexic lacks all the nutrients necessary to interact effectively with these hormones. Estrogen supplements, in particular, also pose the problem of inducing periods in patients. The latest research indicates that supplemental estrogen, which in the past was routinely prescribed for anorexics (usually in the form of birth control pills) to improve bone health, is of little help. Estrogen also induces periods in patients whose self-starvation has caused amenorrhea, making it impossible for doctors to tell whether an eating-disordered patient has gained enough weight to protect her bones. For both these reasons, many physicians no longer prescribe estrogen to anorexics.

Relatively high intakes of calcium and vitamin D are usually recommended for the anorexic, even though research indicates that she cannot make use of these nutrients to build bone until she has returned to a healthy weight and has resumed menses. Standard advice for anorexics is to take 1,500 mg per day of calcium (healthy teens need 1,300 mg per day). Vitamin D is recommended at a dose of 400 IU per day; this is twice the usual recommended intake. There is no benefit to higher doses of calcium and vitamin D, and in fact large doses stress the body and interfere with the absorption of other nutrients.

Osteoporosis medications such as Fosamax® show some promise in helping restore bones in anorexic patients. Although these drugs are currently being tested for anorexics, they are not yet routinely pre-scribed for them. Only weight gain, and the better nutrition it requires, can reliably improve the bone density of eating-disorder sufferers. Your goal as parents of an anorexic child should be to improve nutrition and restore weight as quickly as possible.

Fertility Issues

Researchers have still not determined to what extent a bout of anorexia during childhood or adolescence will have on future fertil-ity. Although ample research has shown that adult anorexia, if not reversed, is likely to lead to infertility, there are numerous reports of severely low-weight, even chronic, anorexics becoming pregnant.

Because of these contradictory data, little is gained by telling young anorexics (who often worry that they might not be able to have chil-dren) that they will face infertility as adults. Instead, they should be assured that if their disorder is treated and resolved, they can expect to bear children if they want to.

My patient Nellie was not assured of this, but instead was told by a school nurse that she was ruining her chance of ever having a fam-ily, thanks to her eating disorder. In response, Nellie's eating became even more self-destructive. When we discussed the issue, she told me, "If I can't have kids, I might as well be really thin."

Handled sensitively, however, the question of an eating disorder's effect on future fertility can sometimes be used as motivation to turn around the disorder.

Angela has suffered from anorexia for all of her teenage years, and as a result, has never had a period. Now, as a senior in high school, she is acutely aware that she eventually wants children, but she wor-ries that her disorder may affect her chances of doing so. She and I are focusing on the natural desire that someday she will have healthy children to help her get motivated to increase her weight.

Another fact that can be used as motivation to end a course of an-orexia before a teenager reaches adulthood is that there is evidence of higher rates of premature and low–birth weight births among babies born to mothers with a long history of anorexia.

It is important to guard against giving a sexually active anorexic teen the impression that her present condition, including lack of periods, is a guarantee that she will not get pregnant. Even amenorrheic girls with anorexia can become pregnant if they do not practice birth control. Despite the lack of periods, the bodies of these girls will occasionally and unpredictably create a hormonal environment that allows pregnancy.

Blood Values

The most common blood work findings are leukopenia (low white blood cell count) and mild anemia (low iron count), and, in rare cases, thrombocytopenia (low platelet count).

Usually, when lab tests reveal these abnormal blood values, the anorexic feels no symptoms. Yet almost immediately upon resumption of adequate food intake, and even before she necessarily begins gaining weight, she feels noticeably warmer, much more energetic, and exhibits improved skin color. Tonya was thrilled to have me feel how warm her hands had become since she started improving her diet. Warm hands are a good sign your child is moving in the right direction.

As an anorexic's condition worsens, her daily life is more likely to be affected by these hematologic changes and the cardiac symptoms we have described. She will most likely notice fatigue, weakness, dizziness, and the inability to exercise at former levels. Jill was a dancer who also liked to jog and play tennis. As her anorexia worsened, she increased her exercise in an attempt to burn off more and more calories and fat. She recognized how serious her problem was when eventually she didn't want to go to dance class, turned down offers to play Frisbee, and had to walk instead of run her usual jogging route.

I notice regularly the difficulty my anorexic patients have with even mild exercise. My former Dartmouth College office was on the third floor of a turn-of-the-century building. Though my anorexic patients usually declined to use the elevator, those formerly athletic girls were exhausted and out of breath after climbing three flights of stairs.

I remember my patient Jill who was delighted when her nutrition and weight recovery allowed her to climb those stairs with ease. Soon she was back to a fairly rigorous, but not excessive, exercise schedule of no more than an hour a day.

As in Jill's case, the changes in blood values and cardiac function that we have described are secondary to malnutrition, and improve almost immediately with better nutrition and weight gain.

Parents should also be aware, however, that even in severe cases of anorexia, blood values can be normal and cannot, therefore, be used as a proof of adequate nutrition. Sometimes lab values improve before your child has reached a safe, healthy weight. This is often confusing to parents whose eating-disordered child may point to improved lab findings as proof that they need not continue to gain weight. I remind parents that though their child looks and reports feeling energetic, if she remains too thin, she is still not cured and remains at risk for anorexia-related health problems. This can be a difficult juncture for some parents because their child seems to have regained her health while remaining "fashionably" thin. Your child's pediatrician or your family doctor can help you assess whether your child is at a truly healthy weight.

Fluid and Cholesterol Imbalances

Anorexics are often dehydrated from restricting their fluid intake, undereating, and sometimes misusing diuretics, all of which are reflected in an elevated blood urea nitrogen (BUN) reading.

Although anorexics usually have low cholesterol levels, abnormally high levels are not uncommon. Some researchers suspect these abnormally high cholesterol levels are related to the effects of starvation on the liver. Without adequate nutrition, the liver, which both makes and metabolizes cholesterol, is unable to break down cholesterol properly. High cholesterol levels are also thought to be caused by starvation-induced abnormalities in estrogen, thyroid, and other hormones.

Whatever the cause, high cholesterol is most likely to occur in acute anorexia, and is much more common in children and adolescents with anorexia than in adult patients.

High cholesterol associated with anorexia usually disappears either with weight restoration or over many years of chronic anorexia. Also important to this problem is that anorexics should not be treated for high cholesterol levels with standard low-fat and low-calorie diets, an approach that would only worsen the patient's malnutrition and likely raise her cholesterol levels even higher. Like other findings associated with anorexia, as the patient recovers, abnormally high cholesterol levels, along with the abnormal liver function tests that often accompany them, return to normal.

If your very thin child is found to have high cholesterol, anorexia is a likely cause, particularly if previous tests have found cholesterol to be normal and there is no family history of high cholesterol. You should be careful how this information is passed on to your child since it may trigger even more stringent restrictions. It is helpful to tell your child that the heart problems anorexics face are unlike the kinds of heart problems some adults have; malnutrition can dangerously shrink and weaken her heart, but she is certainly not suffering from the hardening of the arteries some adults develop on long-term, high-fat diets.

Instead of reducing dietary fat to lower cholesterol as an adult might be advised, the anorexic child needs to increase fat intake and actually reduce consumption of fruits and vegetables (which fill their stomachs and make it difficult to eat anything else) to achieve a lower cholesterol level.

One of my patients, Allison, was told by her psychiatrist, "I think you should know that your cholesterol is above normal." Allison, whom I was treating for severe anorexia, immediately removed the little bit of fat that remained in her diet and proceeded to lose more weight, ever more certain that this was the healthy thing to do. I had to inform Allison, her doctor, and her parents about the anorexia and cholesterol connection and reassure them that fat was not only okay, it was necessary to add it to her diet before she could start to make progress. Allison has made a hard-won recovery and is now in graduate school.

Nutrient Imbalances

Low levels of magnesium, zinc, and phosphate are sometimes found among malnourished anorexics. Low levels of magnesium contribute to osteoporosis and can sometimes lead to cardiac arrhythmias, and low phosphate can contribute to weakness and fatigue. One of the unfortunate consequences of low zinc is a decrease in taste sensitivity. Anorexics often complain that food just does not have any taste to them, which further reinforces their unwillingness to eat. Though the anorexic may be losing calcium from her bones, calcium blood levels are usually normal. The anorexic who purges is at an even higher risk for potassium problems than a bulimic.

The elevated serum carotene levels, or hypercarotenemia, found in many anorexics often results in a yellowish cast to the patient's skin. This is thought to be a consequence of the malnourished liver's inability to metabolize vegetable pigments.

Hormonal Imbalances

Anorexia affects the body's hormonal balance in profound ways. Some hormone levels are lowered while others are elevated. Hormones are necessary for the development of healthy bones, growth, and the onset of puberty and maintaining a healthy energy level and mood. Hormones responsible for adolescent sexual maturation—estrogen in girls, testosterone in boys, and luteinizing hormone (LH) and follicle-stimulating hormone (FSH) in both girls and boys—tend to be lowered in anorexics. These neuroendocrine findings show how hormonally the anorexic adolescent regresses to the level of a prepubescent girl or boy.

Cassie was graduating from high school, yet she had never had a period. Her anorexia began just as she was about to go through puberty, and she had only recently sought treatment for it. Because the anorexia had prevented normal maturation, her body looked like that of a young girl's—she was barely five feet tall and showed very little breast development. Her doctors were worried about the health of her bones and her ability to have children.

Thyroid function tests are occasionally abnormal in anorexics, a finding that confirms researchers' observations that starvation sets the body's basal, or resting, metabolism at a lower level to conserve energy. Lowered thyroid hormone levels, like slowed heart rate, cold intolerance, dry skin, and constipation, are part of the body's effort to keep functioning even as it is vastly undernourished.

The malnutrition of anorexia can cause metabolic changes that may be picked up on standard thyroid function tests. These lab findings are sometimes misinterpreted as a condition known as euthyroid sick syndrome, when actually the changes are due to starvation. The thyroid hormone treatment usually prescribed for euthyroid sick syndrome will not correct an anorexic's abnormally functioning thyroid—only weight restoration will. Hormone replacement, in fact, may cause further weight loss because it raises the metabolism. Another reason not to give anorexics thyroid hormones is that they are known to abuse them in an effort to lose even more weight.

Brain Abnormalities

Anorexic patients sometimes suffer impairments in their ability to think clearly, known as "cognitive deficits." Examples of these deficits include attention/concentration difficulties, impaired automatic processing, difficulty problem solving, inflexibility, poor planning, and lack of insight.

These characteristics account in part for the difficulty of treating entrenched anorexia. Erin, thirteen, had a vacant, spacey look and difficulty carrying on a coherent conversation. She seemed unable to summon the energy even to project her voice, which made her responses to my questions bare whispers. Many of my patients are extremely bright, and Erin was no exception. So it was surprising that she could not remember simple statements made just minutes before in our sessions. Erin seemed immobilized by her eating disorder, unable to make use of any of the strategies that I or her therapist suggested. She remained focused on only one thing: not eating. She refused to let her parents watch her eat and drank so much diet soda that her doctor was worried she was washing critical electrolytes (minerals essential to maintaining the body's water and pH balance) from her body. Erin also had a harder time being honest than most of my patients. After several sessions, she confessed that she had been flushing her meals down the toilet.

The inflexibility of the anorexic is often striking to parents. Their formerly easygoing child now has to have everything just so, and flies into a rage if minor things don't go right.

Kelsey's mother was being run ragged by her increasingly persnickety daughter. Kelsey complained and obsessed about everything from her clothes and the noise level in the house, to, of course, the food that her mother made and served. Kelsey's mom also noticed how her daughter fell apart if plans had to be unexpectedly changed. All of these were things she used to handle with ease before she lost weight. Now Kelsey, who once had time to help her younger siblings in the morning, has trouble just getting herself ready for school.

In severe cases of anorexia, brain changes can place patients in danger of harming themselves, although self-harming behaviors such as cutting or burning are more common among bulimic patients. Sometimes self-harm is unrelated to brain changes, and can even precipitate anorexia or bulimia. Children engaged in these kinds of behaviors should be monitored closely by a physician or psychologist.

My patient Elizabeth, at twelve years old, weighed only sixty pounds. During our first session, she staged a tantrum, locked herself in the restroom, and would not come out, despite the pleading of her mother. Finally, we had to call a security guard to get her out of the restroom. Elizabeth's condition had made tantrums like this a common behavior of hers. Her parents had to lock up all toxic cleaning supplies because Elizabeth regularly felt suicidal enough to drink them.

Most experts believe that cognitive impairments such as those of Erin, Kelsey, and Elizabeth are related to metabolic and endocrine abnormalities associated with malnutrition, and that they improve with refeeding and weight gain. These patients may also be suffering from obsessive-compulsive or other psychiatric disorders that the emotional stress of the eating disorder has brought to the fore. If the types of problems we describe in these three cases do not begin to resolve with weight gain, you should see that your child gets a psychological evaluation; your child may benefit from counseling and/or medication.

Suicide in both anorexia and bulimia is a major cause of death. Chronic eating disorders, obsessive-compulsive disorder symptoms, drug abuse, and major depression all increase the risk for suicide or attempted suicide.

It is also possible, however, that some of these cognitive deficits may be connected to the structural changes in the brains of anorexics that have been detected by researchers in recent years, although there is as yet no clear scientific proof of this link.

Critical Areas

The need for swift and aggressive treatment of an eating disorder is underscored by two areas in which the damage may not be completely reversible: bone mass changes and brain abnormalities. Though there is some recovery in these areas with weight gain, recent research casts doubt on any guarantee of a full recovery. Bone loss due to anorexia can occur in as little as six months and even bouts of anorexia as brief as three months have been associated with brain changes. These findings on bone mass changes and brain abnormalities make early recognition and aggressive treatment essential for young people.

Refeeding Complications

The relatively brief but dangerous period when an anorexic first begins to eat or be fed again is known as "refeeding." Before we go further, we want to stress that only severely malnourished and underweight anorexics who are refed rapidly are at risk for the refeeding problems we describe. Our hope is that your child's eating disorders will be turned around well before any of these complications become an issue. We discuss them here largely because they illustrate how dangerous anorexia can become.

Because rapid refeeding is almost impossible to achieve without tube feeding (liquid meals fed through a tube, which runs through the nose and into the stomach) or total parenteral nutrition (TPN; that is, liquid nutrition given directly into a large vein), refeeding complications are generally only seen in the hospital settings where tube feeding or TPN are administered to save a severely emaciated anorexic's life.

Tube feeding, moreover, which was once routinely used to treat anorexia, and TPN (a more medically complicated method of refeeding) are now rarely used for eating-disordered patients, and instead are reserved for life-threatening cases of chronic food refusal. Today, treatment is more focused on getting the anorexic to choose to eat, not simply ensuring she is receiving adequate nutrition.

In the rare instances when refeeding complications do occur, they can lead to severe myocardial dysfunction (heart muscle problems) and sometimes seizures. The severely malnourished heart, weakened and reduced in size, can also have difficulty managing the sudden increase in blood flow caused by refeeding. Although the health of the heart quickly improves with adequate nutrition, if refeeding is done too quickly, the heart can fail.

Refeeding can also result in acute dilation of the stomach, characterized by the sudden onset of abdominal pain, nausea, vomiting, and persistent abdominal distention. Often this phenomenon can be treated by inserting a nasogastric tube, which allows the removal of foods and fluids. In extremely rare cases, surgical intervention is called for to prevent a rupture of the stomach, which is nearly always fatal.

Anorexia in the refeeding stages has also been associated with acute pancreatitis.

Are Your Child's Lab Findings Too Good to Be True?

Often, the need for such aggressive treatment is masked initially by the time it takes for lab findings to reflect serious consequences of anorexia. The lowered metabolic rate of anorexics that we have described is thought to be one reason that laboratory assessments of anorexics, despite the fact that they are starving, often will appear normal in many respects. It is important, however, that you as parents not be lulled into thinking your child is fine because the lab tests are normal. Laboratory values may be okay for quite some time and then suddenly take a dramatic turn for the worse. Children and teens with anorexia should have regular medical monitoring (routine screening blood tests, measures of heart rate and blood pressure) because, as we have said, anorexia can cause physical complications in every organ system in the body.

Medical Monitoring vs. Full Workups

Regular medical monitoring should not be confused with excessive medical tests, which aim to find a medical reason to explain the eating-disordered child's symptoms. Ongoing medical monitoring alerts parents and professionals to serious impending problems. It is most important when the anorexic is not making at least slow, steady progress or is gaining too quickly and might be at risk for the refeeding complications we discussed.

Chapter 29

Symptoms and Complications of Binge Eating Disorder and Bulimia

Chapter Contents

287

Section 29.1

Complications Associated with Binge Eating Disorder

The problems associated with binge eating are related to obesity. Since people consume so many calories in a short period of time, and generally do not burn them off, they tend to put on a lot of weight. Obesity is one of the biggest health problems in this country. As many as three hundred thousand people die from the complications of obesity annually.

Common problems of the obese and overweight include:

- certain types of cancers;

- diabetes;

- gallbladder disease;

- heart disease;

- high blood pressure or hypertension;

- high cholesterol levels.

People with binge eating disorder are also more subject to some psychiatric illnesses. They have been found to have higher risk of the following illnesses:

- anxiety;

- panic disorder;

- personality disorders;

- major depression;

- alcoholism;

- drug abuse.

There are societal issues and social prejudice which work against people with obesity. For example, some jobs have weight limits, thus keeping out people with weight problems. Airlines and buses have seats which are "one size fits all."

There are also economic drawbacks to being obese or overweight. People need to buy special clothes, or even shop in different stores, and the clothing is more expensive. Some people need to purchase first-class seats on airlines to be comfortable. Some people need to purchase specially made furniture for their homes or offices. Health-care costs are more expensive. Purchasing life, health, and disability insurance is more expensive because overweight people are considered greater risks.

One of the criteria for people with binge eating disorder is for them to feel remorseful or embarrassed over their behavior. In addition, we live in a society where "thin is in," so the results of years of binge eating can cause a person with binge eating disorder to isolate herself from the rest of family and friends. The emotional distress over the behavior causes people with binge eating disorder to hide their behavior. It is very rare for an individual to seek help for her eating behavior, despite the emotional pain that it causes her.

Section 29.2

Medical Symptoms and Complications Associated with Bulimia

Excerpted from *The Parent's Guide to Eating Disorders*, by Marcia Herrin, EdD, MPH, RD, and Nancy Matsumoto (Gürze Books: Carlsbad, CA, 2007). © 2007 Gürze Books. Reprinted with permission.

Many of the symptoms of bulimia and anorexia overlap, especially among anorexics who purge. For ease of reading, we have separated the symptoms of bulimia from those of anorexia. But readers should understand that the following symptoms and lab findings described for bulimics also apply to purging anorexics. Extremely low-weight patients are more likely to experience the most dire consequences outlined here than those whose weight remains within a normal range.

Electrolyte and Mineral Imbalances

As we have said, in many ways the physiology of eating disorders is still a mystery to experts. Electrolyte imbalances, which can be detected by blood tests, are a case in point. Electrolyte imbalances are common among bulimics, since vomiting can cause them to lose valuable minerals. Yet for unknown reasons, not all bulimics develop these imbalances.

Electrolyte disturbances, most often in the form of severely low potassium levels, can cause a wide range of symptoms ranging from muscle weakness (bulimic patients may notice that they feel weak and tired), constipation, cloudy thinking, and, in severe cases, cardiac arrhythmias that can cause sudden death. Often, however, eating-disorder patients report feeling fine, despite dangerously low potassium levels, and exhibit a sense of well-being that can be misleading.

In cases of dangerously low potassium levels, oral supplements or intravenous solutions are often prescribed to protect heart function, although these measures are short-term fixes that cannot solve the problems caused by repeated purging. Although over-the-counter potassium supplements are available, we urge you not to attempt independently to correct your child's potassium imbalance because supplemental potassium can easily reach toxic levels. Restoring potassium levels must be undertaken under the supervision of a medical professional who can do frequent lab tests. If potassium is not restored properly, the patient is at a high risk for potentially fatal heart problems. One practical solution available to you at home is to encourage your child to eat potassium-rich foods. Almost all foods contain some potassium; fruits and vegetables are particularly good sources. Just helping your child to stop purging and to begin to eat a normal array of foods in normal amounts will go a long way in maintaining healthy potassium levels.

Even when potassium levels are normal, however, you cannot assume that a child is not purging. Many patients manage to maintain normal potassium levels despite significant purging. If, however, potassium is low and there is no other medical explanation, it is almost certain that the patient is either vomiting or abusing laxatives or diuretics.

Purging also throws the body's acid-base balance off-kilter, which is reflected in another type of electrolyte disturbance, elevated bicarbonate levels in the blood. These laboratory values of low potassium and elevated bicarbonate levels could, to the unsuspecting or inexperienced doctor, incorrectly indicate a kidney problem, not surreptitious vomiting.

Although elevated serum bicarbonate is not as serious as the low potassium that can accompany purging behaviors, it is something that can be tested for, and is a much more reliable marker than potassium for purging behaviors. For this reason, some doctors order a serum bicarbonate test when they suspect purging, even though potassium levels are normal.

The important point to remember about purging is that lab and physical changes and serious medical problems are more likely to occur when a child or adolescent is at a very low weight. The normal or overweight child is protected to a certain extent simply because their bodies are healthier and stronger than the malnourished anorexic's.

Glandular Abnormalities

Sometimes the salivary glands, located below the ear and along the lower jawbone, may become visibly swollen, leading to the "chipmunk" cheeks of the bulimic. Parents may recognize this look since these parotid glands are those that are affected by mumps. The exact cause of this symptom is somewhat of a mystery. One theory is that the glands become irritated by regurgitated stomach acid that leaks through a duct in the throat. Another is that they are overstimulated to produce enzymes to digest binged foods. It is likely that both theories are true.

291

The swollen parotid glands of bulimics may secrete abnormally high levels of amylase, an enzyme that digests carbohydrates. Elevated amylase levels, however, may also indicate a problem with the pancreas, such as pancreatitis or pancreatic gallstones. Blood tests can determine whether the high blood levels are from the salivary glands or the pancreas. Although it is rare, acute pancreatitis has been reported in connection with bulimia as well as in anorexia in the refeeding stage.

Dental Problems

Repeated vomiting among bulimics and purging anorexics will inevitably lead to serious dental problems. An increase in cavities or extreme sensitivity of the teeth to heat and cold are often the first dental complications. The teeth may become chipped and ragged looking (especially if a spoon is used to induce vomiting) and the front teeth can lose their natural shine as the enamel, battered by repeated exposure to gastric acid, softens. The lingual, or backside of the front teeth, which faces the tongue, and the occlusal, or the flat top of molars, also lose their enamel and begin to take on a yellowish hue. As the enamel becomes thinner and thinner, you can see through it to the dentin, or core of the tooth. In severe cases, even the dentin is eroded as well, and the pulp of the tooth is exposed. This is extremely painful, and the tooth usually dies as a result.

The gums of bulimics are often sore and may even bleed, usually the result of "toothbrush trauma." In their efforts to clean their teeth and mouths after vomiting, bulimics will often brush their teeth vigorously immediately after purging, adding significantly to existing dental damage. Some bulimics have such naturally resilient teeth that despite significant purging, it takes longer than usual for damage to occur. At first, my patient Kerrie told me how odd it made her feel to hear her dentist compliment her on her wonderful teeth and their apparent health. She and I knew that she was throwing up regularly, yet even her own dentist saw no dental signs of bulimia. A good report from your child's dentist doesn't necessarily mean that your child is not purging.

In bulimics who have been vomiting for about four years or longer, dental fillings, which are more resistant to the effects of gastric acid than dental enamel, are likely to project above the surface of the teeth as the enamel around them erodes. Dental cavities may increase, probably because of the exposure to sugary binge food combined with the softening effect vomiting has on tooth enamel.

If you suspect your child has an eating disorder, you should alert your child's dentist at the earliest opportunity. The dentist can look for any telltale signs of purging, and if such signs are present, can discuss preventive measures available to protect the teeth. Protective measures include using a fluoride or a baking soda rinse, or rinsing with water after purging rather than brushing (which can damage teeth softened by stomach acid). Your child can also minimize erosion of their dental enamel by avoiding acidic foods, such as citrus fruits or juices and even diet or regular colas.

If your child is having difficulty giving up purging, talk to your dentist about the possibility of dental sealants to protect her teeth from stomach acids. Sealants, which were developed to protect the teeth of children prone to cavities, are clear coatings that dentists bond into the grooves of teeth that are particularly subject to decay. While sealants clearly are protective, some dentists are reluctant to use them as they may reduce the bulimic's incentive to recover. Another problem is that sealants are difficult to apply well on the teeth that need them the most. If they are poorly applied, they can make dental hygiene more difficult for the patient.

An alternative to sealants that dentists prefer to use is custom-made, fluoride-filled dental trays (similar to mouth guards or the cosmetic teeth-whitening trays now used by dentists) that actually protect the teeth from direct contact with purged stomach fluids and improve the resistance of the enamel to acid dissolution.

Another advantage of enlisting your dentist in your cause is that your child may be more willing to listen to him or her talk about the high risk of future dental problems than you. Hearing from a dental authority that the appearance and health of their teeth may be permanently affected by purging can have quite a positive impact on the child who is just starting to experiment with purging.

Throat and Esophageal Problems

Chronic, self-induced vomiting leads to a number of problems that result from the sensitive tissues of the throat coming in contact with harsh stomach acid. Swallowing may become painful or difficult. Hoarseness and a chronic sore throat are common.

Bulimics who frequently self-induce vomiting will experience a diminished gag reflex. Because of this, or because in some cases bulimics are not able to "learn" to throw up easily, they may resort to forcefully stimulating their throats to induce vomiting. They may use elongated objects to do this. I have even had two patients who after accidentally swallowing either a toothbrush or a spoon have had to have the "instrument" surgically removed. Behaviors such as this can sometimes lead to injuries to the surfaces of the back of the throat, which can in turn become infected.

Libby, a college student, told me how embarrassed and scared she was to tell her roommate that she needed to go to the emergency room because she had swallowed her toothbrush. Once there, she was chagrined to overhear a doctor asking a group of interns if they could identify the object in her x-rays. None of them could; they had never heard of bulimics going to such lengths to purge.

Bulimics run the added risk of rare but potentially fatal complications such as tears in the esophagus from frequent vomiting. Tears are indicated when there is blood in the vomit. Although it is only in rare cases that the presence of blood indicates a life-threatening esophageal rupture or a tear serious enough to require immediate medical attention, any blood in the vomit should be taken seriously, and the child should be seen promptly by a medical professional. At the very least, the presence of blood in the vomit indicates significant purging.

Most bulimics find the presence of blood disturbing, something of a wakeup call telling them of the seriousness of their situation. Parents can use this opportunity to open a dialogue about the gravity of future problems if the bulimia is not addressed. Marta was sure she was dying when she first noticed traces of blood in the toilet bowl after she had vomited. Her parents made sure she was evaluated by a physician known for her work with eating-disordered patients.

Seeing a doctor with a special expertise in eating disorders is valuable in many different ways. When another of my patients, Bess, noticed blood in her vomit, her family doctor minimized the blood by saying, "It just looks like a lot of blood because it is diluted in water," and noted that Bess had only microscopic abrasions in her throat that were nothing to worry about. Though this is often true in such situations, this physician missed a golden opportunity to get her to see the seriousness of her eating disorder.

Hand and Eye Problems

Bulimics who vomit by manually stimulating the gag reflex may develop calluses or scars on the backs of the fingers and across their knuckles from repeated contact with the teeth. Here again, experienced doctors will recognize these marks as "Russell sign," named after the researcher, Gerald Russell, who first described it in 1979.

Eight months after she stopped purging, Sophie told me that one of the best things about her recovery was that she no longer had to make sure to keep her hands out of view. While she was bulimic, Sophie worried that eventually someone would figure out she was bulimic from how red and inflamed the backs of her hands had become.

Vomiting, and the increased pressure on the eyes that it causes, is the likely source of burst blood vessels in the eyes of bulimics and purging anorexics. Known as conjunctival hemorrhages, this reddening of the eye is usually transient; and although scary-looking, it is not dangerous. As with esophageal tears, such hemorrhages can present an opportunity for you to discuss the disorder with your child, sometimes even providing the excuse your child has been looking for to accept help from you.

One of my patients suffered another more serious consequence from forcible vomiting: a retinal detachment, which required laser surgery to repair.

Another eye-area symptom is petechiae. These small red dots are caused by minute amounts of blood that escape into the skin around the eyes when vomiting is forcefully induced.

Lucy's reddened eyes were the first clue her parents had that she was engaged in self-induced vomiting. They knew that she was anorexic, but Lucy told me she was a master at hiding the evidence of her purging and had successfully kept that part of her disorder a secret. Then her mother confronted her about her hemorrhages and wondered "out loud" if Lucy could possibly be vomiting. Lucy confessed immediately, relieved she could finally allow her parents to help her with her purging habit.

Gastrointestinal Problems

Vomiting or chronic abuse of laxatives can result in gastrointestinal bleeding. Persistent vomiting can also cause the problem of spontaneous regurgitation, or reflux. Frequent purging causes the lower esophagus to relax, making it easy for the contents of the stomach to rise up into the throat or even into the mouth. When the bulimic leans over after eating, or burps, for example, sometimes for no apparent reason, she will spontaneously vomit.

Many bulimics experience this reflux as extreme heartburn. The esophagus becomes inflamed, which can, in serious chronic cases, progress to precancerous changes in the esophagus.

Another complication that requires immediate attention is gastric rupture, which occurs when the stomach becomes so full it literally bursts. Sometimes an extremely large binge cannot be purged because it changes the pressure in the gut, making it impossible to vomit. Lisa had to be rushed to the emergency room one weekend after bingeing on a big bowl of chocolate chip cookie dough. The dough expanded in her stomach, causing it to rupture.

Bowel Problems

Bulimics who chronically abuse laxatives may become dependent on them to stimulate bowel movements. As the colon stretches and loses its muscle tone, sufferers may experience chronic and severe constipation and an uncomfortable sense of fullness and even pain. In severe cases of longstanding laxative abuse, adult patients have been known to permanently lose bowel function and be doomed to life with a colostomy bag.

Fluid Imbalances

The feeling of emptiness and even the changes in body weight patients experience after self-induced vomiting and/or laxative or diuretic abuse convinces them that they have rid their bodies of binge calories. In fact, however, their main achievement is a temporary reduction in body fluid. Researchers have proven that the stomach and intestines retain significant calories in spite of self-induced vomiting. Laxatives rid the body of only about 10 percent of calories consumed, and diuretics have no effect whatsoever on caloric retention. The chronic purger, however, is often convinced that she is losing weight because she feels lighter after purging. She eventually discovers that purging does not rid her body of all the calories consumed during bingeing, and that the ironic fate of most bulimics is weight gain.

Purging can sometimes even cause the exact opposite effect that the anorexic or bulimic desires. Chronic vomiting and laxative or diuretic abuse leads to dehydration. Dehydration, in turn, stimulates the body's renin-aldosterone system, which helps the kidneys regulate the body's fluid and electrolyte balance. The result is "rebound water retention," where the kidneys begin to reabsorb fluid to make up for what was lost by purging. A vicious cycle begins in which the fluid and electrolyte losses of purging cause the body to hold on to even more water and electrolytes. The bulimic feels as if she is "retaining" water, which, in fact, she is. This is a situation that might tempt the bulimic to try a different form of purging, such as diuretics, when previously she may have used self-induced vomiting or laxatives. The dehydration continues or worsens, and the cycle starts over again.

Diuretics are rarely used by children and young adolescents because they are less likely to be aware that diuretics can dramatically affect body weight by causing loss of fluid. Younger patients, just by virtue of being younger, are also less likely to have access to prescription diuretics. Most young patients who do abuse diuretics take over-the-counter brands such as Aqua-Ban® and Diurex®, which their mothers may have on hand for premenstrual water retention. I advise parents not to keep diuretics and laxatives in easy view in the family medicine cabinet.

Abusing diuretics signals a serious problem that should be addressed immediately. Nonprescription pills, in and of themselves, are not very effective, and consequently, rarely cause health problems; what they can do, however, is confound the doctor's assessment of a patient's urinalysis by masking indicators of chronic vomiting. Doctors often routinely check the urine of bulimic patients. Simple tests can show if the patient is chronically vomiting. If the patient is using diuretics, however, the diuretics change urine chemistry, resulting in false normal readings. If you or your child's doctor suspects diuretic abuse, urine can be tested for this.

Prescription diuretics are far more dangerous than over-the-counter brands, sometimes causing weakness, nausea, heart palpitations, frequent urination, constipation, and abdominal pain. Chronic use can permanently damage the kidneys, potentially leading to a lifetime of dialysis. Parents or any adults, for that matter, should not leave their prescription medications in view or in reach of children, in order not to tempt a susceptible child. Several patients have told me that they helped themselves to Grandpa's or Great Aunt Annie's prescription diuretics.

Kidney and Pancreatic Problems

Purging can lead to impaired kidney function caused by chronic dehydration and low potassium levels associated with purging or the abuse of diuretics. As we noted, chronic abuse of diuretics has caused some patients to require dialysis.

Acute pancreatitis has been reported in connection with bulimia as well as in anorexia in the refeeding stage. With bulimia, pancreatitis is thought to be caused by the irritation of the pancreas by repeated bingeing and chronic diuretic abuse. With anorexia, pancreatitis is associated with malnutrition, although why it sometimes occurs during the refeeding stage is not well understood.

Menstrual Irregularities, Fertility, and Pregnancy

Menstrual irregularities or amenorrhea (cessation of menstrual periods) can occur among girls with bulimia, although it is unclear whether these symptoms are due to malnourishment, weight fluctuations, or emotional stress. Underweight bulimics are most likely to have menstrual irregularities.

If untreated, bulimia, like anorexia, may result in infertility for women of childbearing ages. Studies show that up to 60 percent of women seeking help through infertility clinics are suffering from either chronic, longstanding anorexia or bulimia. Remarkably, most recovered anorexics and bulimics are able to have healthy children.

For former eating-disordered patients who do become pregnant, pregnancy itself can stir up old eating-disordered behaviors, particularly bingeing and purging.

Paula came to see me years after I had treated her as a teenager for anorexia and bulimia. She had recovered, finished college, and now was married and pregnant with her first child. Paula felt at risk for a relapse after a serious bout of morning sickness landed her in the hospital. She and I decided to return to a food plan tailored to meet the increased nutrient needs of pregnancy. Paula delivered a beautiful baby girl, and I saw her several more times after that because she just wanted to be sure she was on the right track.

Eating-disordered patients who, unlike Paula, have not been able to shake their disorder before pregnancy have higher-than-average rates of miscarriages, premature births, and low birth-weight infants.

A Word about Ipecac

Although bulimics rarely make regular use of syrup of ipecac, experimentation with this common, nonprescription emetic (which many families have in their medicine cabinets as a precaution in case a toddler accidentally ingests a poison) is not unusual. As many as 28 percent of bulimics have experimented with ipecac, which is believed to have contributed to singer Karen Carpenter's untimely death from an eating disorder in 1983.

Progressive weakening of skeletal muscles and heart problems have resulted from the abuse of ipecac. The cardiac problems are the most serious, in some cases resulting in sudden death. Cardiac involvement, which can be detected by an electrocardiogram (EKG), is indicated by difficult breathing, rapid heart rate, low blood pressure, and arrhythmias. Early signs of ipecac toxicity are weakness, aching, chest pain, gait abnormalities, tenderness, and stiffness, especially in the neck. Ipecac is particularly dangerous because it builds up in the body; doctors warn patients that taking it regularly, or even with some frequency, means they are building up a lifetime cumulative dose.

We advise parents who no longer have toddlers in the house to get rid of their supply of ipecac. As little as three standard one-ounce-sized (30 ml) bottles of ipecac, even if taken in small doses over a long period of time, are toxic enough to be fatal. If you suspect your child has used ipecac, an electrocardiogram, an echocardiogram, and a thorough medical evaluation are in order.

Brain Abnormalities

There has been far less research done among bulimics than among anorexics on the subject of cognitive impairment. One research group did, however, find impaired cognitive performance in chronic bulimics. Brain-imaging studies have also shown some structural changes in some but not all tested bulimics.

Insulin Refusal: A Dangerous Temptation for the Diabetic

Unfortunately, eating disorders are becoming increasingly common among insulin-dependent diabetic adolescents who have figured out that when they stop using insulin or reduce their dose, they lose weight. If a diabetic does not take insulin, then the basic cellular fuel—sugar—cannot enter the body's cells and is excreted into the urine. Although the diabetic may continue to eat normally, her cells, in effect, starve and weight loss results. Most children, before they are diagnosed with diabetes, lose weight for this very reason.

The diabetic who fails to take insulin can suffer serious long-term consequences, including vision and heart and related circulation problems. In the short term, avoiding insulin can result in abdominal pain, nausea, blurred vision, headache, and general malaise. Diabetics with eating disorders have been found to have a higher rate of early eye, kidney, and nerve damage than do diabetics without eating disorders.

Chapter 30

Eating Disorders and Infertility, Pregnancy, and Breastfeeding

An estimated 0.5 percent to 1 percent of females thirteen to eighteen have anorexia. Another 1 to 3 percent are bulimic and many researchers believe these conditions are seriously underreported.

Self-starvation and the resulting nutritional deprivation wreaks havoc on their young, developing, and often, arrested bodies. They often have no periods. Their bones are brittle. Their estrogen and thyroid levels are imbalanced.

Then they grow up and want to have children.

As these girls grow into their would-be peak reproductive years, they may have married and now want children. Fertility, though, is elusive to women who have struggled with eating disorders all of their adolescence.

As a reproductive specialist and professor at the University of Texas Medical School at Houston in the departments of Internal Medicine and Obstetrics, Gynecology and Reproductive Sciences, Dr. Shahla Nader sees patients who are referred by other physicians who cannot figure out what is wrong.

After taking an in-depth health history she will ask the patient, "Do you consider yourself to have an eating disorder?" The patients usually say yes if they do. Nader's goal is to replace the hormones and help the patient correct her body weight.

"Eating Disorders and Infertility, Pregnancy, and Breastfeeding," reprinted from *HealthLeader,* www.uthealthleader.org. Produced by The University of Texas Health Science Center at Houston, © 2003. Reviewed by David A. Cooke, M.D., FACP, October 2010.

Nader explains that women have to have a certain critical level of body weight for the very sensitive internal clock, located in the brain's hypothalamus, to work. If a young woman is starving, she will not reproduce.

"A woman comes to me, wanting to get pregnant, but has amenorrhea—no menstrual flow. Sometimes being underweight is the reason," obstetrician/gynecologist Pamela D. Berens observes. Just a 5 percent weight gain may bring back her monthly cycle and ovulation.

It is important for Berens to know if the underlying reason for the patient's weight loss is an eating disorder, which she says must be fixed, with the patient gaining weight for six to twelve months, before becoming pregnant.

"Gaining weight is more effective than using fertility drugs. If a drug were used to make her ovulate and she became pregnant, but the eating disorder was not under control, she would be dealing with those symptoms throughout her pregnancy and not gaining weight properly. This in turn has a potentially negative effect on the growth of the fetus," says Berens, who is an associate professor in the Department of Obstetrics, Gynecology and Reproductive Sciences at the medical school.

It is best for the expectant mother to gain weight throughout her pregnancy (usually twenty-two to twenty-six pounds if she is at her ideal body weight when she becomes pregnant). A woman with an eating disorder history should be seen frequently during her pregnancy to be sure she is gaining weight each trimester.

"A woman who does not gain weight properly could have a low birthweight baby that is growth-restricted or even stillborn," Berens warns. "I try to explain to my patients that it is not a good thing to have a petite baby, who is poorly grown and undernourished."

New mothers are under increased physical strain and sleep deprivation under the best of circumstances. Their emotions may be turbulent as they settle in to a new hormonal rhythm. Eating disorders that might have been under control during the pregnancy may rear mightily after childbirth, right when nutritional value is crucial for mom and nursing child.

It is imperative for the new mother to be in control of any eating disorder symptoms while she is breastfeeding. "New mothers who are weight-conscious will immediately notice that one of the benefits of breastfeeding is that it uses up lots of the mom's calories—usually five hundred to six hundred a day," comments Berens, who has successfully helped many patients who have come to her wanting to get pregnant. However, those calories must be replaced to keep both mother and child healthy.

Women with diagnosed eating disorders are urged to confide their issues to their doctors before trying to get pregnant. Treatment options and support groups are available.

Chapter 31

Eating Disorders and Oral Health

At first glance, the mouth of a person with an eating disorder appears normal, but a closer look inside may reveal serious problems: erosion on the surfaces of the teeth, abscesses on the gums, glandular enlargement of the cheeks, and a chemical change in the saliva.

Frequently, it is the dentist who is the first doctor to diagnose a patient with an eating disorder. All these changes are caused by the lack of proper nutrition and the acid from self-induced vomiting.

Don't Be Fooled by the Smile

"These changes are most obvious on the back surfaces of the upper teeth, as well as those along the gum line and the chewing surfaces. The loss of tooth structure in these areas frequently causes sensitivity to hot and cold and can even result in the development of abscesses," explains Dr. Catherine M. Flaitz, dean of the University of Texas Dental Branch at Houston. "When there is significant destruction, the pulp or nerve of the tooth can become damaged and require root canal treatment and crown restorations."

Self-induced vomiting can cause trauma in the mouth, depending on what the person puts in her mouth to induce regurgitation:

───────────

"Hideous Secret: Eating Disorders and the Mouth," reprinted from *Health-Leader*, www.uthealthleader.org. Produced by The University of Texas Health Science Center at Houston, © 2003. Reviewed by David A. Cooke, M.D., FACP, October 2010.

- If fingers are used regularly, a callous forms on the backs of the hands due to the repeated rubbing of the fingers against the upper teeth.

- Fingernails can scratch the roof of the mouth.

- The person can also get tears in the corners of the mouth from exaggerated opening.

- Others get bruises or ulcers in the roof of the mouth or tonsil area from the pressure or from the object that is used to induce vomiting.

With loss of enamel from erosion, the teeth become thinner, smooth, and glassy in appearance. These changes are usually seen after two years of binge eating and purging. With time, significant tooth erosion can develop, causing the teeth to yellow and become brittle. This deterioration of the enamel, which is the outer layer of the tooth, cannot be regenerated—once lost, it is gone forever. As the enamel wears off, the teeth appear yellow or amber in color.

Acid Overdose

"These conditions are caused by acid in the mouth from self-induced vomiting, carbonated drinks, and increased amounts of fruits that are consumed to cause diarrhea," Flaitz says. It is the citrus fruits— oranges, lemons, grapefruit—that do the most damage if eaten in large amounts. Tomatoes are highly acidic, also. Hard candies that are artificially fruit flavored can also cause significant damage because the flavoring is acidic and the candy slowly dissolves in the mouth.

Bleaching Makes It Worse

If young people with eating disorders notice that their teeth are turning darker, they may try to whiten their smiles with over-the-counter bleaching agents. These products not only won't improve the color of eroding teeth, but might further wear away enamel. Bleaching products will cause eroding teeth to be more sensitive and darker in color because the second layer of the tooth, dentin, becomes exposed.

Dry Mouth

Another change is in the saliva. For some, there is a decreased amount, but for everyone the consistency thickens and cannot dilute, cleanse, and neutralize the inside of the mouth as it did before. "To neutralize the inside of the mouth, we recommend the patient rinse with water either alone or containing a fourth teaspoon of baking soda. Another option is to rinse with an antacid," she explains.

Chewing sugarless gum helps stimulate saliva and promote the natural re-mineralization or re-hardening of teeth. The use of topical fluorides helps to decrease sensitivity and prevent cavities from forming.

To correct the damage done inside the mouth, the dentist can cover the teeth with restorations or crowns to help prevent further damage.

It Gets Worse

Even more changes take place inside the mouth:

- The lining thins and pales due to a poor diet and anemia.

- Sores in the mouth result from a vitamin deficiency or from injuries by objects that are used to induce vomiting.

- Swelling of the glands in the cheeks is seen in 10 percent to 50 percent of bulimics who binge and purge.

- Facial enlargement occurs, depending on the length of time a person has been purging. The exact cause is unknown but might be related to chronic stimulation of the glands.

Other possible head and neck problems from eating disorders are hair loss from nutritional deprivation, chapped lips and very dry skin from dehydration, and very fine fuzzy hair growth on the face.

"These changes are very disconcerting for a young person obsessed with their body image," Flaitz observes.

Chapter 32

Eating Disorders and Osteoporosis

What Is Anorexia Nervosa?

Anorexia nervosa is an eating disorder characterized by an irrational fear of weight gain. People with anorexia nervosa believe that they are overweight even when they are extremely thin. According to the National Institute of Mental Health, an estimated 0.5 to 3.7 percent of females have anorexia nervosa. Although the majority of people with anorexia are female, an estimated 5 to 15 percent of people with anorexia are male.

Individuals with anorexia become obsessed with food and severely restrict their dietary intake. The disease is associated with several health problems and, in rare cases, even death. The disorder may begin as early as the onset of puberty. The first menstrual period is typically delayed in girls who have anorexia when they reach puberty. For girls who have already reached puberty when they develop anorexia, menstrual periods are often infrequent or absent.

What Is Osteoporosis?

Osteoporosis is a condition in which the bones become less dense and more likely to fracture. Fractures from osteoporosis can result in significant pain and disability. Osteoporosis is a major health threat

"What People with Anorexia Nervosa Need to Know about Osteoporosis," National Institute of Arthritis and Musculoskeletal and Skin Diseases, National Institutes of Health, January 2009.

307

for an estimated forty-four million Americans, 68 percent of whom are women.

Risk factors for developing osteoporosis include the following:

- Thinness or small frame

- Family history of the disease

- Being postmenopausal and particularly having had early menopause

- Abnormal absence of menstrual periods (amenorrhea)

- Prolonged use of certain medications, such as those used to treat lupus, asthma, thyroid deficiencies, and seizures

- Low calcium intake

- Lack of physical activity

- Smoking

- Excessive alcohol intake

Osteoporosis often can be prevented. It is known as a silent disease because, if undetected, bone loss can progress for many years without symptoms until a fracture occurs. Osteoporosis has been called a childhood disease with old age consequences because building healthy bones in youth helps prevent osteoporosis and fractures later in life. However, it is never too late to adopt new habits for healthy bones.

The Link between Anorexia Nervosa and Osteoporosis

Anorexia nervosa has significant physical consequences. Affected individuals can experience nutritional and hormonal problems that negatively impact bone density. Low body weight in females causes the body to stop producing estrogen, resulting in a condition known as amenorrhea, or absent menstrual periods. Low estrogen levels contribute to significant losses in bone density.

In addition, individuals with anorexia often produce excessive amounts of the adrenal hormone cortisol, which is known to trigger bone loss. Other problems, such as a decrease in the production of growth hormone and other growth factors, low body weight (apart from the estrogen loss it causes), calcium deficiency, and malnutrition, contribute to bone loss in girls and women with anorexia. Weight loss, restricted dietary intake, and testosterone deficiency may be responsible for the low bone density found in males with the disorder.

Studies suggest that low bone mass (osteopenia) is common in people with anorexia and that it occurs early in the course of the disease. Girls with anorexia are less likely to reach their peak bone density and therefore may be at increased risk for osteoporosis and fracture throughout life.

Osteoporosis Management Strategies

Up to one-third of peak bone density is achieved during puberty. Anorexia is typically identified during mid to late adolescence, a critical period for bone development. The longer the duration of the disorder, the greater the bone loss and the less likely it is that bone mineral density will ever return to normal.

The primary goal of medical therapy for individuals with anorexia is weight gain and, in females, the return of normal menstrual periods. However, attention to other aspects of bone health is also important.

Nutrition. A well-balanced diet rich in calcium and vitamin D is important for healthy bones. Good sources of calcium include low-fat dairy products; dark green, leafy vegetables; and calcium-fortified foods and beverages. Supplements can help ensure that people get adequate amounts of calcium each day, especially in people with a proven milk allergy. The Institute of Medicine recommends a daily calcium intake of 1,000 mg (milligrams) for men and women, increasing to 1,200 mg for those age fifty and older.

Vitamin D plays an important role in calcium absorption and bone health. It is synthesized in the skin through exposure to sunlight. Food sources of vitamin D include egg yolks, saltwater fish, and liver. Many people obtain enough vitamin D by getting about fifteen minutes of sunlight each day; others may need vitamin D supplements to achieve the recommended intake of 400 to 600 International Units (IU) each day.

Exercise. Like muscle, bone is living tissue that responds to exercise by becoming stronger. The best activity for your bones is weight-bearing exercise that forces you to work against gravity. Some examples include walking, climbing stairs, lifting weights, and dancing.

Although walking and other types of regular exercise can help prevent bone loss and provide many other health benefits, these potential benefits need to be weighed against the risk of fractures, delayed weight gain, and exercise-induced amenorrhea in people with anorexia and those recovering from the disorder.

Healthy lifestyle. Smoking is bad for bones as well as the heart and lungs. In addition, smokers may absorb less calcium from their diets. Alcohol also can have a negative effect on bone health. Those who drink heavily are more prone to bone loss and fracture, because of both poor nutrition and increased risk of falling.

Bone density test. A bone mineral density (BMD) test measures bone density in various parts of the body. This safe and painless test can detect osteoporosis before a fracture occurs and can predict one's chances of fracturing in the future. The BMD test can help determine whether medication should be considered.

Medication. There is no cure for osteoporosis. However, medications are available to prevent and treat the disease in postmenopausal women, men, and both women and men taking glucocorticoid medication. Some studies suggest that there may be a role for estrogen preparations among girls and young women with anorexia. However, experts agree that estrogen should not be a substitute for nutritional support.

Part Five

Recognizing and Treating Eating Disorders

Chapter 33

Recognizing Eating Disorder Warning Signs

Chapter Contents

Section 33.1

Physiological Symptoms and Warning Signs

"Symptoms and Warning Signs," *Medline Plus Magazine*, National Institutes of Health, Spring 2008.

Anorexia Nervosa

- Emaciation (extremely thin from lack of nutrition)
- Relentless pursuit of thinness; unwilling to maintain a normal or healthy weight
- Distorted body image; intense fear of gaining weight
- Lack of menstruation among girls and women
- Repeatedly weighing him- or herself
- Portioning food carefully, eating only small amounts of only certain foods
- Excessive exercise; self-induced vomiting; misuse of laxatives, diuretics, or enemas

Other symptoms that may develop over time:
- Thinning bones
- Brittle hair and nails
- Dry, yellowish skin
- Growth of fine hair over the body
- Mild anemia and muscle weakness and loss
- Severe constipation
- Low blood pressure, slowed breathing and pulse
- Feeling cold all the time
- Lethargy

Bulimia Nervosa

- Frequently eating large amounts of food (binge eating)
- Feeling a lack of control over the eating
- Compensating for binge eating with self-induced vomiting, misuse of laxatives and diuretics, fasting, and excessive exercise
- Binging and purging in secret; feelings of shame and disgust
- Intensely unhappy with body size and shape despite normal height and weight

Other symptoms include the following:

- Chronically inflamed and sore throat
- Swollen glands in neck and below jaw
- Worn tooth enamel from exposure to stomach acids
- Gastroesophageal reflux disorder
- Intestinal distress from laxative abuse
- Kidney problems from diuretic abuse
- Severe dehydration from purging

Binge Eating Disorder

- Frequently eating large amounts of food (binge eating)
- Feeling unable to control the eating behavior
- Feelings of guilt, shame, and/or distress about the behavior, which can lead to more binge eating

Section 33.2

Behavioral Warning Signs

"Why Do People Develop Eating Disorders?" © 2005 Alliance for Eating Disorders Awareness. Reprinted with permission. For additional information and treatment referrals, visit www.eatingdisorderinfo.org. Reviewed by David A. Cooke, M.D., FACP, October 2010.

Telling Signs of Anorexia

- The individual is constantly complaining about being "fat," "obese," or "huge."
- The individual is very preoccupied with weight, counting calories and fat grams, and dieting.
- The individual is drained and has little energy.
- The individual has begun wearing extremely loose fitting clothing.
- The individual comes up with newfound excuses not to eat such as, "I already ate and I have an upset stomach."
- The individual is extremely defensive about his/her weight.
- The individual is often cold.
- The individual often cooks or bakes food for other people, but refuses to eat the food themselves.
- The individual has started growing fine facial and body hair—a type of fur (lanugo).
- The individual is extremely irritable and has dramatic mood swings.
- The individual tends to be isolated in social situations and/or avoids social gatherings.
- The individual consumes a lot of noncaloric foods such as diet soda, gum, etc.
- The individual's hair is falling out and/or becoming extremely dry and brittle.

- The individual often withdraws from touching others.

- The individual avoids restaurants and eating in front of others.

- The individual's complexion has become pale and his/her skin is extremely dry.

- When the individual looks in the mirror, his/her reflection is like a "funhouse" mirror (distorted).

- Mealtimes have become extremely "ritualistic"—for example, the individual will insist on eating in the same bowl, he/she will cut their food into tiny pieces, he/she will not let the articles of food on the plate touch one another, he/she will keep on moving food around the plate to make it appear as if something has been eaten, etc.

- The individual uses excessive laxatives, diuretics, or diet pills to control weight.

If you answered "YES" to most of the questions listed above, please urge the individual to seek help from a healthcare professional.

Telling Signs of Bulimia

- The individual often goes to the restroom right after meals and remains for an extended period of time.

- The individual feels like he/she does not have control over food.

- The individual hides food in secret locations for use during binges.

- The individual eats a great deal but does not seem to gain or lose a lot of weight.

- The individual takes laxatives and gives himself/herself enemas more than once a week.

- The individual constantly complains about being "fat," "obese," or "huge."

- The individual has bloodshot eyes.

- The individual eats nothing or very little in front of others, and then binges in private.

- Quantities of food seem to mysteriously disappear from their refrigerator and/or pantry.

- The individual tends to have swollen glands in his/her neck and/or face.

- The individual has scrape wounds on the back of her/his knuckles (due to the contact between knuckles and teeth to induce vomiting).
- The individual abuses ipecac syrup, laxatives, diuretics, and/or diet pills.
- The individual has started to excessively drink, smoke, abuse drugs, or spend money.
- The individual is extremely defensive when questioned about his/her weight.
- The individual's tooth enamel is eroding and has increased cavities.
- The individual has begun to wear extremely tight fitting, figure revealing clothes.
- The individual will go through times of dramatic weight fluctuations of ten pounds or more within a short period of time.
- The individual tends to be sexually overactive, even quite promiscuous.
- The individual takes numerous trips to grocery stores, convenience stores, etc. in a single day.
- The individual has an enormous preoccupation with body weight and food.
- The individual is constantly complaining of a sore throat.
- The individual alternates between eating massive quantities of food and periods of self-starvation.

If you answered "YES" to most of the questions listed above, please urge the individual to seek help from a healthcare professional.

Telling Signs of Binge Eating Disorder

- The individual feels as if he/she has no control over food.
- The individual's main focus in life is his/her weight and food.
- The individual uses food to help cope with stress, emotional distress, and overcome daily problems.
- The individual's weight is higher than normal and/or is even obese.
- The individual is constantly complaining about being "fat," "obese," or "huge."

- The individual has major mood shifts with no apparent justifications.

- The individual eats nothing or very little in front of others, and then binges in private, keeping a high weight.

- The individual appears to be depressed and/or anxious.

- Quantities of food seem to mysteriously disappear from the refrigerator and/or pantry.

- When the individual is eating, he/she is terrified that they will be unable to stop.

- The individual is extremely defensive when questioned about his/her weight.

- The individual believes that he/she will be a better person if/when they are thinner.

- The individual goes from one diet to the next continuously.

- The individual takes numerous trips to grocery stores, convenience stores, etc. in a single day.

- The individual hides food in secret locations that will be used later for binges.

- The individual resists activities due to shame that is affiliated with his/her weight.

- The individual avoids any sexual activity and/or any emotional intimacy.

- The individual no longer feels full and/or satisfied when eating.

If you answered "YES" to most of the questions listed above, please urge the individual to seek help from a healthcare professional.

Chapter 34

Confronting a Person with an Eating Disorder

Chapter Contents

Section 34.1

How to Approach a Loved One

"How to Approach a Loved One," © 2005 Alliance for Eating Disorders
Awareness. Reprinted with permission. For additional information and
treatment referrals, visit www.eatingdisorderinfo.org. Reviewed by David
A. Cooke, M.D., FACP, October 2010.

How to Help Your Friend

Do's

- Increase your knowledge about eating disorders (request information packets, read books, attend seminars).

- Talk with the person about your concerns in a loving and supportive way. It is important to discuss these issues with honesty and respect.

- Talk with the person at an appropriate time and place—in private, free from distractions.

- Encourage the person to seek professional help as soon as possible. Suggest that she/he see someone who specializes in eating disorders (a physician, therapist, or dietician).

- Be prepared that the person may deny that she/he has a problem. If so, and if she/he refuses to get help, it will be important to tell someone else about your concerns. If your friend is under eighteen, her/his parents need to know immediately.

- Listen with a nonjudgmental ear.

- Talk about things other than food, weight, and exercise.

- Be available when your friend needs someone, but remember, it is okay to set limits on what you can and cannot do.

- Hang in there! It won't be easy.

Don'ts

- Don't try to solve her/his problems or help with the eating disorder on your own. Get help from others.

- Don't confront your friend with a group of people, in front of a group of people.

- Don't talk about weight, food, calories, or appearance. Do not make any comments on what she/he looks like.

- Don't try to force or encourage your friend to eat. Do not get into power struggles.

- Don't let her/his peculiarities dominate you or manipulate you.

- Don't gossip about her/him to others.

- Don't be scared to talk with her/him.

- Don't expect to be the perfect friend—reach out for support when you need it.

- Don't expect your friend to be "cured" after treatment. Recovery can be a long process.

- Don't keep this a secret for your friend. Remember, her/his life may be in danger.

How to Help Your Child

Do's

- Increase your knowledge about eating disorders (request information packets, read books, attend seminars).

- Talk with your child about your concerns in a loving and supportive way. It is important to discuss these issues with honesty and respect.

- Talk with your child at an appropriate time and place—in private, free from distractions.

- Seek professional help as soon as possible. Arrange to see someone who specializes in eating disorders (a physician, therapist, or dietician). You can receive national and international referrals from various eating disorder organizations.

- Be prepared that your child may deny that she/he has a problem.

- Listen with a nonjudgmental ear.

- Talk about things other than food, weight, and exercise.

- Be available when your child needs someone, but remember, it is okay to set limits on what you can and cannot do.

- Hang in there! It won't be easy.

Don'ts

- Don't try to solve her/his problems or help with the eating disorder on your own. Get help from others.

- Don't confront your child with a group of people, in front of a group of people.

- Don't talk about weight, food, calories, or appearance. Do not make any comments on what she/he looks like.

- Don't try to force or encourage your child to eat. Do not get into power struggles.

- Don't blame yourself for what is happening to your child.

- Don't let your child's peculiarities dominate you or manipulate you.

- Don't be scared to talk with your child.

- Don't expect to be the perfect parent—reach out for support when you need it.

- Don't expect your child to be "cured" after treatment. Recovery can be a long process.

- Don't panic: Look for the help you need. It is available.

How to Help Your Student

Do's

- Increase your knowledge about eating disorders (request information packets, read books, attend seminars).

- Talk with your student at an appropriate time and place—in private, free from distractions and other students.

- Encourage your student to tell their parents.

- Encourage your student to seek professional help as soon as possible. Suggest that she/he see someone who specializes in eating disorders (a physician, therapist, or dietician).

- Be prepared that the person may deny that she/he has a problem. If your student is under eighteen, her/his parents need to know immediately.

- Listen with a nonjudgmental ear.

- Talk about things other than food, weight, and exercise.

- Be available when your student needs someone, but remember, it is okay to set limits on what you can and cannot do.

- Hang in there! It won't be easy.

Don'ts

- Don't try to solve her/his problems or help with the eating disorder on your own. Get help from others.

- Don't confront your student in front of the class.

- Don't talk about weight, food, calories, or appearance. Do not make any comments on what she/he looks like.

- Don't try to force or encourage your student to eat. Do not get into power struggles.

- Don't gossip about her/him to others.

- Don't be scared to talk with her/him.

- Don't forget to reach out for support when you need it.

- Don't expect your student to be "cured" after treatment. Recovery can be a long process.

- Don't keep this a secret for your student. Remember, her/his life may be in danger. If she/he is under eighteen, her/his parents need to know immediately.

Section 34.2

How to Approach Your Student: A Guide for Teachers

"Guidelines for Helping a Student," © Rebecca Manley, M.S., Multi-service Eating Disorder Association (MEDA), 1996. Reprinted with permission. For additional information, contact MEDA at 866-343-6332, or www.medainc .org. Reviewed by David A. Cooke, M.D., FACP, October 2010.

Prepare yourself for your talk. Gather general information before you talk to the student. Find out about the resources for help in your school and community without revealing the identity of the student. Speak in an anonymous way with the school nurse/physician, health educator, and administration to find out if there is any school policy about students with eating disorders (such policies are more likely to be in place at boarding schools). Find out what the ramifications might be for participation in classes and sports. Read about eating disorders if you need more information. Always talk privately with her before letting others know about the student by name, even if you strongly believe she is at risk. You can bring in other individuals later, but you risk the student's trust if you talk about her without her knowing.

Do other students know? The student you approach may want to know whether you noticed her or whether other students came to you about her. If other students do come to you, discuss with them whether they want their conversation with you to be confidential. You need to respect their request and reassure them that they did the right thing by communicating their concern. Tell them that you will follow through on their approach to you and put their concern in the hands of responsible adults who will do their best to help. Check to see if any student who approaches you is also worried about herself, and offer her the same kind of advice. Avoid getting involved in long talks with the concerned students about the at-risk student.

Plan with care. It is best to be able to offer your student a strategy for securing help. Locate a quiet, safe, and private place to talk. Plan ahead so you'll have the amount of time you'll need to talk and be sure that you won't be interrupted or overheard. Begin by telling the student that you are concerned about her and gently offer some specific observations about her emotional wellbeing or lack thereof. For example: "You seem (really) unhappy and preoccupied/anxious/ fidgety/distant/jumpy/angry, and I'm worried about you." If her performance has dropped in class or sports, give her specific observations. For example: "You don't seem to be having any fun anymore, you're pushing yourself too hard, you don't raise your hand anymore, you're working out so hard that it looks like you might be injuring yourself, your energy's depleted, your grades are dropping." As you talk, communicate about what is going on inside her. Listen to what she says without making any judgments, interpretations, or promises that you will get very involved in her recovery.

Offer a few observations about her behavior to explain why you think she has an eating disorder. For example, "I see you skip meals, I watch you leave class and run to the bathroom, I hear you talk all the time about being afraid of being fat, what you ate, how much you're going to exercise, etc." Don't try to make a diagnosis or do therapy. Do let her know that you have some sense that she may have an eating disorder and she needs to get help to evaluate this. If you have found out your school policy concerning participation in sports, let her know it in the most reassuring way possible. "As far as I know, our school has a policy that you will still be able to play sports and do all activities unless participating would be dangerous to you."

Your student may feel threatened by your discovery or observations. She may deny that she has a problem or get upset. If she gets upset or mad, stay calm. Don't panic or get angry. Don't get into a "Yes you do/ No I don't " power struggle here. Give her space to respond, listen to her, and ask her to listen to you. Remind her that teachers tell students when they are worried about them. If she insists that she doesn't have a problem, or she can stop on her own, you can say something like, "You know how it is with alcoholism and denial. The addiction makes it hard to see you have a serious problem and that you need help. I'm worried you're trapped in a similar kind of situation. I'm really worried about you, and even though I hear what you're saying, I think you are really struggling and you need help stopping. I believe in you and I know you deserve to get help and get better." If she has tried to get better on her own and hasn't succeeded and is ashamed, let her know that it is very hard to recover without help and that this is not a weakness or failure on her part. You may need to approach a student more than once before she will agree to get help.

Offer the name of a referral and offer to go with her if you feel comfortable doing so. Let the student know you'll touch base with her to follow up. Ask if it's okay for you to let the referral person know to expect to be hearing from her. In a few days, or whatever seems to be the right amount of time, check in with the student and ask if she contacted the person. Follow up with the referral person and then continue to be supportive of the student as you would with any other student. Avoid comments about food, exercise, or appearance.

If she refuses help, tell her again the specifics of why you are concerned, and if needed, your belief that something further must be done. Don't prolong a conversation that is going poorly. Do get consultation from a professional. Depending on what the professional says, the age of the student, and the degree of risk, you may decide to approach the student again and tell her that you talked to the professional. Stay calm and avoid sounding like your mission is to rescue or cure her, but also let her know you are concerned that she has a serious problem and it would be irresponsible for you not to try to help. Eating disorders are serious physical and psychological problems, but not usually emergencies. However, if your student is fainting, depressed, suicidal, or otherwise in serious danger, get professional help immediately. "I don't care if you're mad at me. Teachers don't let students suffer in danger and isolation."

Section 34.3

What to Do When You Think Your Friend Has an Eating Disorder

"I Think My Friend May Have an Eating Disorder. What Should I Do?"
November 2007, reprinted with permission from www.KidsHealth.org.
Copyright © 2007 The Nemours Foundation. This information was provided
by KidsHealth, one of the largest resources online for medically reviewed
health information written for parents, kids, and teens. For more articles
like this one, visit www.KidsHealth.org, or www.TeensHealth.org.

Signs of Eating Disorders

In our image-obsessed culture, it can be easy for teens (and adults,
for that matter) to be critical of their bodies. Normal concerns about
body image can cross the line and become eating disorders when a person starts to do things that are physically and emotionally dangerous—
things that could have long-term health consequences.

Some people go on starvation diets and can become anorexic. Others
go on eating binges and then purge their bodies of the food they've just
eaten through forced vomiting, compulsive exercise, taking laxatives,
or a combination of these (known as bulimia).

Although eating disorders like anorexia and bulimia are far more
common in girls, guys can get them, too. So how do you know if a friend
has an eating disorder? It can be hard to tell—after all, someone who's
lost a lot of weight or feels constantly tired may have another type
of health condition. But some of the signs that a friend may have an
eating disorder include:

- Your friend has an obsession with weight and food (more than
  general comments about how many calories he or she eats in a
  day). It might seem like your friend talks about food, weight, and
  being thin and nothing else.

- Your friend knows exactly how many calories and fat grams are in
  everything that he or she eats—and is constantly pointing this out.

- Your friend feels the need to exercise all the time, even when
  sick or exhausted.

- Your friend avoids hanging out with you and other friends during meals. For example, he or she avoids the school cafeteria at lunch or the coffee shop or diner where you usually meet on weekends.

- Your friend starts to wear big or baggy clothes. Lots of people wear baggy clothes as a fashion statement, but someone who wears baggy clothes to hide their shape might have other issues.

- Your friend goes on dramatic or very restrictive diets, cuts food into tiny pieces, moves food around on the plate instead of eating it, and is very precise about how food is arranged on the plate.

- Your friend seems to compete with others about how little they eat. If a friend proudly tells you she only had a diet soda for breakfast and half an apple for lunch, it's a red flag that she could be developing an eating disorder.

- Your friend goes to the bathroom a lot, especially right after meals, or you've heard your friend vomiting after eating.

- Despite losing a lot of weight, your friend always talks about how fat he or she is.

- Your friend appears to be gaining a lot of weight even though you never see him or her eat (people with bulimia often only eat diet food in front of their friends).

- Your friend is very defensive or sensitive about his or her weight loss or eating habits.

- Your friend buys or takes laxatives, steroids, or diet pills.

- Your friend has a tendency to faint, bruises easily, is very pale, or starts complaining of being cold more than usual (cold intolerance can be a symptom of being underweight).

What to Do

If a friend has these symptoms and you're concerned, the first thing to do might be to talk to your friend, privately, about what you've noticed. Tell your friend that you're worried. Be as gentle as possible, and try to really listen to and be supportive of your friend and what he or she is going through.

It's normal for people with eating disorders to feel guarded and private about their eating problems. Try not to get angry or frustrated. Remind your friend that you care.

330

People with eating disorders often have trouble admitting—even to themselves—that they have a problem. Trying to help someone who doesn't think he or she needs help can be hard. Many people feel successful and in control when they become thin, but those with eating disorders can become seriously ill and even die. If your friend is willing to seek help, offer to go with him or her to see a counselor or a medical expert.

If your concerns increase and your friend still seems to be in denial, talk to your parents, the school guidance counselor or nurse, or even your friend's parents. This isn't easy to do because it can feel like betraying a friend. But it's often necessary to get a friend the help he or she needs.

Eating disorders can be caused by—and lead to—complicated physical and psychological illnesses. You can support your friend by learning as much as you can about eating disorders. Your friend's body image and behavior may be a symptom of something else that's going on. Many organizations, books, websites, hotlines, or other resources are devoted to helping people who are battling eating disorders.

Being a supportive friend also means learning how to behave around someone with an eating disorder. Here are some ways to support a friend who is battling an eating problem:

- Try your best not to talk about food, weight, diets, or body shape (yours, your friend's, or even a popular celebrity's).

- Try not to be too watchful of your friend's eating habits, food amounts, and choices.

- Try not to make statements like, "If you'd just eat (or stop working out so much), you'll get better."

- Focus on your friend's strengths—that he or she has a great smile, is helpful and friendly, or good at math or art.

- Try to avoid focusing on how your friend looks physically.

Most important, remind your friend that you're there no matter what. You want to help him or her get healthy again. Sometimes you'd be surprised how asking simple questions such as "what can I do to help?" or "what would make you feel better?" can lead to a great conversation about how you can help your friend heal.

Chapter 35

Diagnosing Eating Disorders

Chapter Contents

Section 35.1

Identifying Eating Disorders

"Eating Disorders," © 2010 A.D.A.M., Inc. Reprinted with permission.

Diagnosis

The first step toward a diagnosis is to admit the existence of an eating disorder. Often, the patient needs to be compelled by a parent or others to see a doctor because the patient may deny and resist the problem. Some patients may even self-diagnose their condition as an allergy to carbohydrates, because after being on a restricted diet, eating carbohydrates can produce gastrointestinal problems, dizziness, weakness, and palpitations. This may lead such people to restrict carbohydrates even more severely. It is often extremely difficult for parents as well as the patient to admit that a problem is present.

Screening Tests

Various questionnaires are available for assessing patients. The Eating Disorders Examination (EDE), which is an interview of the patient by the doctor, and the self-reported Eating Disorders Examination-Questionnaire (EDE-Q) are both considered valid tests for assessing eating disorder diagnosis and determining specific features of the individual's condition (such as vomiting or laxative use).

Another test is called the SCOFF questionnaire, which can help identify patients who meet the full criteria for anorexia or bulimia nervosa. (It may not be as accurate in people who do not meet the full criteria.)

SCOFF Questionnaire

- Do you make yourself Sick because you feel uncomfortably full?

- Do you worry you have lost Control over how much you eat?

- Have you recently lost more than One stone's worth of weight (fourteen pounds) in a three-month period?

- Do you believe yourself to be Fat when others say you are too thin?

- Would you say that Food dominates your life?

Answering yes to two of these questions is a strong indicator of an eating disorder.

Measuring Body Mass Index

A doctor will evaluate a patient's body mass index (BMI). The BMI is the measurement of body fat. It is derived by multiplying a person's weight in pounds by 703 and then dividing it twice by the height in inches (BMI calculators are available online.):

- A healthy BMI for women over age twenty is 19 to 25.

- Those over 25 are considered overweight; those over 30 are considered obese.

- Those under 17.5 are considered to be at risk for health problems related to anorexia. (However, young teenagers can have lower BMIs without necessarily being anorexic.)

For example, a woman who is 5'5" and weighs 125 pounds has a healthy BMI of 21. A woman at the same height who weighs 90 pounds would have a dangerously low BMI of 15.

Diagnosing Bulimia Nervosa

A doctor generally makes a diagnosis of bulimia if there are at least two bulimic episodes per week for three months. Because people with bulimia tend to have complications with their teeth and gums, dentists can play a crucial role in identifying and diagnosing bulimia.

Diagnosing Anorexia Nervosa

Generally, an observation of physical symptoms and a personal history will confirm the diagnosis of anorexia. The standard criteria for diagnosing anorexia nervosa are:

- the patient's refusal to maintain a body weight normal for age and height;

- intense fear of becoming fat even though underweight;

- a distorted self-image that results in diminished self-confidence;

- denial of the seriousness of emaciation and starvation;
- the loss of menstrual function for at least three months. The doctor then categorizes the anorexia further:
- Restricting (severe dieting only)
- Anorexia bulimia (binge-purge behavior)

Diagnosing Complications of Eating Disorders

Once a diagnosis is made, a doctor will check for any serious complications of starvation and also rule out other medical disorders that might be causing the anorexia. Tests should include:

- a complete blood count;
- tests for electrolyte imbalances;
- test for protein levels;
- an electrocardiogram and a chest x-ray;
- tests for liver, kidney, and thyroid problems;
- a bone density test.

Section 35.2

Suggested Medical Tests in Diagnosing Eating Disorders

Excerpted from "Navigating the System: Consumer Tips for Getting Treatment for Eating Disorders," © 2008 National Eating Disorders Association. For more information, visit www.NationalEatingDisorders.org.

The most important first step is to have a complete assessment. This includes a medical evaluation to rule out any other physical cause for the symptoms, to assess the impact the illness has had to date, and to determine whether immediate medical intervention is needed. See the following for specific tests. Equally important is the mental health assessment, preferably by an eating disorder expert to provide a full diagnostic picture. Many people with eating disorders have other problems as well including depression, trauma, obsessive-compulsive disorder, anxiety, or chemical dependence. This assessment will determine what level of care is needed (inpatient, outpatient, partial hospital, residential) and what professionals should be involved in the treatment.

Recommended Laboratory Tests

Standard

- Complete blood count (CBC) with differential

- Urinalysis

- Complete metabolic profile: sodium, chloride, potassium, glucose, blood urea nitrogen, creatinine, total protein, albumin, globulin, calcium, carbon dioxide, aspartate transaminase (AST), alkaline phosphates, total bilirubin

- Serum magnesium

- Thyroid screen (T3, T4, thyroid stimulating hormone [TSH])

- Electrocardiogram (ECG)

Special Circumstances

Fifteen percent or more below ideal body weight (IBW):

- Chest x-ray
- Complement 3 (C3)
- 24 creatinine clearance
- Uric acid

Twenty percent or more below IBW or any neurological sign:
- Brain scan

Twenty percent or more below IBW or sign of mitral valve prolapse:

- Echocardiogram

Thirty percent or more below IBW:

- Skin testing for immune functioning

Weight loss 15 percent or more below IBW lasting six months or longer at any time during course of eating disorder:

- Dual energy x-ray absorptiometry (DEXA) to assess bone mineral density
- Estradiol level (or testosterone in males)

Criteria for Level of Care

Inpatient

Medically unstable:

- Unstable or depressed vital signs
- Laboratory findings presenting acute risk
- Complications due to coexisting medical problems such as diabetes

Psychiatrically unstable:

- Symptoms worsening at rapid rate
- Suicidal and unable to contract for safety

Residential

- Medically stable so does not require intensive medical interventions
- Psychiatrically impaired and unable to respond to partial hospital or outpatient treatment

Partial Hospital

Medically stable:

- Eating disorder may impair functioning but not causing immediate acute risk
- Needs daily assessment of physiological and mental status

Psychiatrically stable:

- Unable to function in normal social, educational, or vocational situations
- Daily bingeing, purging, severely restricted intake, or other pathogenic weight control techniques

Intensive Outpatient/Outpatient

Medically stable:

- No longer needs daily medical monitoring

Psychiatrically stable:

- Symptoms in sufficient control to be able to function in normal social, educational, or vocational situations and continue to make progress in recovery.

Chapter 36

Choosing an Eating Disorders Treatment Facility or Therapist

Chapter Contents

Section 36.1

Steps in Choosing the Right Treatment Facility

"Steps in Choosing the Right Treatment Facility," by Angela Picot, PhD,
Eating Disorders Recovery Today, Fall 2008, Volume 6, Number 4.
© 2008 Gürze Books. Reprinted with permission.

If you have made the critical decision to pursue a higher level of care to treat an eating disorder, it is important to carefully consider your options. Every individual has different needs and not all treatment centers are the same. There is a wide range of orientations, interventions, services, and specialties unique to each center.

Step One: Determine Level of Care

The first step is for you and the treatment team (any therapist, psychiatrist, nutritionist, or internist with whom you currently receive services) to determine the most appropriate level of care. If you do not currently have a treatment team, schedule a thorough clinical assessment with a therapist who specializes in the treatment of eating disorders for recommendations.

If you need more support than individual outpatient therapy can provide, consider an intensive outpatient or partial hospitalization program, which typically offer daily four to eight hours of psychotherapy and meal support with periodic medical monitoring. If you are in need of medical intervention or require stabilization in a safe, contained environment prior to beginning more intensive therapy, a two- to three-week inpatient stay may be the best choice. If symptoms have persisted despite other interventions, consider a residential treatment center, where the typical length of stay is one to three months.

Step Two: Specific Issues

The next step is to think about other issues, in addition to the eating disorder, that might need to be addressed in treatment. For instance, do you suffer from depression or anxiety? Do you have a history of trauma? Are you battling substance abuse problems? Many centers have special groups, treatment interventions, and trained therapists to help address these and other co-occurring conditions. This will help narrow down your choices. A general internet search is often sufficient for research, although there are other resources that offer a list of treatment programs by state.

Step Three: Ask Questions

Once you have a list of possible choices, it is time to more deeply explore each specific program. Here are some questions to consider:

- What is the orientation of the program? (i.e., Is it a twelve-step model? Is there a spiritual component? Is there behavioral and nutrition therapy?)

- How much time is spent in group and individual therapy? What is the staff-to-participant ratio?

- What types of experiential therapies are offered? (i.e., art, movement, equine)

- Is there a physician on staff? What happens if I need immediate medical attention or medical monitoring?

- Are psychiatric services available and what is the treatment perspective?

- Is there a family or marital therapy component?

- What are the possibilities for discharge planning? (i.e., Does the program have options for step-down level of care or transfer back to the referring providers?)

- Will the program communicate with my existing team to ensure continuity of care?

- Can they provide statistics regarding number of patients treated in the past year, their ages and clinical characteristics, and short-term and long-term outcomes?

Step Four: Insurance and Availability

Call each center and ask about availability and insurance. Some have a wait-list, so anticipate that it might be several weeks before admission is possible. Most centers will take your insurance information and check benefits to determine if reimbursement is possible.

The billing departments will typically work in advance to determine a payment plan. Some programs offer discounted rates or scholarships based on need. Some require payment up front for a certain length of stay, while others use a pay-as-you-go model. Even if you don't think that your insurance will cover a certain program, call to see what type of plan can be arranged.

Step Five: Make a Decision

A number of treatment centers around the country provide high-quality services. It is worth the time and effort to select the one that will be the best fit for you. Be sure to talk to your treatment team and support system when making this decision. Keep in mind that any intensive treatment should be followed up by an appropriate aftercare plan. Congratulations on taking this important step in your recovery.

Section 36.2

Finding a Therapist

Eating disorders are extremely complex disorders that can be life threatening. It is important to seek the help of a qualified professional to assist you in the recovery process. Having a good support system of friends and loved ones is extremely helpful, but it is vital to have a professional to help and guide you.

Locating a Therapist

One of the best ways to locate a therapist is through a recommendation from someone that has a problem similar to yours and has had a good experience with that particular therapist. Since it is unlikely that your acquaintances will have a similar problem and be willing to tell you about their therapy, it is good to have other options.

For other potential therapists, you can contact a professional referral service. These can be found listed under "Mental Health" in your phonebook, or under the specific heading of the type of professional for which you are searching. Professional organizations maintain referral lists of qualified therapists. For instance, you could look up an organization for psychiatrists or psychologists. These organizations have the benefit of being able to help you find the appropriate match according to your specific type of problem and the therapist's expertise. If a therapist receives any complaints, the referral service is available to evaluate and resolve the dispute. If consistent problems occur, the therapist will be removed from the service. As most of the referral services require that the therapists maintain the highest level of professionalism, a therapist from a referral service has of necessity been exposed to extra screening.

Do not just accept the first therapist that you talk to. Wait for at least three therapists to return your call. The fact that your call is returned quickly does not imply that he or she is a good therapist. It may be preferable to see a therapist that is busy and popular. However, if a therapist does call you back quickly then that does not mean anything bad. Give yourself at least a day and a half to call three therapists to talk to them on the telephone, and evaluate whether you find a sense of rapport.

Additional Certification

Be careful to protect yourself. Just because someone says they are a therapist does not mean that they have had any training. People can call themselves a therapist, a psychotherapist, an analyst, a counselor, a marriage counselor, an eating disorder specialist, or a sex therapist and not have had any formal training. Although very uncommon, it is nevertheless possible to practice as a psychiatrist in the United States without having obtained any specialized training more than a medical license.

The term "psychologist" is regulated by law (in many states) which means that if a person says they are a psychologist, then that means that they have to be licensed in the state in which they practice. Again be careful because some therapists say they are a psychologist because they have a Ph.D. after their name (which means they are referred to as "doctor") but they are in fact licensed to practice under a specialty other than psychology. Thus, a person with a Ph.D. in psychology from their graduate training may actually be state licensed as a marriage counselor. In some states, a marriage counselor can practice without being licensed. So how do you protect yourself? By asking the following questions:

345

- To a psychiatrist: Have you had residency training in psychiatry and are you board certified by the American Board of Psychiatry and Neurology (more than one-third are board certified).

- To a psychologist: Are you licensed *as* a psychologist? If not, under what license do you practice and what is your training?

- To any other therapist: What is your license, degree, and training?

Before Calling the Therapist

First decide if you want a same-sex therapist or one of the opposite sex. If you are apprehensive about therapy then choose the sex of the therapist with whom you feel most comfortable.

Next, find out how much you can afford for therapy. If therapy is once a week, then figure out how much you can afford to pay for four sessions in a month. If you have insurance, then contact your carrier and obtain in writing what they cover; i.e., if you have to see a specific therapist on their list, or if you have to see a particular type of therapist. Ask the carrier how much they pay for each office visit, and how many sessions they pay for. Also, ask about annual and lifetime payout limits.

Now you are ready to contact the therapist.

Questions to Ask on the Phone

Ask the potential therapist if he or she has a few minutes to talk to you about therapy. If he or she is not available at that moment, then ask when you can call at a more convenient time. If you discover that they are too busy for this brief introductory talk, you may want to ask whether they are accepting new clients and when the first available appointment could be made. If it is too long until you can get an appointment and you feel the need to be seen immediately then ask for a referral to another therapist. The average wait is less than a week although rarely, with very busy therapists, it can be up to six months, so check with the therapist.

Does the therapist limit his or her practice to a particular type of client? Does the therapist do family or couples therapy if necessary? What type of therapy does he or she use? What type of experience, training, and license does the therapist have? Will the therapist read your history before you go to your first session? How long are the sessions, and how often does the therapist generally schedule sessions? In addition, of course, what is the fee and will the therapist accept your insurance and how are co-payments handled? (co-payments are the amount that you have to pay beyond the insurance payment.) You can ask the therapist about a "sliding fee scale," which means that the fee may "slide" or vary according to your ability to pay or your monthly income.

Has the therapist ever had a license revoked or suspended; has he or she ever been disciplined by a state or professional ethics board and would he be willing to discuss it? (You can call the state licensing board to check out his or her license, credentials, and any ethical violations).

Tell the therapist that you want to talk to a few other potential therapists and you will call back if you decide to make an appointment. Give yourself some time to think over and digest your feelings about the telephone conversations. Then choose a therapist and make an appointment for an initial trial session. The first session should be used to help you decide if you *want* to work together.

After You Have Left Your First Session

Assess carefully your reaction to how it felt. Was the therapist open to the manner in which you presented your history? Did you get a sense that you could be comfortable with this therapist? Did you feel a sense of connection with the therapist? Remember that each therapist creates a different environment and you have to decide if the atmosphere felt right to you. Do you feel that you will be able to trust this therapist? Did the therapist push you to reveal things that were uncomfortable too quickly? Were your needs listened to? Did the therapist behave in a professional manner? Did you feel comfortable about the goals that you two were able to set? Did your therapist tell about how therapy works and were you able to set some goals?

What Does the Therapist Expect of You?

This varies from therapist to therapist but usually you are expected to:

- Show up on time for appointments. Unlike other doctors that may keep you waiting for an appointment or that may accept you even if you show up late, a therapist has a specific hour set aside for you. If you are late, then you are missing time that was reserved for you. The therapist has no obligation to make the session run late because you showed up late. Most likely, the therapist will have another client waiting to start at the beginning of the next hour. The therapist should not take telephone calls or attend to any business other than yours during your therapy session.

347

- Cancel appointments in advance so the therapist can reschedule (usually twenty-four to forty-eight hours). Usually therapists charge the full fee for missed appointments that are not canceled in advance because you are paying for the therapist's time that was allotted for you. Insurance will not pay for missed appointments.

- Share your perceptions and feelings as openly and honestly as you can. This involves taking the risk of sharing your deepest fears and concerns—this will help you to make progress quickly.

- Actively work on your issues with your therapist. Some people come into therapy with the attitude, "I'm here, now fix me," when in actuality the process has to be one of both of you working together.

- Complete any "homework" which was assigned. (Homework is designed to help the benefits of therapy to extend beyond the therapy hour.)

- Think about and reflect on your therapy between sessions. Be ready to discuss thoughts that you have about the previous sessions or any insights that have come to you since your last session with the therapist. You may even want to start keeping a journal of your experiences. If you have tried but cannot come up with any thoughts about the therapy then that is understandable.

- Discuss with the therapist when you feel that you are finished with therapy *before* actually stopping.

If you follow these guidelines, you are not only living up to the expectations of therapy; you are also putting yourself in the best position to get the most out of the experience.

What Not to Expect

Do not expect a miracle cure from your therapist. Your problems have been with you for a long time and long-established patterns can take a while to change. Do not expect your therapist to be your friend outside of the therapy session. This can lead to complications with your therapy and should be avoided. You may wonder why your therapist does not acknowledge you in public. This is because your therapist wants to keep your relationship confidential. If you make the first move to say hello, then the interaction would likely be much different.

Also do not expect your therapist to attend parties or other functions. Some therapists will come to significant life milestones such as a graduation or marriage, but other therapists believe that it is not appropriate. Talk to your therapist about your feelings concerning these matters.

What to Watch Out For

If you feel that the therapist is setting goals for you which are based on what the therapist considers is important for you to change and these goals are not your own, then be wary. At times, therapists will unwittingly introduce their own unresolved issues, which influence their treatment decisions. This is something to watch out for. For instance, if you mention that you are in an unhappy marriage and yet you are going to therapy to get over stage fright, and the therapist says you have to work on your marriage first, then he is a therapist to avoid. That therapist may be dealing with unresolved personal relationship issues, which are influencing his or her judgment about your treatment. This is rare, but it is something to be aware of.

Never let the therapist perform any action or ask you to do anything that is against your morals and values. If a therapist ever asks you to do something unacceptable and does not respect your wishes then leave immediately. Therapists are in a position of power and at times try and wield that power by saying "I know what is best for you." As with any profession, there are a small percentage of bad therapists who will abuse this power. Remember, never do anything that is against your values.

A therapist should never touch you without your permission. Some therapists will put their hand on your shoulder once they know you to offer support, but if such a gesture makes you uncomfortable then tell the therapist. If he or she does not respect your wishes then leave immediately.

If you ever have a particular problem or disagreement with your therapist, it is vital to bring this out in the open. Disagreements will inevitably arise; this is part of the therapy process. You should watch out for therapists who do not listen to your concerns or apologize for mistakes.

Unprofessional Behavior

Therapists are expected to uphold the moral and legal standards of the community. Clients should be treated with dignity, respect, and fairness.

The following are behaviors that are not ethical for a therapist:

- Any sexual approach is unprofessional for a therapist. Asking you to remove any of your clothes, or touching you in any way without your permission is unethical. Having romantic encounters or even asking to see you outside of therapy is also unethical. Be wary of therapists who try to elicit help from you for their own problems or charities or outside business interests. Therapists may bring up personal anecdotes to assist with your therapy, but the focus should not change to dealing with the therapist's problems.

- The therapist may give you a reduced fee to help to accommodate your financial situation. When your situation improves it is customary to re-evaluate the circumstances and possibly pay the therapist's regular fee. But the therapist cannot increase his normal fees just because he believes you can afford a higher fee.

Though these situations are rare, if you believe that your therapist behaved in an unprofessional manner then discuss this behavior with the professional ethics committee of your state licensing board.

Types of Therapy

Cognitive/behavioral therapy. Treatment approach based on the theory that people's emotions are controlled by their opinions and views of the world. The therapist uses various techniques of talk therapy and behavioral prescriptions to alleviate negative thought patterns and belief systems. The therapist helps patients by teaching them to view their thinking as a type of behavior that they can bring under conscious control, ending in positive results.

Eclectic therapy. There are many well-defined schools of psychotherapy each with an organizing philosophy, procedures, and therapeutic techniques. A therapist that uses "eclectic therapy" combines various techniques of "pure schools of thought" to create an eclectic way of doing therapy. Different therapeutic schools have strengths and weaknesses that proper blending of technique may be able to even out.

Family systems. Family systems therapists focus on how an individual patient exists and has existed within the social group that they associated with (i.e., the family being a primary social group). They focus on the concept that no individual's problems can be made sense of without also looking at how these problems fit into the larger scheme of their family system, the family system being the complex arrangement of relationships within one's family. Family systems therapists believe that only by addressing the problems within the family system can the individual problems and behaviors be solved. Marriage and family therapists (MFT) often use these techniques.

Gestalt therapy. Gestalt therapy uses a humanistic approach to psychotherapy. The approach proceeds from the idea that people are born to be spontaneous and whole in their beings but lose this awareness over time as they interact with others (and experience shame, guilt, etc.). The result of this loss of wholeness is a perception of the self as split (into mind and body, self and other, thinking and feeling, etc.). The Gestalt therapist works with his or her client to get back to a more holistic state of being. To do this the therapist frequently bypasses rational thinking processes and makes direct emotional appeals to the client who otherwise would be cut off from those emotions. One famous technique for doing this is called the "empty chair" (Reference: Mark Dombeck, Ph.D., January 1, 2000. Collection: Mental Health).

Psychoanalysis. Therapy based on the concept that mental health problems are a result of past conflicts which patients have pushed into the unconscious. The therapist meets three to five times a week with the patient to help identify and resolve the patient's past conflicts that have given rise to their current mental health issues.

Psychodynamic. Based on the principles of psychoanalysis, this therapy is less intense. This type of therapy is generally provided once or twice a week over a shorter time span. This type of therapy is based on the premise that human behavior is determined by one's past experiences, biological/genetic components, and one's current reality. It recognizes the significant effects that emotions and unconscious motivations can have on one's mental state and human behavior.

Section 36.3

Questions to Ask When Considering Treatment Options

"Questions to Ask When Considering Treatment Options" © 2005 National Eating Disorders Association. For more information, visit www.National EatingDisorders.org. Reviewed by David A. Cooke, M.D., FACP, October 2010.

There are many differing approaches to the treatment of eating disorders. No one approach is considered superior for everyone, however, it is important to find an option that is most effective for your needs. The following is a list of questions you might want to ask when contacting eating disorder support services. These questions apply to an individual therapist, treatment facility, other eating disorder support services, or any combination of treatment options.

1. What is your experience and how long have you been treating eating disorders?

2. How are you licensed? What are your training credentials? Do you belong to the Academy for Eating Disorders (AED)? AED is a professional group that offers its members educational training every year. This doesn't prove that individuals are up-to date, but it does increase the chances.

3. What is your treatment style? Please note that there are many different types of treatment styles available. Different approaches to treatment may be more or less appropriate for you dependent upon your individual situation and needs.

4. Do you or your facility have a quality improvement program in place or regularly assess the outcome of the treatment provided?

5. Are you familiar with either the American Psychological Association (APA) guidelines or Britain's National Institute for Health and Clinical Excellence (NICE) criteria for the treatment of eating disorders?

6. What kind of evaluation process will be used in recommending a treatment plan?

7. What kind of medical information do you need? Will I need a medical evaluation before entering the program?

8. What is your appointment availability? Do you offer after-work or early morning appointments? How long do the appointments last? How often will we meet?

9. How long will the treatment process take? When will we know it's time to stop treatment?

10. Are you reimbursable by my insurance? What if I don't have insurance or mental health benefits under my health care plan? It is important for you to research your insurance coverage policy and what treatment alternatives are available in order for you and your treatment provider to design a treatment plan that suits your coverage.

11. Ask the facility to send information brochures, treatment plans, treatment prices, etc. The more information the facility is able to send in writing, the better informed you will be.

With a careful search, the provider you select will be helpful. But, if the first time you meet with him or her is awkward, don't be discouraged. The first few appointments with any treatment provider are often challenging. It takes time to build up trust in someone with whom you are sharing highly personal information. If you continue to feel that you need a different therapeutic environment, you may need to consider other providers.

Section 36.4

Encountering Treatment Resistance

It is very common, indeed it is one of the hallmarks of the illness, that patients resist treatment. Parents and family members often find themselves arguing with the patient trying to convince him or her of the seriousness or the facts of the illness. While friends and families see an illness causing damage and pain often the patient remains convinced the situation is under control. Patients often hide symptoms and trick family and even doctors into believing things are better than they are. This is especially frustrating when the patient is able to maintain other parts of life, like work and athletics and academics, at a high level at the same time believing one can ingest calories from smells or that food is unnecessary.

It is very important that families know that eating disorder patients are often "anosognosic." They are blocked in their own minds from seeing the gravity of the illness or the risk of the behaviors. This is a condition similar to that found in certain brain injuries, but is reversible. With full nutrition and normalized eating and behaviors the patient can regain self-awareness and engage in therapy and learning that nurture insight and motivation.

Regardless of age, families should not delay treatment while waiting for insight or motivation, or settle for treatment that only addresses insight and motivation without also including medical treatment and restoration. Whether the patient is able to understand or not, the family can do everything possible to facilitate treatment. In other words, the level of resistance ought not guide treatment decisions.

Families should be aware that resistance to treatment can come in many forms including hiding food, faking weights, self-harm, verbal and physical attacks on caregivers, false or distorted stories to authorities, threats of suicide and self-harm, actual suicide and self-harm. Keeping patients and other family members safe while refusing to enable eating disorder behavior is the highest priority during eating disorder recovery. Patients and siblings need to know that the anxiety and resistance of the patient will neither delay care nor will it be allowed to harm anyone. As difficult as recovery is, delayed recovery is harder. Although early intervention and firm boundaries in the home can be enough to contain resistance it may also be necessary to use inpatient care when situations arise that the family cannot handle safely at home. The time a patient is hospitalized is an opportunity for the family to create safe boundaries for after discharge.

"Some patients lash outward during the necessary anguish of recovery, some suffer invisibly, but the pain is there. When parents and caregivers react with anger, or with avoidance, we can inadvertently aid the illness. Our confident, optimistic, firm support is so important in helping our children feel safe," says Laura Collins, F.E.A.S.T. executive director.

One tool for families to use when trying to understand eating disorders is to "separate the illness from the patient." This concept has many names, including "narrative" therapy and "externalization," and can be very helpful to caregivers. By seeing the actions and reactions of the patient as belonging to "ED" or "the illness," the parent can be freed from anger at the loved one and ally with the patient being held hostage and out of sight by this malignant condition. Anger, frustration, bargaining, arguing, moral pressure, fear: all of these may be set aside when a parent knows they are not dealing with the loved one directly, but through the illness. The love a parent feels, as well as the optimism, need not be dependent on a loving or insightful response. By not taking the resistance, anger, and desperation of the patient personally, a caregiver is also free to make decisions based on the patient's needs and not his or her words.

Chapter 37

Determining the Type of Treatment Needed

Chapter Contents

Section 37.1

Levels of Care

Levels of Care

Please note: Eating disorders develop in men, women, girls, and boys. For ease in reading, we have used "she" and "her" in the text below.

The term "level of care" refers to the intensity of services provided by a treatment setting. Which level of care is appropriate for a patient is determined at the time of her initial diagnosis and subsequently whenever a change in her condition may warrant a transition to a different level. Settings include acute care hospitalization, residential care, partial hospitalization, and various intensities of outpatient treatment. Many individuals need time in more than one level of care.

In evaluating what treatment setting will best meet the patient's needs, a number of factors are considered:

- Is she medically stable?

- How severe are her abnormal eating behaviors?

- What is her psychological status? Does she have psychiatric problems that co-exist with her eating disorder?

- How well does she function at school or work and in other activities?

- How motivated is she to recover from her disorder?

- Is there a treatment program in her geographic area that will meet her needs?

- Does she have health insurance?

- Does the insurance cover treatment for an eating disorder?

Continuity of Care

As an individual improves, a less intensive level of care may become appropriate. For example, it is not unusual for a treatment team to recommend that a patient attend partial hospitalization following her discharge from a residential treatment center. Going to a less structured setting can be stressful for an individual, perhaps making her vulnerable to a setback. The change becomes all the harder if she will have one or more new providers. If it is not feasible for a patient to keep the same clinicians when she changes level of care, it is important for her discharge team to ease her transition by communicating with her new providers and by arranging for her to meet them.

Acute Care Hospitalization

Inpatient treatment is appropriate when a patient's safety is at risk:

- Heart rate: Less than 40 beats per minute (b.p.m.) for adults. For children and adolescents, less than 50 b.p.m. during the day and less than 45 b.p.m. at night.

- Blood pressure: Less than 90/60 mmHg for adults and less than 80/50 mmHg for children and adolescents.

- Orthostatic blood pressure changes: Greater than 20 b.p.m. rise in heart rate or greater than 10 mmHg fall in blood pressure.

- Body temperature: Less than 97 degrees Fahrenheit.

- Dehydration.

- Electrolyte imbalance.

- Severe depression, suicidality.

- Weight : Less than 85 percent of healthy body weight generally. Rapid weight loss may indicate hospitalization even if weight is not less than 85 percent.

- A rapid weight drop in an adolescent or child with an eating disorder may be an indication for hospitalization even if the amount of weight lost is not extreme. Children who do not take in enough food or fluid are quite vulnerable to dehydration and—in comparison to adult patients—may be at risk of medical compromise from a proportionately smaller decline in weight.

- Patient cannot modify abnormal eating habits without staff support during and after meals. Severe, frequent purging may necessitate hospitalization even if lab tests show no significant problems.

Inpatient Services

Inpatient care, which generally lasts from several days to a couple of months, focuses on medical monitoring and management of complications resulting from the eating disorder. Whether the patient is admitted to a medical or psychiatric unit is highly individualized. Based on the results of periodic laboratory testing, intravenous fluids may be needed to stabilize the patient's electrolytes.

Inpatients who are underweight work with a registered dietitian to restore their nutritional health. Many have pursued thinness at all cost and feel unduly anxious about ingesting foods that they consider "unsafe." A key component of hospital programs is positive reinforcement for progress toward healthy behaviors. One-on-one psychotherapy offers the patient empathy and helps motivate her to participate in her program. Nursing staff is instrumental in supporting and encouraging individuals during meals and snacks. Some hospital units provide group therapy sessions, giving patients opportunities to share their feelings with each other and with staff. Family education support groups are often available as well.

Discharge planning is based not on weight status alone, but rather on a combination of variables, including how motivated the patient is to follow her nutrition program. Individuals discharged to outpatient care after gaining weight in the hospital may be at risk of relapse if they have not made emotional progress in support of recovery.

Residential Care

Residential care is appropriate for patients who are not in dire medical straits but require the support and supervision of a twenty-four-hour program in order to reduce their abnormal eating behaviors. Most residential facilities have a comfortable, informal feel rather than the less personal atmosphere of a hospital. Many patients entering residential centers weigh less than 85 percent of what their doctors recommend—although individuals of all weights may require residential care—and struggle with unwelcome, relentless thoughts about food or body size. Treatment plans include medical monitoring and are tailored to meet each resident's needs. Nursing staff provides support during meals and snacks.

Residents participate in individual and family therapy as well as in a variety of groups that are designed to help them manage their unhealthy thoughts, feelings, and behaviors. Led by mental health professionals, these group meetings focus on topics such as relaxation techniques, assertiveness training, peer relationships, family life, self- and body-acceptance, coping with change, or handling free time. In addition, many residential and hospital programs bring in registered arts therapists to run groups in drawing, painting, sculpture, music, dance, or drama. For adolescent patients who are missing a number of days of middle or high school, residential facilities often offer academic curricula.

Length of stay in residential care varies from a month to a year or longer, though thirty to sixty days is most common. Most patients make progress but may not recover from their eating disorders during residential treatment and thus need well-planned aftercare either in partial hospitalization or in an intensive outpatient program; which of these two follow-up settings is appropriate depends upon the patient's level of improvement, what services will now meet her needs, geographic factors, and insurance considerations.

Partial Hospitalization

Partial hospitalization, also called day treatment, is suitable for patients who do not require twenty-four-hour care but are not ready for outpatient programs. Individuals entering this level of care may be quite absorbed in negative thoughts about calories or weight and need structure in their day in order to refrain from unhealthy behaviors. Partial hospitalization programs, which are often part of an inpatient or residential facility, consist of up to eight hours of structured activities, including support and encouragement during meals and snacks. Individuals commute to treatment from home or perhaps from transitional housing units affiliated with a residential center. In recommending partial hospitalization, the physician considers how many days a week the patient needs to attend in order to derive optimal benefit.

For an individual to make good use of partial hospitalization, she needs to be able to participate in groups, which constitute a major part of the program. Led by mental health professionals, these group discussions focus on topics such as women's or men's issues, adjusting to change, relaxation methods, family or peer relationships, expressing feelings, managing free time, and body appreciation. Arts-based therapies and instruction in meal planning, cooking, and grocery shopping may also be available. Participation in some groups is shared with individuals on the inpatient unit.

Patients who attend day treatment also have appointments with various members of their treatment team, which is likely to include an individual or family therapist, a primary care physician, and a nutrition counselor. Collaboration among treatment providers is essential. Time spent at the partial hospitalization level ranges from a week to a few months. Having made progress in day treatment, an individual is generally well enough for intensive outpatient or outpatient care.

Outpatient Treatment

Intensive outpatient treatment is appropriate for individuals who need some structure from health professionals in order to refrain from abnormal behaviors and work toward feeling more at peace with themselves. As an example of intensive outpatient treatment, evening programs offering supervised dinner followed by group therapy are often helpful to those who work or go to school during the day. In addition to attending a structured program, the individual in intensive outpatient care meets with the various members of her treatment team, which may include a psychotherapist, a psychopharmacologist, a primary care physician, and a registered dietician.

Generally, individuals stay at the intensive outpatient level for a couple of weeks to a few months. As they move beyond the need for staff support during meals and snacks, they will continue to require management and monitoring on an outpatient basis. With further progress, they can begin to meet with the members of their professional team less frequently. Some individuals with anorexia nervosa may need outpatient psychotherapy for years.

References

American Psychiatric Association (APA). *Practice guideline for the treatment of patients with eating disorders*. 3rd ed. Washington (DC): American Psychiatric Association; 2006 Jun. 128 p. [765 references].

Berman, M.I., Boutelle, K.N., Crow, S.J. A case series investigating acceptance and commitment therapy as a treatment for previously treated, unremitted patients with anorexia nervosa. *European Eating Disorders Review*. (In press).

Bewell, C.V., Carter, J.C. Readiness to change mediates the impact of eating disorder symptomatology on treatment outcome in anorexia nervosa. *International Journal of Eating Disorders*. 2008; 41: 368–71.

Bowers, W.A., Ansher, L.S. The effectiveness of cognitive behavioral therapy on changing eating disorder symptoms and psychopathology of 32 anorexia nervosa patients at hospital discharge and one year follow-up. *Annals of Clinical Psychiatry*. 2008; 20: 79–86.

Crow, S., Peterson, C.B. Refining treatments for eating disorders. *American Journal of Psychiatry*. 2009; 166: 266–67.

Crow, S., Peterson, C.B., Swanson, S.A., Raymond, N.C., Specker, S., Eckert, E.D., Mitchell, J.E. Increased mortality in bulimia nervosa and other eating disorders. *American Journal of Psychiatry*. (In press).

De Young, K.P., Anderson, D.A. Prevalence and correlates of exercise motivated by negative affect. *International Journal of Eating Disorders*. (In press).

DiVasta, A.D., Feldman, H.A., Quach, A.E., Balestrino, M., Gordon, C.M. The effect of bed rest on bone turnover in young women hospitalized for anorexia nervosa: a pilot study. *Journal of Clinical Endocrinology and Metabolism*. 2009; 94: 1650–55.

Doyle, P.M., le Grange, D., Loeb, K., Doyle, A.C., Crosby, R.D. Early response to family-based treatment for adolescent anorexia nervosa. *International Journal of Eating Disorders*. (In press).

Exterkate, C.C., Vriesendorp, P.F., de Jong, C.A. Body attitudes in patients with eating disorders at presentation and completion of intensive outpatient day treatment. *Eating Behaviors*. 2009; 10: 16–21.

Fittig, E., Jacobi, C., Backmund, H., Gerlinghoff, M., Wittchen, H.U. Effectiveness of day hospital treatment for anorexia nervosa and bulimia nervosa. *European Eating Disorders Review*. 2008; 16: 341–51.

Frisch, M.J., Franko, D.L., Herzog, D.B. Residential treatment for eating disorders. *International Journal of Eating Disorders*. 2006; 39: 434–42.

Frisch, M.J., Franko, D.L., Herzog, D.B. Arts-based therapies in the treatment of eating disorders. *Eating Disorders*. 2006; 14: 131–42.

Greenfield, Lauren. *Thin*. New York: Chronicle Books, 2006.

Halmi, K.A. Salient components of a comprehensive service for eating disorders. *World Psychiatry*. 2009; 8: 150–55.

Hay, P.P., Bacaltchuk, J., Stefano, S., Kashyap, P. Psychological treatments for bulimia nervosa and binging. *Cochrane Database of Systematic Reviews*. 2009; 7: CD000562.

Herpertz-Dahlmann, B., Salbach-Andrae, H. Overview of treatment modalities in adolescent anorexia nervosa. *Child and Adolescent Psychiatric Clinics of North America*. 2009; 18: 131–45.

Jones, A., Bamford, B., Ford, H., Schreiber-Kounine, C. How important are motivation and initial Body Mass Index for outcome in day therapy services for eating disorders? *European Eating Disorders Review*. 2007; 15: 283–89.

Kaplan, A.S., Walsh, B.T., Olmsted, M., Attia, E., Carter, J.C., Devlin, M.J., Pike, K.M., Woodside, B., Rockert, W., Roberto, C.A., Parides, M. The slippery slope: prediction of successful weight maintenance in anorexia nervosa. *Psychological Medicine*. 2009; 39: 1037–45.

Lavender, J.M., Jardin, B.F., Anderson, D.A. Bulimic symptoms in undergraduate men and women: Contributions of mindfulness and thought suppression. *Eating Behaviors*. 2009; 10: 228–31.

Masson, P.C., Sheeshka, J.D. Clinicians' perspectives on the premature termination of treatment in patients with eating disorders. *Eating Disorders*. 2009; 17: 109–25.

McHugh, M.D. Readiness for change and short-term outcomes of female adolescents in residential treatment for anorexia nervosa. *International Journal of Eating Disorders*. 2007; 40: 602–12.

Mond, J.M., Calogero, R.M., Anderson, D.A. Excessive exercise in eating disorder patients and in healthy women. *Australian and New Zealand Journal of Psychiatry*. 2009; 43: 227–34.

Pretorius, N., Arcelus, J., Beecham, J., Dawson, H., Doherty, F., Eisler, I., Gallagher, C., Gowers, S., Isaacs, G., Johnson-Sabine, E., Jones, A., Newell, C., Morris, J., Richards, L., Ringwood, S., Rowlands, L., Simic, M., Treasure, J., Waller, G., Williams, C., Yi, I., Yoshioka, M., Schmidt, U. Cognitive-behavioural therapy for adolescents with bulimic symptomatology: the acceptability and effectiveness of internet-based delivery. *Behaviour Research and Therapy*. 2009; 47: 729–36.

Roehrig, J.P., McLean, C.P. A comparison of stigma toward eating disorders versus depression. *International Journal of Eating Disorders*. (In press).

Rothschild, L., Lacoua, L., Stein, D. Changes in implicit and explicit measures of ego functions and distress among two eating disorder subgroups: outcomes of integrative treatment. *Eating Disorders*. 2009; 17: 242–59.

Schaffner, A.D., Buchanan, L.P. Integrating evidence-based treatments with individual needs in an outpatient facility for eating disorders. *Eating Disorders*. 2008; 16: 378–92.

Schmidt, U. Cognitive behavioral approaches in adolescent anorexia and bulimia nervosa. *Child and Adolescent Psychiatric Clinics of North America*. 2009; 18: 147–58.

Slane, J.D., Burt, S.A., Klump, K.L. The road less traveled: Associations between externalizing behaviors and eating pathology. *International Journal of Eating Disorders*. (In press).

Strik Lievers, L., Curt, F., Wallier, J., Perdereau, F., Rein, Z., Jeammet, P., Godart, N. Predictive factors of length of inpatient treatment in anorexia nervosa. *European Child & Adolescent Psychiatry*. 2009; 18: 75–84.

Treasure, J., Sepulveda, A.R., MacDonald, P., Whitaker, W., Lopez, C., Zabala, M., Kyriacou, O., Todd, G. The assessment of the family of people with eating disorders. *European Eating Disorders Review*. 2008; 16: 247–55.

Treat, T.A., McCabe, E.B., Gaskill, J.A., Marcus, M.D. Treatment of anorexia nervosa in a specialty care continuum. *International Journal of Eating Disorders America*. 2008; 41: 564–72.

Wade, T.D., Frayne, A., Edwards, S.A., Robertson, T., Gilchrist, P. Motivational change in an inpatient anorexia nervosa population and implications for treatment. *Australian and New Zealand Journal of Psychiatry*. 2009; 43: 235–43.

Wallier, J., Vibert, S., Berthoz, S., Huas, C., Hubert, T., Godart, N. Dropout from inpatient treatment for anorexia nervosa: Critical review of the literature. *International Journal of Eating Disorders*. (In press).

Weltzin, T., Cornella-Carlson, T., Weisensel, N., Timmel, P., Hallinan, P., Bean P. The combined presence of obsessive compulsive behaviors in males and females with eating disorders account for longer lengths of stay and more severe eating disorder symptoms. *Eating and Weight Disorders*. 2007; 12: 176–82.

Zaitsoff, S.L., Taylor, A. Factors related to motivation for change in adolescents with eating disorders. *European Eating Disorders Review*. 2009; 17: 227–33.

Zeeck, A., Weber, S., Sandholz, A., Wetzler-Burmeister, E., Wirsching, M., Hartmann A. Inpatient versus day clinic treatment for bulimia nervosa: a randomized trial. *Psychotherapy and Psychosomatics*. 2009; 78: 152–60.

Section 37.2

Types of Therapy

"A Brief Overview of Therapies Used in the Treatment of Eating Disorders: A Consumer's Guide," by Patricia Santucci, M.D. © 2008 National Association of Anorexia Nervosa and Associated Disorders (www.anad.org). Reprinted with permission.

There are over four hundred schools of psychotherapy, each claiming a distinct theory and set of treatment techniques. Psychodynamic and cognitive-behavioral therapies probably represent the most widely used.

There is no one definitive form of therapy recommended for eating disorders. Often the therapist will evaluate where the patient is. Some individuals may be very knowledgeable and have had experience with some intervention. For others, therapy is a totally new experience.

Most often a supportive psycho-educational format launches the process. Most therapists will either combine or progress to a cognitive-behavioral or psychodynamic approach. A variety of professionals may collaborate to make sure that medical, dental, and nutritional components are addressed. If this sounds pretty complex, you are correct. Now just to add confusion to the entire picture, assume all these therapies can be done in individual, group, family, couples, and maybe even via the internet! Don't panic. That's why there are professionals out there to help sort out what will work for you.

There are several treatments that hold promise and should be strongly considered. But who gets what and why? Many therapists will take an eclectic approach and combine different forms of therapy in order to develop your treatment plan. Some will work together with a treatment team with professionals providing an area of specialization, such as medication, nutritional counseling, family, or group therapy. Your therapist, however, may have a certain philosophy or be trained in a specific approach. Make sure you ask and understand the goals in treatment. Remember your treatment should always be individualized to meet your needs.

Above all, one of the most important things in therapy is what we call the therapeutic alliance. It's the key to any successful therapy. Some studies have suggested that this therapeutic relationship may be as important, if not more important, than the specific technique in determining outcome. People get well in many ways but one thing is for sure; the relationship of trust and mutual respect serves as a foundation for treatment. You be the judge!

Often individuals have an image in their mind regarding what happens in therapy. Below is a partial list of terms and some additional comments that might be helpful in understanding the various therapeutic approaches. This list is by no means complete or comprehensive, but it may help you be a more informed consumer in order to select an approach that fits you.

It is important to note that formal psychotherapy may be ineffective with starving patients and should not be used alone to treat severely malnourished patients. It may help the patient to become motivated and gain weight, but medical, nutritional, and supportive treatment should be initiated during this stage. Once malnutrition has been corrected and weight gain is starting to occur and the patient no longer acutely medically compromised, various forms of psychotherapy can be very helpful.

Understanding the Language

Bio-psycho-social model: Since the causes of eating disorders seem multiple, this philosophy approaches eating disorders as an interactive process which involves genetic and biological factors, psychological factors, and sociocultural and family factors. This might seem like a shotgun approach—and it is. Eating disordered patients are complex and often have serious and chronic conditions that require various treatments at different stages.

This approach often allows the therapist to bring a variety of different theories and approaches to treatment. Within this broad model, however, treatment can still vary widely. Ask if the therapist has a specific approach and whether there has been training using this approach with eating disorders.

Medical model: Mood disturbances and anxiety states are quite common in eating disorders. The need for nutritionally and medically stabilizing individuals is seen as an important first step.

In anorexia, the assessment for antidepressant medication is often done following weight gain since starvation itself can worsen the symptoms of depression. In addition, there is some evidence that medication should be considered for prevention of relapse for patients who have restored their weight or who continue to show signs of depression or obsessive compulsive problems.

In bulimia nervosa, antidepressant medications are effective for many patients as one component of the initial treatment in combination with therapy. They appear to help with some of the psychological symptoms and also directly decrease the binge/purge cycle. There are a number of other medications that may be useful in the treatment of eating disorders. One should not rely on medication alone for the treatment of eating disorders.

Cognitive behavior therapy (CBT): CBT has been used increasingly in recent years. It is a very directive and time-limited therapy. The therapist and patient work together to identify irrational beliefs and illogical thinking patterns associated with body image, weight, food, and perfectionism. There is a focus on the behavioral components of the illness such as binge eating, purging, dieting, and ritualistic exercise. Outcome studies show that CBT compares favorably with antidepressant medication and is often considered the treatment of choice for bulimics. Its short-term structure with the availability of manuals has made it a useful resource.

Psychodynamic therapy: This is based on the idea that people can achieve greater understanding of the psychological forces that motivate their actions. Insight through psychological exploration then opens up the possibility for change in personality and behavior. The assumption is that the present is shaped and governed by the past. This approach is frequently used for eating disorders when the person is at the appropriate stage to benefit from this type of intervention.

Feminist psychodynamic psychotherapy: This model is based on the assumption that social conditioning of women results in repression of certain needs and aspects. The therapist engages the patient in dialogue that encourages her to find her own truths and have her own voice. The importance of interpersonal relationships and intimacy are a focus. The therapist acts as a resource and doesn't claim to know all the answers, encouraging the open exchange of ideas and fostering the development of self.

Interpersonal therapy: This is a short-term therapy that was initially used to treat depression and modified to treat eating disorders. Individuals are taught to evaluate their interactions with others with an understanding that interpersonal conflicts may not have caused the eating disorder per se but may indeed maintain the disorder. Problem areas, other than the eating disorder, are identified and a treatment contract is formulated. The focus is here and now with less attention paid to the eating disorder behavior and symptoms.

If a patient replied in therapy that her eating was terrible, the therapist would not focus on the details of the disturbed eating behavior but rather the importance of understanding why this had happened. The patient would be asked if it could be related to one of the identified interpersonal problem areas. The expectation is that as one improves interpersonal function, there is improvement of the eating disorder.

Family therapy/marital therapy: There are a variety of approaches to family therapy. Some will view therapy as treatment *with* the family, others as treatment *of* the family. Certainly family therapy should be considered whenever possible, especially for adolescents who still live with their parents and patients still with ongoing conflicts or marital discord. Some have suggested the younger the patient the more significant the use of family therapy. In addition, if the eating disorder patient is a mother, special help should be paid to mothering skills to decrease the risk of transmitting an eating disorder.

Psychoanalysis: In its true form this is the couch therapy. Sessions are usually held four to five times a week, and a completed analysis may take three to five years. The focus is on self-understanding and correction of developmental lags so that there can be reorganization of the personality. Free association and dream analysis occur in this type of therapy. Analysis is not for everyone, being more suitable for individuals at the healthier end of the spectrum.

Focal psychoanalytic psychotherapy: This is a short-term approach where the therapist takes a nondirective approach. No advice is given regarding the eating behavior, symptoms, or problems. The focus is on the meaning of the symptoms in terms of the patient's history and experiences with his or her family.

Dialectic therapy (DBT): Although DBT is a cognitive behavioral treatment, it differs from standard CBT. There is a focus on helping patients to observe and label their emotional reactions to trauma, validation, and acquiring a balance between acceptance and change. This is a fairly new type of approach which is being modified for the treatment of bulimia and binge eating disorder. It holds promise especially for those who have experienced post-traumatic stress or exhibit chronic or severe suicidal behavior because of lack of basic skills for self-regulation.

Supportive psychotherapy: Most forms of therapy will have a supportive component. This approach is different from exploratory work because the goal is not insight—it is lessening of anxiety. Usually this is done through reassurance, advice, bolstering the individual's personal strengths, and encouraging more adaptive defenses.

Nutritional therapy: Nutritional rehabilitation and counseling often will help patients gain weight and stabilize their eating patterns. Depending on the level of training, interest, and expectations by the treatment team, the dietitian often deals with body image, education about nutrition, risk regarding the eating disorder, concerns about weight, and irrational fears related to the eating disorder. Some dietitians will shop for food, help prepare and eat meals with patients and their families.

Psycho-educational therapy: Usually this is included in most treatment so that there is understanding of the definition of the illness, why individuals develop the illness, what predisposes them and what might precipitate the illness. Nutrition, medical issues, sociocultural issues such as the drive for thinness in our society, etc. are often covered.

Addiction model: There is a high prevalence of substance abuse among persons with eating disorders and the likelihood that either condition may precipitate the other. There is much debate as to whether eating disorders are true addictions. There is also a great deal of variability from chapter to chapter and sponsor to sponsor.

The presence of a currently active substance abuse problem does have implications for treatment. Ideally, treatment which focuses concurrently on both the eating disorder and the substance disorder should be attempted in a setting where the staff is competent to treat both.

For patients with anorexia nervosa, treatment which focuses only on a narrow and zealous application of the twelve-step program, or other approaches which exclusively call for abstinence without addressing nutritional, cognitive, or behavioral problems are of concern when used as the sole approach. Many addiction programs, however, will attempt to offer a blended model incorporating the medical model and cognitive behavior therapy.

For patients with bulimia nervosa, considerable controversy exists regarding the role of the twelve-step programs or other approaches that focus exclusively on the need for abstinence when they are the only intervention and do not address nutritional, psychological, or behavioral problems.

Self-help: Self-help may be a valuable first step for treatment. The major goal is to provide support and communication between individuals who are at different stages of recovery. Sometimes family and friends are invited or they may have their own support group. Usually leaders are recovered or volunteer professionals who offer their service at a no-cost basis.

This group becomes a safe place where you can learn about the disorder, share feelings, find someone who has had similar experience, and realize that recovery is possible. With an informal structure, one can attend as needed. In addition, there are now some self-help manuals, online web sites, news groups, and chat rooms focusing on the treatment of eating disorders. In the prevention area, there is an ongoing study of an online self-help form that may help students reduce the risk of developing an eating disorder. While a substantial amount of worthwhile information and support is available, it is important to critique the content.

Expressive therapy: The expression of oneself through the arts is another form of therapy which is useful, particularly when there is difficulty of putting feelings into words. Whether it is dance, movement, art, drama, drawing, painting, etc., these avenues allow the opportunity for communication that might otherwise remain repressed.

Light therapy: Many individuals with seasonal affective disorder (SAD) also have dysfunctional eating. Recent studies have shown that light therapy has improved mood and decreased bingeing and purging. The positive effects can last for about four weeks.

Eye movement desensitization and reprocessing (EMDR): EMDR is a unique form of psychotherapy. It was originally developed in the eighties to help patients with traumatic experiences, recovering memories of past trauma, and post-traumatic stress.

Although an old adage in the eating disorders field warns, "no single treatment approach works for everyone," an interesting new treatment worth considering is developing in the eating disorders field. While traditional treatment of eating disorders has concentrated on individual psychotherapy, Christopher Dare and Ivan Eisler at Maudsley Hospital in London have developed an original family-centered approach. Instead of being criticized as a dysfunctional social unit, the family of the sufferer assumes responsibility for making the patient eat. No one is blamed for having triggered the illness; rather, the illness is treated as a medical condition and the family must care for the sick member.

This family-centered treatment progresses in three distinct phases, in which power shifts from the family back to the patient after she or he reaches an acceptable weight. The first phase focuses on empowerment and eating. The family separates the patient from her or his illness and learns strategies to successfully battle the disease. Placed in the position of a "therapeutic bind," the family is urged to take immediate

371

action, which provokes anxiety; yet this anxiety is balanced by the therapist's acceptance and expertise. Food functions as medicine in the Maudsley method, and the parents act as doctors who administer the feared remedy. For this method of re-feeding to succeed, the parents must establish an alliance and agree to enforce consistent food rules. In order for the patient not to feel like an enemy of the food-wielding parents, she or he is encouraged to turn to siblings for support.

The second phase of treatment starts when the patient complies with the parents' food guidelines and makes steady weight gain. At this point, the parents help their child assume increased responsibility for eating. According to the Maudsley model, once the patient maintains a stable weight of near 95 percent of his or her ideal weight without substantial parental supervision, the patient should begin individual therapy. At this point in their recovery, they can focus on issues and anxieties surrounding adolescence, a life phase that they have avoided by having an eating disorder. They can explore their identity and independence and learn to construct clearer family boundaries.

Despite its unconventional approach of enlisting the family as the primary player in the recovery team, the Maudsley treatment offers some definite benefits. Parents are more likely to resist food manipulation by their child, since they take on active roles in treatment and are instructed by therapists not to tolerate resistance. They are encouraged to offer incentives and support for cooperation. Moreover, since their child's life is in imminent danger, they will expend an enormous amount of energy to successfully coax their child to eat and regain health.

Despite these remarkable outcomes, there are still some crucial factors to examine. Data from Maudsley studies indicates that this treatment is less effective for older adolescents and for adults, along with chronically ill patients, and those who binge and purge. In addition, some families may not be able to put in the enormous time and effort that is required to supervise meals and settle the accompanying food battles. Another variable to consider is the enmeshed parental relationships that eating disordered patients are often involved in. The highly involved parental role in the Maudsley treatment may further exacerbate these dysfunctional patterns. The patient may also experience more difficulty in gaining a sense of autonomy following treatment.

Despite these possible drawbacks, the Maudsley therapy is now gaining popularity with researchers in the United States. Currently, psychologists at the University of Chicago, University of Michigan, Columbia University, and Stanford University are testing this treatment.

Chapter 38

Psychotherapeutic Approaches for Eating Disorders

Chapter Contents

Section 38.1

Psychotherapy and Eating Disorders

Excerpted from "Eating Disorders," © 2010 A.D.A.M., Inc.
Reprinted with permission.

Eating disorders are nearly always treated with some form of psychotherapy. Depending on the problem, different psychological approaches may work better than others.

Cognitive-Behavioral Therapy

Cognitive-behavioral therapy (CBT) works on the principle that a pattern of false thinking and belief about one's body can be recognized objectively and altered, thereby changing the response and eliminating the unhealthy reaction to food. One approach for bulimia is the following:

- Over a period of four to six months the patient builds up to eating three meals a day, including foods that the patient has previously avoided.

- During this period, the patient monitors and records the daily dietary intake along with any habitual unhealthy reactions and negative thoughts toward eating while they are occurring.

- The patient also records any relapses (binges or purging). Such lapses are reported objectively and without self-criticism and judgment.

- The patient discusses the responses with a cognitive therapist at regular sessions. Eventually the patient is able to discover the false attitudes about body image and the unattainable perfectionism that underlies the opposition to food and health.

- Once these habits are recognized, food choices are broadened, and the patient begins to challenge any entrenched and automatic ideas and responses. The patient then replaces them with a set of realistic beliefs along with actions based on reasonable self-expectations.

Interpersonal Therapy

Interpersonal therapy deals with depression or anxiety that might underlie the eating disorders along with social factors that influence eating behavior. This therapy does not deal with weight, food, or body image at all.

The goals are to:

- express feelings;

- discover how to tolerate uncertainty and change;

- develop a strong sense of individuality and independence;

- address any relevant sexual issues or traumatic or abusive event in the past that might be a contributor of the eating disorder.

Studies generally report that interpersonal therapy is not as effective as cognitive therapy for bulimia and binge eating, but may be useful for some patients with anorexia. The skill of the therapist plays a strong role in its success.

Motivational Enhancement Therapy

Motivational enhancement therapy is another form of behavioral therapy that uses an empathetic approach to help patients understand and change their behaviors concerning food. It may be offered in an individual or group setting.

Family Therapy

Because a patient's eating disorder affects the entire family, family therapy can be an important component of recovery. It can help all family members better understand the complex nature of eating disorders, improve their communication skills with one another, and teach strategies for coping with stress and negative feelings. Family-based psychotherapies are also integral parts of nutritional rehabilitation counseling programs, such as the Maudsley approach.

Section 38.2

Your Teen and Cognitive Behavior Therapy

"Your Teen and Cognitive Behavior Therapy," by Chris Haltom,
PhD. © 2010 Eating Disorder Hope (www.eatingdisorderhope.com).
Reprinted with permission.

You have probably heard of cognitive behavior therapy or CBT. Most psychotherapies for teens and adults with eating disorders receive some form of CBT as part of their treatment. Even most family work includes some form of cognitive behavior intervention. The easiest way to understand CBT for eating disorders is to consider the thoughts and behaviors that characterize eating disorders. Then think about the psychotherapy and counseling work required to challenge and change those thoughts and behaviors.

One example of CBT skills taught to those in eating disorder recovery is called "Catch it, challenge it, change it" (Remuda Ranch, 2007). This intervention or skill starts with "catching" a negative, distorted thought related to a particular situation. A typical situation a teen with an eating disorder might react to in a negative fashion is consuming a healthy, well-balanced dinner. She or he might say to her- or himself, "I have eaten dinner and now I am fat and disgusting." "Catching" this toxic thought is the first step. Developing awareness of thoughts present in the mind is a prerequisite skill. For example, someone who has developed this skill might say to themselves, "stop and look at what you are thinking right now."

It is also useful to figure out what feelings a person is experiencing when having a toxic thought. Usually, distorted eating disorder thoughts are associated with uncomfortable feelings like sadness, anger, anxiety, or self-loathing.

After "catching" a self-defeating thought or message the next step is to "challenge" the toxic thought. This is done by stating the untruth of the toxic message. Another alternative is to ask questions that either help discover the truth or help find a more a realistic replacement thought or thoughts. A challenge to the fat-because-of-dinner thought might be, "What is the truth about being fat and disgusting because of eating dinner?" In order to get started a therapist or counselor might first role model this skill by asking your teen a challenge question like "What evidence is there that you are fat and disgusting because you ate dinner?" Later teens are expected to learn to question themselves with their own challenge questions.

Finally, "changing" the thought takes the form of finding a replacement thought or alternative interpretation. It is important that the alternative thought is not pie-in-the-sky positive. The alternative thought needs to be rational, realistic, and believable to the person challenging themselves. For example, when teens tell themselves they are ugly and disgusting because of eating a meal, they often feel shame, embarrassment, and self-loathing. When they give themselves realistic alternatives such as "one meal does not cause people to change their body size or appearance" or "eating a balanced meal will support my recovery" resulting feelings are often positive and self-esteem is improved.

Parents and carers often find it helpful to understand the self-defeating thinking and behaviors their teens are struggling with. Most carers have had the exasperating experience of encountering entrenched, negative beliefs in their children, often realizing that a head-on corrective approach doesn't work. Beliefs like "mayonnaise will make me fat" or "sitting still will make me gain weight" are not so easily caught, challenged, or changed. Developing cognitive-behavior skills takes patience. It takes intentional, incremental identification and challenge of negative thoughts and behaviors unique to each teen struggling with an eating disorder.

Parents and carers often have their own cognitive-behavior retraining to perform on themselves. The incredible stress that eating disorders create in the home can lead to carers having their own negative or unrealistic thoughts. For example, in an effort to entice their child to eat, parents might buy diet foods or allow excessive exercise. This is born out of a desperate belief that these approaches will get their child to eat or stop purging. In turn, it can be hard for parents to accept new beliefs such as "consistent, balanced eating is non-negotiable" or "some foods that the media have labeled 'bad' are fine in moderation." They may find themselves challenged by the knowledge that eating disorders are illnesses, not choices on the part of a willful teen.

Teens with eating disorders may try to negotiate permission to skip or skimp on a meal, delay a meal, or substitute diet foods for regular foods. Parents learn to "catch" their temptation to yield to eating disorder thinking in their offspring. They might "challenge" themselves with the question, "Am I accommodating the disorder?" Finally, parents might "change" their thinking and behavior by saying to their teen, "I am sorry the eating disorder is giving you such a hard time—let's try to work on fighting this together."

Here are some tips for carers about catching, challenging, and changing eating disorder thoughts and behaviors:

- Distorted beliefs about food, eating, weight, and/or size are almost always part of the struggle of those with eating disorders. Read about eating disorders. Ask open-ended (not "yes" and "no") questions to your teen about their eating disorder experience. *Listen to their rev*elations about their inner thoughts

- It is usually best not to directly correct distorted perceptions. Rather, the most effective change occurs when the corrections come from the person with distorted beliefs. You can assist by supporting honest self-reflection and self-questioning.

- Sometimes teens with eating disorders will ask you to correct their toxic thoughts because they are seeking reassurance. For example, a teen might ask, "I am not getting fatter, am I ?" Be careful not to provide reassurance for this kind of obsessive, eating-disorder-driven question. Any reassurance you provide will only temporarily satisfy and will inadvertently reinforce eating disorder thoughts. Distorted thoughts about getting larger may not change until your teen is recovering. However, it is fine to empathize with the anxiety behind a question about size-reassurance or other worries your teen may have.

- Think of your own beliefs about eating disorders, nutrition, body image, weight, and recovery. Try to uncover any distorted or false beliefs, challenge them, and change them. For example, a challenge to the false belief that "It is my fault my daughter (or son) developed an eating disorder" might be "no one is to blame for eating disorders" or "it is an illness and no one caused it."

- An important part of CBT is collaboratively setting goals with both teens with eating disorders and their families. Be involved in setting goals for treatment. By doing so you will establish a strong foundation for cognitive-behavior changes that are lasting.

- As part of goal-setting, continue to provide treatment professionals with *helpful observations* of your teen's thoughts and behaviors at home. This collaborative effort with treatment team members assists in identifying key thoughts and behaviors that need addressing in treatment.

Summary

Cognitive behavior therapy interventions have been adapted for anorexia, bulimia, binge eating, and partial syndrome eating disorders in adolescents. A manualized application of CBT for adolescents with bulimia has been developed (Lock, 2005). Christopher Fairburn and his colleagues have long been providing specialized treatment protocols for those with bulimia and binge eating disorder. It is useful to understand what cognitive behavior therapy is and how it might help your child in treatment.

References

Fairburn, CG, Cooper, Z., and Shafran, R. (2003) Cognitive behavior therapy for eating disorders: a "transdiagnostic" theory and treatment. *Behavior Research and Therapy*, 41: 509–29.

Lock, J. (2005) Adjusting cognitive behavior therapy for adolescents with bulimia nervosa. *American Journal of Psychotherapy*, 59: 267–81.

Remuda Ranch (2007) Recovery skill taught to adolescent clients as part of their residential treatment: Hope skill: "Catch it, challenge it, change it," Changing negative messages.

Wonderlich, S., Mitchell, J., Zwaan, M., and Steiger, H. (2008) *Annual Review of Eating Disorders, Part 2 - 2008*, Academy of Eating Disorders. New York: Radcliffe Publishing.

Section 38.3

Family Therapy: An Overview

"Family Therapy Is Cutting Edge Treatment for a Family Disease," by Abigail H. Natenshon, MA, LCSW, GCFP, © 2010. Reprinted with permission.
Abigail H. Natenshon has been a psychotherapist specializing in eating
disorders for four decades. As the director of Eating Disorder Specialists
of Illinois: A Clinic Without Walls, she has authored two books, *When Your
Child Has an Eating Disorder: A Step-by-Step Workbook for Parents and
Caregivers* and *Doing What Works: An Integrative System for the Treatment
of Eating Disorders from Diagnosis to Recovery.* Natenshon, who is also a
Guild Certified Feldenkrais Practitioner, hosts three informative websites,
including www.empoweredparents.com, www.empoweredkidz.com, and www
.treatingeatingdisorders.com.

Eating Disorders Are Family Diseases

Eighty-seven percent of individuals afflicted with eating disorders
are children and young adults under the age of twenty. As most of these
young people reside at home, side by side with family members and
loved ones, the onset, diagnosis, treatment, and recovery of their eating
disorders can be expected to play out at kitchen tables, behind closed
doors in family bathrooms, in restaurants, and in gymnasiums:

- When young children, teens, and young adults living at home become afflicted with an eating disorder, the entire family system
  becomes affected. Parents, siblings, extended family, friends, and
  loved ones all share in the suffering.

- Unprepared as they may be, parents and family members typically become the primary diagnosticians of an eating disorder.
  Eating disorders are secretive and lethal diseases that rarely
  show themselves in the medical doctor's office. In addition, their
  presence is typically silent in laboratory tests till the latter-most
  dire stages of disease.

- The recovery process essentially happens at home, as well.
  Patients typically spend forty-five minutes a week with their
  therapist or doctor. For the rest, 24/7, children live out their recoveries at home, and within the context of daily living; and that

is as it should be. Parents, families, teachers, coaches, all need to become educated, enlightened, and supported in their efforts to support the child in recovery.

- The most complete and sustainable recoveries happen slowly, gradually, over time, incorporated as they are into daily life functions. This is fortunate in the face of the limited coverage provided through health insurance companies as compared to the duration of most eating disorder treatments.

- In research carried out at the Maudsley Hospital of London, England, there is evidence to show that family treatment is more effective than individual psychotherapy for anorexics living at home who have been ill for less than three years.

- The nature and degree of parental involvement will vary widely with the age and needs of the child, the severity of the disorder and co-occurring conditions, the skills and capacities of the parent, the family therapy skills and welcoming attitude of the treatment team, and the nature and quality of the ever-changing parent/child connection.

- The family-based nature of eating disorders is also relevant to patients who have grown beyond childhood into their adult years. No matter what our age or life stage, we remain products of the system of our family of origin. The effective involvement of family members in the individual patient's recovery from an eating disorder can only enhance the speed, effectiveness, and sustainability of the healing process.

Family Therapy Is the Most Effective Way to Treat Everyone's Needs

Parents and siblings are deeply affected by the presence of an eating disorder within the family system. The potency of the eating disorder typically drives a wedge between family members, isolating the afflicted child from loved ones at the time of his or her greatest need; separating the other siblings from parents who tend to be hyper-focused on the eating disordered child; and at times, creating conflict and guilt between husbands and wives, particularly for those who fail to achieve a "united front" in offering their parental response. Family members need a vehicle through which to understand the complexity of the disease and recovery processes, a forum to communicate their own concerns and needs to the patient and with each other, and the opportunity to learn how best to support the child and the recovery process. They need personal support and bolstering in the face of what typically tends to be an extended, convoluted, jarring, and frustrating recovery process for the entire family. Family therapy provides that vehicle.

Therapists treating eating disorders must be vigilant and respectful of the power of the family system in eradicating (or possibly sustaining) disease, tapping into the family system as a most powerful resource. The individual child's efforts to make recovery changes are facilitated and enhanced not only by a family that understands the recovery process, but by family members who are committed to making their own parallel personal changes to accommodate the needs and requirements of the changing child and family system. In instances where a child's resistance to recovery may be extreme, changes made within the wider family system can be sufficient to evoke required change in the afflicted family member. The potential for the family unit to facilitate change is far greater than the sum of its parts; children heal more completely, more sustainably, and more effectively when families are enabled to become constructively involved. Clear communication becomes enhanced, and in becoming direct, eradicates the risk for confidentially breeches and privacy rights infringements. Moreover, children who learn to function and communicate more effectively within the context of their family carry these valuable interpersonal skills into their other relationships as well, making life a healthier, happier place to be, both now and in the future.

Eating Disorder Psychotherapists Need to Embrace Parents and Families in Treatment

It is up to the eating disorder psychotherapist to "grow" the relationship between parent and child, for it is within the healthfully bonded connection that the greatest and most effective capacity for healing lies. The healing human connection in eating disorder recovery originates between patient and therapist in a quality therapeutic relationship. The therapist incorporates the willing and able parental unit into a bonding process that enhances parent/child connectedness, accompanied by increased trust, growing autonomy, and the child's increased capacity for healthy individuation and separation; but most significant of all is the patient's healthy reconnection to his or her own re-integrated self, the very benchmark of recovery, healing, and mental health.

Beware of the warnings of misguided health professionals who may imply that eating disorders are caused by parental involvement, which they consider to be controlling interference, in their children's lives. Such a professional might seek to exclude the child's parents from the psychotherapy process in order to protect patient/therapist privilege (confidentiality rights). This kind of advice might indicate a professional unaware of the unique requirements of eating disorder treatment, or the power of the family system to support the child's recovery; he or she may simply be inexperienced in this treatment specialty, unfamiliar with family systems theory, or otherwise uncomfortable treating family groups. Parents need to understand and keep in mind that the best prognosticator of healthy separation is healthy parent-child bonding and secure attachment. The best prognosticator of successful treatment is the practitioner who, in treating the individual, envisions, and is open to engaging, the wider family system as a context for cure. In instances where the patient may be resistant to, or geographically too removed from family involvement, the skilled practitioner will be able to conduct forms of family treatment "in absentia."

It is for the child-patient's therapist to role model loving limit-setting and problem-solving for parents, inspiring and enabling them to become their child's greatest resources as "most valuable players" on the treatment team. In educating and guiding parents to supersede the power of the eating disorder in restoring firm and grounded external values and guidance, parents regain the confidence and know-how they need to become "parental" once again. At the same time, they offer their child an invaluable opportunity to internalize self-regulatory controls; parents and child must both come to understand that the need for parental controls of the severely ill child is temporary, until such time as the recovered individual becomes once again capable of resuming the capacity and responsibility for his or her own self-regulation.

Taking Action

Parents need to act on the knowledge they acquire. Parental involvement may vary from providing:

- ongoing and unconditional support, day in and day out;
- nutritious meals which they prepare and sit down to eat together with the child;
- the monitoring of food intake and symptom management;
- involvement in family treatment to support the child and recovery process and to resolve underlying emotional issues that may be driving the dysfunction.

In summary, when it comes to the treatment and healing of eating disorders, simply loving one's child is not enough.

Section 38.4

Psychotherapeutic Approaches for Bulimia

Excerpted from "Eating Disorders," © 2010 A.D.A.M., Inc.
Reprinted with permission.

Some doctors recommend a stepped approach for patients with bulimia, which follow specific stages depending on the severity and response to initial treatments:

- Support groups may be helpful for patients who have mild conditions with no health consequences.

- Cognitive-behavioral therapy (CBT) along with nutritional therapy is the preferred first treatment for bulimia that does not respond to support groups.

- Drug therapy used for bulimia is typically a selective serotonin reuptake inhibitor (SSRI) antidepressant. A combination of CBT and SSRIs may be effective if CBT alone is not helpful.

Patients with bulimia rarely need hospitalization except under the following circumstances:

- Binge-purge cycles have led to anorexia.

- Drugs are needed for withdrawal from purging.

- Major depression is present.

Psychotherapeutic Approaches and Medications for Bulimia

Psychologic Therapy

Cognitive behavioral therapy (CBT) is the first line of therapy for most patients with bulimia. Interpersonal therapy may be tried if CBT fails. In interpersonal therapy (also known as "talk therapy"), therapists help patients explore how social and family relationships may affect their eating disorder.

Antidepressants

The most common antidepressants prescribed for bulimia are selective serotonin reuptake inhibitors (SSRIs) such as:

- fluoxetine (Prozac®);
- sertraline (Zoloft®);
- paroxetine (Paxil®);
- fluvoxamine (Luvox®).

Studies are mixed, however, on whether SSRIs offer an additional advantage in reducing binge eating compared to CBT. Fluoxetine has been approved for bulimia and is considered the drug of choice, although some studies suggest that other SSRIs work just as well. Other types of antidepressants, such as tricyclics, monoamine oxidase (MAO) inhibitors, and buprorion (Wellbutrin®), carry more risks of side effects than SSRIs and do not appear to be effective for treatment of bulimia.

Antidepressants may increase the risks for suicidal thoughts and actions during the first few months of treatment. In particular, adolescents and young adults should be carefully monitored during this time period for any changes in behavior.

Other Drug Therapy for Bulimia Nervosa

Topiramate

The antiepileptic drug topiramate (Topamax®) has been shown in studies to reduce bingeing and purging episodes in patients with bulimia. However, due to this drug's risk for serious side effects, topiramate should be used only if other medication has failed. In addition, because people tend to lose weight while taking topiramate, it should not be used by patients who have low or even normal body weight.

Section 38.5

Family Involvement Is Key to Helping Teens with Bulimia

Excerpted from "Family Involvement and Focused Intervention
May Be Key to Helping Teens with Bulimia," National
Institute of Mental Health, September 17, 2007.

Family-based treatment for adolescent bulimia nervosa (FBT-BN) is more effective than an individual-based therapy called supportive psychotherapy (SPT) in helping teens overcome bulimia according to a National Institute of Mental Health (NIMH)–funded study. Participants who received FBT-BN also showed faster treatment effects than those who received SPT. The study was published in the September 2007 issue of the *Archives of General Psychiatry*.

Daniel le Grange, PhD, of the University of Chicago, and colleagues randomly divided eighty teenagers with bulimia, ages twelve to nineteen, into two treatment groups, FBT-BN or SPT. FBT-BN, adapted from a similar treatment for teenagers with anorexia nervosa, first focuses on empowering parents to take action and help stop their teenager's bulimia-related behaviors, such as binge eating and purging. The treatment also tries to help parents see that the behaviors are separate from their child. Finally, FBT-BN helps the family address how bulimia affects the teenager's development.

In contrast to the family-based therapy, SPT focuses on the individual and does not specifically address the eating disorder; it was adapted from a similar treatment for adults with bulimia nervosa. SPT aims to help the affected adolescent resolve underlying problems that may have contributed to the eating disorder. The treatment also encourages patients to think about how they are affected by personal issues and what they can do about them in the future. Both groups received treatment for twenty visits over six months and were also reassessed six months following the end of treatment.

Six months after the end of treatment, sixteen of the forty-one participants (39 percent) who received FBT-BN were in remission, compared with seven of the thirty-nine people (18 percent) in the SPT treatment group. For this study, the researchers defined remission as showing no binge eating or other bulimia-related behaviors in the preceding four weeks. The participants who received FBT-BN also showed reductions in all bulimia-related behaviors by mid-treatment, earlier than people who received SPT.

Based on their findings, the researchers suggest that FBT-BN is more effective than SPT for treating adolescents with bulimia. Further study is needed to determine which component of FBT-BN was key to successful treatment, involving the family or focusing on the eating disorder.

Section 38.6

Psychological Approaches for Anorexia

Excerpted from "Eating Disorders," © 2010 A.D.A.M., Inc.
Reprinted with permission.

Psychotherapy

Family therapy is an important component of anorexia treatment, especially for children and adolescents. Adults usually begin with motivational psychotherapy that provides an empathetic setting and rewards positive efforts toward weight gain. After weight is restored, cognitive behavioral therapy techniques may be helpful.

Antidepressants

Studies have not reported benefits for treating anorexia nervosa with selective serotonin reuptake inhibitors (SSRIs), the antidepressants that are often useful for patients with bulimia. A few studies suggest that these drugs could be useful for people with anorexia nervosa who also have obsessive-compulsive disorder (OCD).

The Maudsley Approach

For adolescent and other younger patients in the early stages of anorexia nervosa, the Maudsley approach to "refeeding" may be effective. The Maudsley approach is a type of family therapy that enlists

387

the family as a central player in the patient's nutritional recovery. Parents take charge of planning and supervising all of the patient's meals and snacks. As recovery progresses, the patient gradually takes on more personal responsibility for determining when and how much to eat. Weekly family meetings and family-based counseling are also part of this therapeutic approach.

Chapter 39

Online Intervention May Be Helpful for College Women at Risk for Eating Disorders

A long-term, large-scale study has found that an internet-based intervention program may prevent some high-risk, college-age women from developing an eating disorder. The study, funded by the National Institutes of Health's (NIH) National Institute of Mental Health (NIMH), was published in the August 2006 issue of the *Archives of General Psychiatry*.

The researchers conducted a randomized, controlled trial of 480 college-age women in the San Francisco Bay area and San Diego, California, who were identified in preliminary interviews as being at risk for developing an eating disorder. The trial included an eight-week, internet-based, cognitive-behavioral intervention program called "Student Bodies," which had been shown to be effective in previous small-scale short-term studies. The intervention aimed to reduce the participants' concerns about body weight and shape, enhance body image, promote healthy eating and weight maintenance, and increase knowledge about the risks associated with eating disorders.

The online program included reading and other assignments such as keeping an online body-image journal. Participants also took part in an online discussion group, moderated by clinical psychologists. Participants were interviewed immediately following the end of the online program, and annually for up to three years thereafter to determine their attitudes toward their weight and shape, and measure the onset of any eating disorders.

"College Women at Risk for Eating Disorder May Benefit from Online Intervention," *NIH News*, National Institutes of Health, August 7, 2006. Reviewed by David A. Cooke, M.D., FACP, October 2010.

"Eating disorders are complex and particularly difficult to treat. In fact, they have one of the highest mortality rates among all mental disorders," said NIMH director Thomas Insel, M.D. "This study shows that innovative intervention can work, and offers hope to those trying to overcome these illnesses."

Over the course of a lifetime, about 0.5 to 3.7 percent of girls and women will develop anorexia nervosa, and about 1.1 to 4.2 percent will develop bulimia nervosa. About 0.5 percent of those with anorexia die each year as a result of their illness, making it one of the top psychiatric illnesses that lead to death.

Anorexia generally is characterized by a resistance to maintaining a healthy body weight, an intense fear of gaining weight, and other extreme behaviors that result in severe weight loss. People with anorexia see themselves as overweight even when they are dangerously thin. Bulimia generally is characterized by recurrent episodes of binge eating, followed by self-induced purging behaviors. People with bulimia often have normal weights, but like those with anorexia, they are intensely dissatisfied with their bodies. All eating disorders involve multiple biological, behavioral, and social factors that are not well understood.

The intervention appeared to be most successful among overweight women who had elevated body mass indexes (BMIs) of 25 or more at the start of the program. In fact, among these women in the intervention group, none developed an eating disorder after two years, while 11.9 percent of the women with comparable baseline BMIs in the control group did develop an eating disorder during the same time frame. BMI is a reliable indicator of a person's body fat by measuring his or her weight and height.

The program also appeared to help women in the San Francisco Bay area who had some symptoms of an eating disorder at the start of the program, such as self-induced vomiting; laxative, diet pill, or diuretic use; or excessive exercise. Of those in the intervention group with these characteristics, 14 percent developed an eating disorder within two years, while 30 percent of those with these characteristics in the control group developed an eating disorder during the same time frame.

The authors suggest that the intervention helped these high-risk women become less concerned about their weight and shape, while also helping them understand healthier eating and nutrition practices.

"This is the first study to show that eating disorders can be prevented among high-risk groups," said lead author C. Barr Taylor, M.D., of Stanford University. "The study also provides evidence that elevated weight and shape concerns are causal risk factors for developing an eating disorder," he added.

The study suggests that relatively inexpensive options such as internet-based interventions can have lasting effects on women at high risk of developing an eating disorder. However, the authors note that the results cannot be generalized widely because there were differences in the women's baseline characteristics and treatment responses between the two sites used in the study.

Also, the rate at which the women stuck with the program was very high—nearly 80 percent of the online program's web pages were read—suggesting that the participants were unusually motivated. "Women who are less motivated may be less likely to participate in or stick with this type of long-term intervention," added Taylor.

In addition, women with restricted or no access to computers would not be able to benefit from an online intervention program. However, the authors conclude that such internet-based programs may be a good first step in a diligent program designed to screen women for potential eating disorder risks.

Chapter 40

Pharmacotherapy: Medications for Eating Disorders

Please note: Eating disorders develop in men, women, girls, and boys. For ease in reading, we have used "she" and "her" in the text below.

Treatment for an eating disorder generally includes primary care, nutrition counseling, psychotherapy, and medication. An individual's primary care physician or psychopharmacologist evaluates what kind and dosage of medication is appropriate for her. Although no known medication is a cure-all for eating disorders, several drugs have emerged as helpful to individuals with these illnesses. In fact, many of the medications traditionally prescribed to relieve the symptoms of anxiety and depression are now used to treat eating disorders.

For individuals with bulimia nervosa, the choice is generally a type of antidepressant called a selective serotonin reuptake inhibitor (SSRI). Often prescribed in combination with psychotherapy, SSRIs are better tolerated and generate fewer side effects than the "older" antidepressants (tricyclic antidepressants and monoamine oxidase inhibitors [MAOIs]). Prozac® (fluoxetine), the only medication approved by the U.S. Food and Drug Administration for the treatment of bulimia nervosa, is an SSRI. So are Lexapro® (escitalopram), Luvox® (fluvoxamine), Paxil® (paroxetine), and Zoloft® (sertraline). Patients start on a low dose, which is increased gradually, as tolerated. SSRIs generally take up to six weeks to become effective, so individuals should not expect improvement immediately.

"Pharmacotherapy," © 2010 Harris Center for Education and Advocacy in Eating Disorders at Massachusetts General Hospital (http://www.massgeneral .org/harriscenter). Reprinted with permission. All rights reserved.

SSRIs are valuable not only for their potentially positive effects on the mood problems and anxiety that often accompany bulimia nervosa but also because they tend to help relieve the urge to binge eat. Complex and not well understood, the mechanisms through which SSRIs reduce binge eating are a topic of ongoing research. Located near the pituitary gland toward the base of the brain, the hypothalamus is a structure that regulates a number of functions, including appetite and weight. Key to this regulatory activity are neurotransmitters, so named because they transmit information from one neuron (brain cell) to another. The chemicals norepinephrine and dopamine are neurotransmitters; another is serotonin, which manages mood, anxiety, and satiety (the sense that one has eaten enough) and is probably dysregulated in eating disorder sufferers.

The last decade has seen the development of new antidepressants that can be helpful in the treatment of eating disorders. One of these is Effexor® (venlafaxine), which blocks the reuptake of serotonin and norepinephrine. Others include tetracyclic compounds such as Ludiomil® (maprotiline—blocks norepinephrine reuptake) and Remeron® (mirtazapine—may enhance noradrenergic and specific serotonergic activity). Sometimes it is necessary for a patient to try several antidepressants or dosages before finding one that is therapeutic.

In 2004, amid concerns that antidepressants increase the risk of suicide in children and adolescents, the U.S. Food and Drug Administration issued a "black box warning" advising clinicians that young patients on these medications needed close monitoring. Subsequently, a major review of many studies revealed that the risk of suicidal thoughts and behaviors among children and adolescents on antidepressants is much lower than originally thought. The prescribing physician provides education about the safety and potential benefits of antidepressants so that young patients and their parents can make thoughtful, informed decisions.

For the treatment of binge eating disorder (BED), antidepressants often improve mood and help with binge suppression, but don't necessarily lead to weight loss. Several other medications are now under study for use with this disorder, and early results sound promising. One is Meridia® (sibutramine), an appetite suppressant belonging to a new family of medications approved by the U.S. Food and Drug Administration for the treatment of obesity. Testing of sibutramine as a possible medication for BED has demonstrated decreases in binge eating, body weight, and depression. Also under investigation is the specific norepinephrine reuptake inhibitor Strattera® (atomoxetine), which is used for the treatment of attention-deficit hyperactivity disorder. A short-term trial of Strattera in patients with BED resulted in lower body weight and less binge eating. A third potential medication for BED is the anticonvulsant drug Topamax® (topiramate), which can reduce the frequency of binge eating and promote weight loss and may also be useful for patients with bulimia nervosa. Some patients with BED need to try a series of medications in order to determine what is most effective.

Many individuals with anorexia nervosa are treated with antidepressants and seem to tolerate them well. Although SSRIs tend to ease the anxiety, low mood, and obsessive-compulsive thinking that go along with this illness, they do not lead to weight gain or keep patients who have gained weight in the hospital from relapsing post-discharge.

For those with severe anorexia nervosa who continue to deny that they have a problem, medications such as Zyprexa® (olanzapine) can be helpful. Originally formulated for the treatment of schizophrenia, these atypical antipsychotic drugs are likely to allay the relentless obsessions, compulsions, and agitation that often occur in anorexia nervosa and may permit some weight gain.

Benzodiazepines such as Ativan® (lorazepam) or Klonopin® (clonazepam) can help quell the anxiety that is frequently experienced in eating disorders. A number of patients benefit from the combined use of a benzodiazepine and an SSRI. Ativan is short acting compared to some SSRIs and can be useful right before meals to increase an individual's ability to take in food.

BuSpar® (buspirone) is an anti-anxiety medication that differs chemically from the benzodiazepines and tends to be less sedating. It takes about two to four weeks for this medication to become effective. Buspar can be therapeutic to individuals with eating disorders who struggle not only with anxiety but also with depression. Sometimes Buspar is prescribed in combination with an SSRI.

For eating disorder sufferers who do not find antidepressants helpful there is the anticonvulsive medication Neurontin® (gabapentin), which exerts a therapeutic effect on anxiety and mood. Neurontin can be taken in conjunction with an SSRI.

Continued research into the genetics of eating disorders and into the biology of neurotransmitters is paving the way for the development of new medications for the treatment of these illnesses. Building on current knowledge, further studies are likely to enhance the ability of clinicians to predict which patients will respond to (which) antidepressants. In addition, research is underway to determine how to best use medication in conjunction with psychotherapy.

References

Bissada, H., Tasca, G.A., Barber, A.M., Bradwejn, J. Olanzapine in the treatment of low body weight and obsessive thinking in women with anorexia nervosa: a randomized, double-blind, placebo-controlled trial. *American Journal of Psychiatry.* 2008; 165: 1281–88.

Bridge, J.A., Iyengar, S., Salary, C.B., Barbe, R.P., Birmaher, B., Pincus, H.A., Ren, L., Brent, A. Clinical response and risk for reported suicidal ideation and suicide attempts in pediatric antidepressant treatment: a meta-analysis of randomized controlled trials. *Journal of the American Medical Association.* 2007; 297: 1683–96.

Capasso, A., Petrella, C., Milano, W. Pharmacological profile of SSRIs and SNRIs in the treatment of eating disorders. *Current Clinical Pharmacology.* 2009; 4: 78–83.

McElroy, S.L., Guerdjikova, A., Kotwal, R., Welge, J.A., Nelson, E.B., Lake, K.A., Keck, P.E., Jr., Hudson, J.I. Atomoxetine in the treatment of binge-eating disorder: a randomized placebo-controlled trial. *Journal of Clinical Psychiatry.* 2007; 68: 390–98.

McElroy, S.L., Guerdjikova, A.I., Martens, B., Keck, P.E. Jr., Pope, H.G., Hudson, J.I. Role of antiepileptic drugs in the management of eating disorders. *CNS Drugs.* 2009; 23: 139–56.

Powers PS, Bruty H. Pharmacotherapy for eating disorders and obesity. *Child and Adolescent Psychiatric Clinics of North America.* 2009; 18: 175–87.

Reinblatt, S.P., Redgrave, G.W., Guarda, A.S. Medication management of pediatric eating disorders. *International Review of Psychiatry.* 2008; 20: 183–88.

Walsh, T., Kaplan, A., Attia, E., Olmstead, M., Parides, M., Carter, J., Pike, M., Devlin, M., Woodside, B., Roberto, C., Rockert, W. Fluoxetine after weight restoration in anorexia nervosa. *Journal of the American Medical Association.* 2006; 295: 2605–12.

Wilfley, D.E., Crow, S.J., Hudson, J.I., Mitchell, J.E., Berkowitz, R.I., Blakesley, V., Walsh, B.T; Sibutramine Binge Eating Disorder Research Group. Efficacy of sibutramine for the treatment of binge eating disorder: a randomized multicenter placebo-controlled double-blind study. *American Journal of Psychiatry.* 2008; 165: 51–58.

Chapter 41

Nutritional Support: A Key Component of Eating Disorders Treatment

Please note: Eating disorders develop in men, women, girls, and boys. For ease in reading, we have used "she" and "her" in the text below.

Available in hospital, residential, and outpatient settings, nutritional support is a key part of eating disorders treatment and is generally the province of the registered dietician, in collaboration with the medical physician and psychotherapist. Nutrition counseling is generally provided on a one-to-one basis, and the frequency of meetings varies based on patient need.

Ambivalence about engaging in treatment is common among eating disorder sufferers and ranges in intensity. The individual with anorexia nervosa, bulimia nervosa, or eating disorders not otherwise specified (EDNOS) typically dislikes having abnormal eating behaviors but is afraid to give them up. She is apt to approach nutrition counseling cautiously, perhaps insisting that she is already knowledgeable about healthy eating and doesn't need to see a dietician. Yet there is more to learn from nutrition counseling than patients initially realize. Although information about the basic food groups is included, so are meal planning and the kinds of support and perspective that foster healthier, more realistic attitudes about food and weight. A positive rapport with a dietician can be instrumental in an individual's journey to health.

First, the dietician obtains information from the patient and often, from her family. How long has she been attempting to lose weight? What specific foods is she eating? Is she a vegetarian? Does she engage in purging behaviors? Which kind(s) and how often? Is she involved in sports and other physical activities? How frequent and intense are her workouts? For the patient who is severely underweight, nutritional restoration is urgent in order to prevent or correct medical complications. Using growth charts where applicable and communicating with the other professionals on the team, the dietician establishes a healthy weight range for the individual and sets out to help her reach it.

Central to nutrition counseling is the theme of eating balanced meals, which means drawing from all of the food groups. Healthy eating pyramids can serve as guides to planning daily meals. In learning about the roles of proteins, carbohydrates, and fats the individual begins to appreciate why an adequate intake of all these components is essential for fuel and health. Chances are the underweight individual has had trouble seeing her needs for food realistically. Thus, the dietician talks about energy expenditure as it relates to nutrition and weight, explaining that the patient's intake of nutrients is below the recommended levels. And just as the heart, lungs, kidneys, and liver require a baseline level of nutrition in order to function efficiently, so too does the brain. Such topics can lead to valuable dietician-patient discussion about physical and psychological changes associated with starvation.

Genes, the dietician emphasizes, play an important role in determining size and shape. The body is healthiest in its genetically programmed weight range (also called set-point weight) and strives to stay there. Eating habits and exercise do impact weight but to a much lower degree than many people realize. An underfed body tries to protect itself against starvation by slowing its metabolism (rate of energy production) and this adaptive mechanism can gradually lead to vital sign abnormalities and other physical symptoms. Psychological signs of starvation include increased depression and relentless thoughts about food, calories, and weight that can interfere with concentration. The message that improved nutrition will help diminish these painful food obsessions helps motivate some individuals to modify their eating habits.

Misconceptions about food and weight are common. For example, it is not unusual for a patient to equate dietary fat with body fat. To address this, the dietician explains that calories that develop into fat derive from a combination of foods, not just from fatty ones. It is not unusual for an individual to deem some foods "good" and others "bad" based on fat or carbohydrate content. The truth is that there are no such categories. Yet many individuals, whether or not they have eating disorders, see dieting as normal and expected. Thus, dieticians often devote considerable attention to the reasons why dieting is counter-productive, and why it is important to eat three balanced meals plus snacks each day.

Other topics that may be covered in nutrition therapy include the recognition of hunger and fullness cues, difficulties eating in social situations, and the vicious cycle involved in bingeing and purging. Cognitive behavioral interventions that are introduced in individual or group therapy can be used in nutrition counseling. Thus, the patient practices reframing her negative food and body thoughts into positive, life-affirming ones that can help inform behavior change. Through empathy and through facilitating reflection about the advantages and disadvantages of disordered eating, the dietician aims to improve the patient's readiness to change so that she can regain her health and go on to lead a full and productive life.

References

Anonymous. Position of the American Dietetic Association: Nutrition intervention in the treatment of anorexia nervosa, bulimia nervosa, and other eating disorders. *Journal of the American Dietetic Association*. 2006; 106: 2073–82.

Cockfield, A., Philpot, U. Feeding size 0: the challenges of anorexia nervosa. Managing anorexia from a dietician's perspective. *Proceedings of the Nutrition Society*. 2009; 68: 281–88.

Robinson-O'Brien, R., Perry, C.L., Wall, M.M., Story, M. Neumark-Sztainer, D. Adolescent and young adult vegetarianism: better dietary intake and weight outcomes but increased risk of disordered eating behaviors. *Journal of the American Dietetic Association*. 2009; 109: 648–55.

Chapter 42

Recovery from an Eating Disorder

Chapter Contents

Section 42.1

Defining What It Means to Be "Recovered"

"Defining What It Means to Be 'Recovered,'" by Anna M. Bardone-Cone, PhD, and Christine R. Maldonado, MA, *Eating Disorders Recovery Today*, Summer 2008, Volume 6, Number 3. © 2008 Gürze Books. Reprinted with permission.

It is not surprising that some individuals with eating disorders feel hopeless and defeated during the therapeutic process of treatment. They are often presented with grim outcome statistics and an uncertain prognosis. Some of the most common questions asked of health professionals are: "Will I get better? How will I know I've recovered?"

Professionals are hard pressed to give clear answers and with good reason. Within the field, there is debate and no consensus on how to define recovery. Is it enough to restore to an appropriate weight and begin menstruating again (i.e., physical recovery), but still be having eating disordered thoughts (i.e., psychological recovery)? Other improvements may be behavioral (e.g., cessation of restriction, excessive exercise, bingeing, and purging), and social (e.g., ability to create and maintain meaningful relationships and be successful in school or work).

To understand these different aspects, our research lab at the University of Missouri embarked on an in-depth study by interviewing over ninety girls and women who had had an eating disorder at one point in their lives, and who had been seen at a primary care facility in Missouri for their eating disorder concerns. Participants self-reported on their current stage of recovery; those who identified themselves as "recovered" described why they felt that way, with most of them reporting at least four years of recovery. The remaining portion of this section will shed light on what the women who considered themselves recovered (and who no longer met eating disorder criteria) had to say about how they see themselves in recovery. Their voices, while distinct, revolve around common themes that we have grouped as physical, psychological, behavioral, and social.

Physical Recovery

Physical recovery is usually assessed via weight restoration and the return of menses. However, what passes as adequate weight for one individual (e.g., in terms of body mass index [BMI] or percentile of ideal weight) may not be sufficient for everyone else. Perhaps in physical recovery, in particular, more individualized definitions are needed. Interestingly, no women volunteered weight gain or menses as a way they knew they were healthy, although, per measured weight and height, all had achieved a BMI of at least 18.5. While BMI was assessed in this study as a contributing indicator of eating disorder status, there are clear limitations in relying on BMI to measure health. One woman did refer to being "able to listen to [my] body's signals," suggesting that one aspect of physical recovery focused on being in tune with one's body.

Psychological Recovery

Themes of decreased obsessions related to weight and food were often present in this stage. The women spoke of decreased mental energy going toward the eating disorder:

- "Not battling it every day."
- "Other things preoccupy my mind, not food."
- "Not obsessed with calories/food grams."
- "No obsessive thoughts about food/excessive exercise."
- "Doesn't consume my time or thoughts."

In some exceptional cases, women endorsed a clean split with eating disordered thinking: "I never even contemplate bingeing/purging," and "I no longer have a fear of food or the need to control it." In other cases, the women acknowledged some eating disordered thoughts but appeared confident in their abilities to respond positively: "I can stop myself from thinking and doing things when I know that they're not the best for me."

There were expressions of comfort with eating and an absence of guilt: "I don't feel bad about what I eat. I am satisfied with how I eat," and "I eat anything without feeling guilty." In addition, there was a separation between food and a stress response in comments such as, "I don't overeat because of stress," suggesting the use of other coping mechanisms. Indeed, one woman explicitly stated that she knew she was recovered since she does not "have to use food as a coping mechanism." There were also degrees here—for example, one woman reported being able to eat all foods "with little or no guilt" most of the time, rather than always feeling guilt-free.

Although not as frequently referenced, some women reported that holding positive attitudes toward their bodies was an indication they were healthy. Their statements included "being satisfied with [myself] and the way God made [me]," and being "content with my body."

Behavioral Recovery

While behavioral change has generally been a well-accepted and utilized index of recovery, it is inspiring to hear what these women volunteered. Regarding eating, they said:

- "No restricting meals."
- "No bingeing/purging."
- "Giving up counting calories."
- "I am able to eat all kinds of food without reservations or regret."
- "I can eat whatever I want to."
- "Eat normal meals daily."
- "Eat out."
- "Eat anything without having urges."
- "I used to pick food apart, but now I eat like normal."

Some felt that no longer needing a rigid eating structure or meal plan was an index of recovery. This notion is perhaps best captured by the woman who said, "I eat what I want, when I want." Others acknowledged that behavioral change was more a matter of degree, citing "not as restrictive," rather than absolute change. Women also pointed to differences in exercise: "[I am] not trying to burn off every calorie I eat . . . [I] exercise normally."

Social Recovery

This stage has arguably received the least attention from the research and medical community. Most often eating disorders develop in adolescence and young adulthood, causing disruptions in social growth and expected developmental milestones. For example, the individual's unhealthy behaviors often co-occur with social withdrawal, impeding more mature and intimate relationships. The following are some comments made by recovered women regarding these aspects.

One woman mentioned "being able to eat in front of people," which in many cultures is central to developing and maintaining relationships. Without this ability, individuals with eating disorders miss out on opportunities to "do lunch" with family and friends and, undoubtedly, foster relationships. Another woman pointed out the ability to now "take advice of those close [to me]." Acknowledging loved ones' concerns and considering their advice may reflect repaired relationships, including renewed trust. Lastly, one woman volunteered, "focusing on 'life' and [my] personality." For this woman, and no doubt for others, recovery means regaining a sense of self and life experience that is not wrapped up in an eating disorder.

Concluding Remarks

Based on these voices and what is known among researchers and clinicians, recovery is both about what is absent (e.g., no binge eating, no obsessions) and what is present (e.g., ability to eat whatever one wants, happiness with life). For some, current life is experienced as if there never was an eating disorder; for others, there may be reminders or "scars," such as occasional restriction or urges, but now with new coping skills. To paraphrase Dr. James Lock: "Recovery may be when life replaces the eating disorder." One young woman poignantly reflected this during the interview. While she answered questions, she relayed that the eating disorder felt far away. She could recall details and remembered the pain, but it was like a distant dream and very separate from her current life.

As researchers continue to grapple with defining recovery, both in general terms and with an eye toward individualization, the goal is to apply the information so as to give everyone the best chance at the fullest life possible.

Section 42.2

Self-Soothing Skills: Essential for Recovery

"Self-Soothing Skills: An Essential Tool of Eating Disorder Treatment and Recovery," by Jacquelyn Ekern, MS, LPC. © 2010 Eating Disorder Hope (www.eatingdisorderhope.com). Reprinted with permission.

Eating disorders such as anorexia, bulimia, binge eating disorder, and compulsive overeating are complex disorders with many contributing factors. Biological, social, spiritual, and physical factors are all involved in the development and continuation of an eating disorder. There are no simple answers to overcoming an eating disorder, but there are many helpful recovery tools that a person can develop to become healthier and to lessen the need to rely on disordered eating behaviors to comfort or distract them from themselves. One significant tool is learning to self soothe oneself.

The ability to self-soothe is one of the most essential tools a person can use in an eating disorder recovery treatment regimen. Self-soothing is also beneficial in treating related dual diagnosis issues like addiction and other compulsive behaviors that are often co-occurring with eating disorders. What is self-soothing? Where do people learn how to do it? How is it done? Why is important? And, perhaps most importantly, why is this skill worth developing in an eating disorder recovery treatment plan?

The skill of self-soothing can be acquired by developing a kind and gentle approach to oneself. Those adept at comforting themselves know how and when to rest, to cut themselves some slack. They are kind and gentle with themselves, loving themselves unconditionally and treating themselves with all the respect and care they deserve. Who doesn't want more of that good stuff?

Throughout infancy and childhood, people seek comfort from their primary caregivers. If the caregivers do a good enough job responding to the child's emotional and physical needs, then the child is generally off to a good start in developing a healthy sense of self. But, often the caregivers are unable or unwilling to fully meet the needs of the infant or child. The child then must develop self-soothing techniques on their own to comfort themselves. This is where the favorite blanket, stuffed animal, or thumb sucking come into play. These types of attempts at self-comfort are useful to the infant and child as they make sense of their needs and desires and how to get those needs and desires met.

As people mature throughout their lives, they develop more sophisticated coping skills and ways to comfort themselves. Some of these skills are helpful, some are not. A few helpful skills include distractions such as participating in fun activities, being with friends, and taking up a hobby. These and other diversions can be great coping skills for distracting oneself from their uncomfortable feelings. Prayer, practicing mindfulness, and exercise can also help in dealing with stress and anxiety. Some of the unhealthy ways people seek to soothe themselves are by practicing eating disorders, addictions, compulsive behaviors, and other self-destructive patterns.

Learning and practicing effective self-soothing skills may be one of the most important aspects of an effective eating disorder treatment plan. Here are some suggestions to consider when developing personalized coping skills for a life of recovery and hope:

- **Mindfulness:** Tune into the five senses and be in the moment. Feel the pressure of your body sitting on the chair, smell the scents in the room, listen to the birds outside, look at a beautiful picture on the wall, taste the vibrant flavors of a strawberry.

- **Distractions:** Read good books, go to the movies, play sports, play board games, have some good 'ole fun and leave the worrying for another day.

- **Bubble baths:** A candlelit bubble bath is one of the best comforts this life has to offer! Indulge! It is well deserved.

- **Music:** Play your favorite songs and CDs. Listen to the music closely. Experience the music. Observe how it feels.

- **Journal:** Writing down thoughts and feelings is a cathartic opportunity to express churning emotions and think through situations. This also provides a window into new insights and revelations.

- **Tea:** Have a tea ceremony! Make a cup of tea or a hot chocolate. Put it in a favorite mug or adorable teacup, heat the water in a kettle on the stove, breathe deeply, and enjoy the process of making a cup of tea. Then, enjoy the treat.

- **Exercise:** Take a leisurely walk or a brisk run. This is an excellent way to use up some intense emotional energy or stress. Swimming, bicycling, and yoga are also great forms of exercise that can impart a sense of wellbeing and hence comfort.

- **Wear comfortable clothes:** Put on the most cozy pair of sweats and fuzzy slippers, loose is good! Allow the body to feel the soft sensation of cotton or silk against the skin.

- **Talk:** Talk it out. Talk about the feelings, thoughts, and observations with a trusted friend or therapist. It is comforting to feel understood, in and of itself. Additionally, the burdens may seem less draining when they are shared with another.

- **Get into nature:** Spend some time gardening, observing the beauty of the trees that may line the street, seek out local parks and arboretums to enjoy the beauty of nature.

Learning to self-soothe oneself can be difficult. Life is hectic, stressful, and sometimes frantic; eating disorders are often developed, in part, to deal with these burdens. To help soothe and lessen these difficulties, implement this essential tool. It will be beneficial and rewarding when used as an integral part of an eating disorder recovery treatment plan.

Section 42.3

Overcoming Negative Thoughts

"Eating Disorder Recovery and Overcoming Negative Thoughts,"
by Jacquelyn Ekern, MS, LPC. © 2010 Eating Disorder Hope
(www.eatingdisorderhope.com). Reprinted with permission.

Eating disorder treatment and recovery requires a paradigm shift in thinking. If one chooses recovery, then one must begin to examine their internal dialogue and irrational conclusions about themselves and life, in general. Anorexia, bulimia, binge eating disorder, and compulsive overeating are often signs of a troubled internal relationship with oneself. Understanding the importance of the messages we give ourselves leads many to desire a more positive internal dialogue.

Resolution of uncomfortable feelings and regrettable behaviors directly improves the quality of your life. The theory of cognitive behavior therapy empowers you to use your God-given logical thinking capacity to improve your life.

Using cognitive behavior therapy can inspire hope, self-esteem, and empowerment within you. Here are the common thinking errors identified by this theory, developed by Dr. Aaron Beck (he earned his Ph.D. in psychiatry from Yale University in 1946).

Arbitrary inference. This means to jump to conclusions without a factual basis for your determination. It means to expect the worst, when that is generally not the way things turn out. Actually, things more often than not turn out somewhere in the middle of our highest and lowest expectations.

Selective abstraction. Only focusing on one piece of information and not taking the whole story into account. This means to select only parts of the whole picture to focus on. When we actually process things more logically, it makes sense to take in the whole picture and not just an isolated incident.

Overgeneralization. To apply a negative paradigm about ourselves or our lives to every aspect of our lives. For example, to say "I always lose" is an overgeneralization. No one always loses. Heck, out of millions of little sperm competing for an egg, you are the one that made it! So, this is one success that already contradicts the "I always lose" theory. I bet you can come up with more winning scenarios in your life that refute irrational generalizations like this.

Magnification and minimization. To view a situation as all good or all bad. Rather than appreciating that both good and bad exist in most human experiences. For example, I may focus on the poor economy and feel depressed and anxious about finances. But, if I do not solely focus on the economy, but also appreciate my stable employment, savings account, and retirement plans, then I may find I feel more peaceful and less panicked.

Labeling and mislabeling. "I am a fat pig." Ouch! Name-calling is never okay and least of all toward oneself in our internal dialogue. No human being is a pig, and this is a ridiculous label to call oneself when it is exposed to rational thinking.

Another indication of this thinking error is when one allows past experiences to determine our self-esteem today. People change, evolve, and grow. A failure in one's past does not mean that you cannot be successful now. It just means that you're human, like the rest of us.

Personalization. This means to take things personally. Someone else in a bad mood does not mean it is your fault! Someone else letting you down does not mean you are bad. We must remain clear on what is

409

about us and what is not. Quite often, others' behaviors and attitudes are about them, and don't even involve us.

Polarized thinking. Seeing life and ourselves in black and white is a common thinking error. Not much is that simple! Try to recognize it when you are viewing a situation in extremes and choose to moderate your view. For example, not getting an A on a term paper is disappointing when you have worked hard and done your best. However, one grade and even one class does not determine your academic success overall.

Conclusions

The wonderful thing about recognizing and correcting these irrational thinking errors is that it empowers the individual struggling with an eating disorder to begin taking care of themselves emotionally. They learn self-soothing skills through thinking things through in a more balanced way, thus lessening their need to practice disordered eating to cope.

Section 42.4

Relapse Prevention

"Relapse Prevention: Once Is Enough," by Catherine Pearte, Elizabeth Wack, and Stacey Tantleff-Dunn, PhD, *Eating Disorders Today*, Spring 2007, Volume 5, Number 2. © 2007 Gürze Books. Reprinted with permission.

Preventing relapse is a critical component for treating anorexia nervosa (AN) and bulimia nervosa (BN). While the onset of these disorders can be devastating to both the patient and the patient's family, diagnosis often marks the beginning of an insidious cycle of recovery and relapse. This cycle occurs in approximately one-third of patients, with relapse beginning as early as seven to fifteen months after initial recovery.

Relapse can be described as the manifestation of symptoms after a period of recovery. Symptoms of relapse include weight loss, compensatory behaviors, and deviant attitudes regarding weight and shape. For example, AN patients who initially restricted their caloric intake sometimes develop bulimic symptoms during relapse. Because of the psychological distress and the threat of mortality posed by eating disorders, scientific attempts have been made to predict and prevent relapses that have become all but characteristic of the chronic course of eating disorders.

Researchers have recently begun to emphasize the importance of identifying factors that may predispose patients to relapse. Although the symptoms of AN and BN sometimes overlap and can be treated with the same psychological and pharmacological approaches, factors that contribute to relapse are different in patients with AN as opposed to BN.

Relapse Risk Factors for AN

- Early age of onset
- Lower desired weight
- Duration of illness
- History of suicide attempts
- Obsessive behaviors
- Bingeing before the end of treatment

- Treatment at a nonspecialized clinic
- Previous treatment for an eating disorder
- Absence of treatment during follow-up

Relapse Risk Factors for BN

- Low motivation for treatment
- Absence of treatment during follow-up
- Stressful or difficult circumstances
- Anxiety, nervousness, or depression

Therapies, Medication, and Technology

The gravity of the medical and psychological consequences left in the wake of eating disorders have spurred researchers to conduct trials using specialized therapies, medication, and technology to determine how to best protect patients from relapse. However, there is limited research available to attest to the success of any particular relapse prevention strategy. Several studies have concluded that individuals who remain in therapy after recovery fare better than those who do not receive ongoing therapy. The continuing support of a mental health care professional is important for sustaining patients through the very difficult initial weeks of recovery wherein adjustment to new routines and, in the case of AN, the additional weight, can be a frightening, lonely, and overwhelming ordeal.

Antidepressants

Although research indicates that antidepressant medication may be beneficial in the treatment of a variety of eating disorders, there is less scientific support for the efficacy of antidepressant medications, specifically Prozac® (fluoxetine), in relapse prevention. A 2006 study did not find any difference in relapse rates after fifty-two weeks among patients who were receiving cognitive-behavioral therapy between those who in addition took Prozac and those who in addition took a placebo.[1] This is a particularly disappointing finding considering that if antidepressants were found to be effective in preventing relapse, partially recovered BN and AN patients who often experience high levels of depression could use the medication to jointly alleviate depressive symptoms and lower their likelihood of recurring eating disturbance.

Text Messaging

Medication and psychotherapy are the most common techniques employed in an effort to prevent relapse, but relapse prevention also has been attempted in a rather creative manner, utilizing a particularly prevalent and accessible form of technology: cellular phones. One study was conducted in which researchers tested the feasibility of using text messaging as a form of aftercare communication aimed at preventing the return of bulimic symptoms in patients recently discharged from a treatment facility.[2]

Participants were asked to send a weekly text message to their treatment team addressing five questions about their symptoms and mood state. In return, the team responded each week with advice and support. Although its impact on relapse rates has not yet been assessed, patients expressed that the text messaging made them feel supported post-treatment. More research on the efficacy of this and other innovative approaches is needed.

An Integral Component

Although there has been some effort in the scientific community to identify risk factors and fight relapse directly, there is minimal success documented in the current literature. The medical and psychological consequences of chronic, long-term eating disorders highlights relapse prevention as an integral component in the treatment of eating disorders and an important subject for further scientific investigation.

References

1. Walsh, T.B., Kaplan, A.S., & Attia, E. (2006). Fluoxetine after weight restoration in anorexia nervosa: A randomized controlled trial. Journal of the American Medical Association, 295(22), 2605–12.

2. Bauer, S., Percevic, R., & Okon, E. (2003). Use of text messaging in the aftercare of patients with bulimia nervosa. *European Eating Disorders Review*, 11(3), 279–90.

Chapter 43

Insurance Coverage for Eating Disorders Treatment

Finding the medical coverage for treatment of an eating disorder can be a real challenge, but having a plan makes it much easier to find the treatment you need.

1. Get an assessment so the diagnosis will be established. You will need an assessment so the disorder and its associated mental and physical problems can be properly diagnosed and documented.

2. Do you have mental health benefits? If you have insurance, you may also have mental health benefits. Often these benefits include an amount for hospital or residential treatment and an amount for outpatient treatment as well. Nearly all health policies include major medical benefits, which are typically much greater than the mental health benefits. Some companies provide employee assistance programs (EAPs), and appropriate care is sometimes available through these programs. Read the booklet that comes with your insurance policy or call the phone number on your insurance card and ask about your benefits.

3. Obtaining your benefits. Although you may have what appear to be adequate benefits, the next issue is whether or not you can use them to obtain appropriate care. The three major types

of health insurance policies are: indemnity, preferred provider organizations (PPOs), and health maintenance organizations (HMOs). Very few people have indemnity policies, but they are usually the most comprehensive and have the greatest flexibility. PPOs are usually much more flexible than HMOs. There is usually a deductible (a portion of the charge from the hospital, residential treatment center, or care provider that you pay). And, especially in the case of HMOs, there are reviewers (often untrained clerical personnel) who decide how much of your benefits will be available to you when a diagnosis is made. This decision may be made based on idiosyncratic rules that do not reflect current evidence-based treatment approaches and often do not reflect the consensus of professionals.

4. Determine healthcare providers. It is also important to determine what the treatment center or care provider will need to help you obtain those benefits. This is not always easy to determine in advance. Ask your insurance company to send you a list of providers. If your professionals are on the list, call these professionals and let their office personnel know the results of your assessment, including the diagnoses, the type of treatment recommended and where it will be given, and estimated length of treatment.

If Your Provider Does Not Provide the Recommended Treatment

1. If your insurance benefits do not match the recommended treatment: For example, if you have anorexia nervosa of the binge/purge type, and residential treatment is recommended for sixty days, your insurance benefits may only cover ten days of residential treatment. In this case, first try calling your insurance company and ask to obtain your major medical benefits. It is logical to turn to major medical benefits because the semi-starvation that results from anorexia nervosa is a physiological complication and if untreated will likely result in hospitalization on a medical floor in a general hospital, which will ultimately be very expensive. Eating disorders are medical illnesses and it is worthwhile to mention this fact to your insurance company. Typically, however, this will not result in any change on their part. The next step is to contact the personnel department of the company that purchases the insurance.

Remember that insurance coverage is called a "benefit" but in fact it is a part of the compensation to the worker who has the insurance policy. Insurance coverage is not a gift from the employer. Furthermore, the insurance company is supposed to hold the funds paid by the employer on behalf of the employee and dispense them according to rules set down by the employer. Thus, the employer can decide to fire the insurance company (and ultimately the HMO or PPO). The important point to remember is that it is actually your employer (or the employer of the person who has the insurance) who has power over what benefits are provided from the HMO or PPO. Thus, your personnel department can be helpful. You may find that the insurance company blames the employer or the employer blames the insurance company. Since the employer pays for the insurance benefits (which can include hiring an intermediary HMO), ultimately (although not immediately), the employer can choose to change insurance companies.

2.   Despite your best efforts, your insurance company and personnel department are not helpful. Although it is tempting to give up at this point, other steps can be taken. First, let your insurance company know that you have decided to call the insurance commissioner and then call him. When you speak with the commissioner, tell him what has been recommended, what steps you have taken to obtain treatment, and the results of these attempts. Follow this up with a letter explaining the difficulties. Keep a copy of this letter for your files. If the insurance commissioner is not helpful, the next step is to contact your senators and congressmen and congresswomen. If they aren't helpful, contact the governor.

3.   When efforts to obtain care by contacting your legislators and the governor are not effective, self-help groups may be the answer. For example, the National Eating Disorders Association may be helpful (603 Stewart Street, Suite 803, Seattle, WA 98101, Referral Phone: 800-931-2237 Office: 206-382-3587).

4.   Try creative solutions. Some families have been able to access help by contacting their attorney if benefits are available through an insurance company but the benefits are not available. Other families have gotten their insurance companies to make appropriate decisions by contacting the local newspaper or magazines and describing their plight. Others have called local help programs on radio and television.

417

5. Determine if you can afford care if your insurance company will not pay for it. Once you know what care is recommended, who should provide it, and where this care should be provided, find out the stated total charges from the institution and/or professionals providing the care. Assess your own financial resources and negotiate a fee/ charge you can afford.

If You Have Medicare or Medicaid Benefits

Although many hospitals and treatment centers accept Medicare and/or Medicaid, many have no staff members with experience in treating eating disorders. If the treatment center is a mental health center, which is funded in part by county, state, or federal funds, you can sometimes ask that appropriate care be provided and sometimes there are personnel at the center who are familiar with the treatment of eating disorders.

When You Have No Money or Insurance Benefits

Treatment programs do exist for people who have no money or benefits, but they are often hard to locate. Some agencies that receive public funds do provide treatment, and sometimes that treatment is outstanding. Another way to obtain treatment is through community agencies—sometimes treatment is provided at no cost or with a sliding scale fee. Counseling centers and student health services are another option if your patient is a student on a college or university campus. To get treatment at these locations, you usually pay a student health fee with your tuition.

Many departments of psychiatry within medical schools have low-fee clinics run by psychiatric residents (medical school graduates who have had two or three years of their psychiatric training and are supervised by experienced faculty members). Call the department of psychiatry within the medical school and ask if they have low-fee clinics run by residents and if they will accept a patient with an eating disorder. Be sure to ask about sliding-scale fees and ask about what supervision the medical resident has available to him or her.

No-Fee Research Treatments

Sometimes treatment can be obtained through a research program. For example, periodically Columbia University in New York has openings for patients willing to be part of an ongoing research program for patients with anorexia nervosa. The program is the Eating Disorders Clinic at New York State Psychiatric Institute at Columbia Presbyterian Medical Center in New York City. To ask about the program, call the research assistant at 212-543-5739.

A research study may be underway at a college or university near you, and the newspaper may run announcements of these programs. It is important to remember that although there may be no fee for part of the treatment, there may be fees for certain non-research portions of the study, and there are inclusion and exclusion criteria.

Final Thoughts

Keep trying to get better and trying to locate people to help you. Although you will encounter many barriers to accessing appropriate professional treatment, if you are committed to recovering, it can usually be accomplished. Care providers themselves are energized when patients want to recover and can often help you find the help you need. Many primary care physicians and pediatricians are relentless in trying to find help for their patients and your interest in recovery will encourage them to help you.

Facts to Know When You Seek Insurance Coverage

- Your eating disorder diagnosis

- Other psychiatric disorders

- Physiologic complications of the eating disorder

- Level of care recommended: outpatient, inpatient, partial hospitalization, intensive outpatient

- Anticipated duration of recommended treatment

- Professionals needed and their required expertise

Chapter 44

Living with Someone Who Has an Eating Disorder

Living with Someone with an Eating Disorder

Living with somebody with an eating disorder can often leave you feeling frustrated and helpless. It's not always easy to feel certain about what you can do to help the person you care about. Here are some ideas for anybody living with someone experiencing an eating disorder—from parents and siblings to grandparents, children, and partners:

- **Encourage the person to seek professional help:** Overcoming an eating disorder can be very difficult without assistance, so accessing professional help is an important goal.

- **Encourage the person to recognize their other skills and attributes:** Use your knowledge of the person to encourage them to see the positive effects change can bring.

- **Keep communication positive and open:** Take time to talk about a variety of topics. Focusing on the eating difficulties creates a stressful environment which may result in the person withdrawing from contact with you. The use of laughter and humor is a great communication tool.

"Living with Someone with an Eating Disorder," "How Family and Friends Are Affected," "For Parents," and "For Siblings," © 2009 Eating Disorders Foundation of Victoria. Reprinted with permission. For additional information and resources, visit www.eatingdisorders.org.au.

- **Take the focus off food and weight:** The person with the eating disorder is already overfocused on food and weight issues.

- **Mealtimes should not become a battleground:** Frustrations and emotions need to be expressed but not at mealtimes; this is already likely to be a difficult time.

- **Accept limitations in your responsibilities:** The support and encouragement of family and friends is vital, however it is the person with the eating disorder's responsibility to take the necessary steps toward recovery.

- **Promote independence:** The person with the eating disorder has the right to lead an independent life and make decisions for themselves and in their own time. This can be difficult especially if the person is a child, adolescent, or quite sick, however, recovery often involves the person learning to become more self-sufficient.

- **Set boundaries:** If someone is behaving in a way that is difficult for you, it is okay to let them know that their behavior is not acceptable. Only set boundaries you can enforce.

- **Do things as you usually would:** The person with the eating disorder needs to learn to co-exist with food and with other people, rather than others learning to co-exist with the eating disorder. Try not to make any changes to mealtimes, food shopping, outings, topics of conversation, or other interests.

- **Separate the person from the disorder:** Remind yourself the person's behavior is often a symptom of the eating disorder rather than a reflection of their character.

- **Enjoy things together:** It is important not to let the eating disorder become the focus of the family or relationship. Continue to enjoy things together that you have always done.

- **Build the person's self-esteem:** Try and focus on their positive behaviors rather than the more destructive ones.

- **Spend time with other members of the family or friendship group:** The person with the eating disorder is important, but no more so than other people. Try to avoid a situation where siblings or partners feel neglected.

- **Accept your limitations as a family member or friend:** You cannot deal with all the problems associated with the disorder.

Your role as a family member or friend is unique and something that a therapist can't be, just as the therapist's role is something a family member or friend can't take on.

- **Become informed:** Information about eating disorders, recovery stories, developing coping strategies, and attending support groups can be useful. There are many resources and books written for families and friends.

- **Look after yourself:** Get as much support and information as you need. Support groups, relatives, friends, counselors, telephone support lines, and other professionals may be useful. Looking after yourself is as important as looking after the person with the eating disorder.

- **Be patient:** Eating disorders are complicated and recovery can take some time. Sometimes it's important to remind yourself that the person does not want to be unwell, but they lack the ability to overcome the disorder quickly. There is no specific timeframe for recovery.

How Family and Friends Are Affected

Parents, siblings, partners, friends, extended family, work colleagues, and others often experience many different feelings as they learn to cope with the effects of the eating disorder on the person and on their own lives. The strain of living with the eating disorder can create tensions and divisions within the family. Each person involved will be affected in different ways. Common reactions include:

- Confusion about:
  - the eating disorder and recovery process;
  - why this has happened;
  - the best way to handle the illness in the family, partnership, or friendship circle, etc.;
  - knowing what to say and how to say it;
  - how to support the person.
- Grief and anger about:
  - loss of the person's mental and physical health;
  - change in the person's behavior, denial of problem, and/or refusal to get help;

423

- the difficulties or changes the eating disorder is creating in the family, partnership, or friendship circle;

- not being able to make the person well;

- loss of time alone and/or with other family members/friends;

- loss of trust for the person who may behave deceptively;

- feeling a loss for the person who may have lost sight of their goals and ambitions.

- Guilt or fear about:

  - being responsible for the eating disorder;

  - not recognizing the eating disorder earlier;

  - not providing effective support and help that is required to promote recovery;

  - that the person may not recover.

For Parents

Discovering that your child has an eating disorder can be an extremely confusing, frustrating, and painful experience. It is an extremely difficult role for parents to play as they feel they need to maintain a strong demeanor in order to provide the support and love necessary in caring for a child with an eating disorder. Parents often feel distraught, helpless, guilty, defeated, confused, and exhausted.

In addition to the suggestions outlined in "Living with Someone with an Eating Disorder," the following list provides recommendations to help parents manage their child's eating disorder in a way which promotes their recovery:

- Communication is essential both in promoting your child's recovery, as well as ensuring the eating disorder does not take over the lives and interactions of everybody in your family. Being aware of how each person in the family communicates with each other is important. Calm, clear, concise communication is the best approach with everyone.

- Pursue knowledge and understanding of eating disorders. Becoming informed is a crucial step in best equipping yourself with the skills and strategies for supporting your child. There is a wealth of information available online and in books which will provide background facts about eating disorders. If you are aware of the nature of eating disorders you will be more prepared to handle the changes and challenges that take place throughout a person's eating disorder and recovery experience.

- Role model healthy behaviors and attitudes toward food, weight, and body image. Talk to children about their self-image, offer reassurance that body shapes vary, teach them about the pitfalls of dieting, and role model healthy eating behaviors.

- If you have other children, share what you know about eating disorders, including strategies on how to best support their brother or sister toward recovery.

- Try not to let the needs of the child with the eating disorder overshadow the needs of siblings. Try to give as much time and attention to siblings as possible. Communication is key in ensuring other siblings understand the eating disorder and are equipped with knowledge in how to best support their sibling. Explain that this is an important time in their sibling's life and that, while you may be directing a lot of your time and energy to the child with the eating disorder, this situation will not be forever and your love for them is just as strong.

- Be aware that the distress of siblings can be very acute and is often hidden so as not to burden parents. Encourage siblings to take part in open communication with you and other people in their support network. Encourage them to express their range of feelings about how they are coping with the situation. In addition, try to ensure other siblings are provided with the opportunity to take part in social or leisure activities which will allow them to pursue their own interests outside of the home.

- Seek support for yourself whenever you are feeling overwhelmed. You may consider going to see a counselor or simply connecting with somebody in your own support network.

- Acknowledge that setbacks are a normal part of recovery. Try to take every day as it comes. While relapses can seem devastating, it is best to view them as an opportunity for your child to learn how to better handle future situations. Each setback overcome will leave the person stronger and wiser and these are all building blocks in the recovery process. Recognition of the triggers or causes of setbacks can be the only way that a person learns about them and learns to anticipate and prepare for them.

- Remember recovery is a process, not an end point—consider recovery as the process of healing, rather than an outcome. Many people want to know when the person they love will be recovered and back to their old selves. For most people, there will be no particular day, event, or marker that will indicate that they are "recovered." Recovery can involve personal discovery, relearning, challenges, achievements, and setbacks. For many people, it is just the beginning of a lifelong process of being more aware of who they are and what is important to them. Often, people won't go back to being their old selves, because their recovery is a positive learning experience resulting in significant personal growth.

For Siblings

When a person develops an eating disorder, it can result in great frustration and distress for brothers and sisters as they deal with their own emotions in seeing somebody they love struggle. Siblings may struggle with the disruption to the regular family routine which often occurs when a treatment program is in place. Mealtimes can become disrupted, which may have an impact on siblings' eating behavior. It is important for parents and siblings alike to be mindful of their own attitude toward food and ensure they maintain a regular, healthy eating pattern.

Below are a few tips for siblings of somebody with an eating disorder:

- Accept that your sibling's illness is not your fault.

- Educate yourself about the type of eating disorder your sibling has, in particular the behavioral changes they might experience. It is better to know the facts of the illness and have a good understanding of what the coming weeks and months may be like. Information can be obtained from your local doctor or community health center, books, or expert websites online.

- Know your brother or sister is very distressed and confused and even though they might not say or show it, they have not stopped caring about you.

- Realize it is the eating disorder that makes your sibling grumpy, moody, angry, and hurtful and that it's not really the person saying or behaving in that way. The eating disorder can override rational behavior and limit your sibling's normal (old) behaviors.

426

- Talk to your friends, parents, or a loved relative (perhaps your grandmother, or an aunt) about your feelings and your fears.

- Try to continue normal sibling activities that you shared before your sibling became ill.

- Respect that it may be difficult for your sibling to talk about what they're going through. Let them know there is no time limit on your support and you're happy to listen and be there whenever they feel ready.

- Enjoy time away from the home environment to recharge and do "normal" activities. It is also important to not let your sibling's illness dominate your thoughts all of the time. As hard as this is, reassure yourself that your sibling will be okay while you're spending some time to yourself.

- Consider seeking professional help for yourself to talk about what you may be feeling and experiencing. You may like to talk to a school welfare worker, a psychologist, or a counselor. By talking to someone you may think about things in a different way. Trained professionals can empower you with skills to better deal with situations.

Part Six

Preventing Eating Disorders and Achieving a Healthy Weight

Chapter 45

Eating Disorder Prevention

Chapter Contents

431

Section 45.1

What Can You Do to Help Prevent Eating Disorders?

"What Can You Do to Help Prevent Eating Disorders?" © 2005 National Eating Disorders Association. For more information, visit www.NationalEating Disorders.org. Reviewed by David A. Cooke, M.D., FACP, October 2010.

Learn all you can about anorexia nervosa, bulimia nervosa, and binge eating disorder. Genuine awareness will help you avoid judgmental or mistaken attitudes about food, weight, body shape, and eating disorders.

Discourage the idea that a particular diet, weight, or body size will automatically lead to happiness and fulfillment.

Choose to challenge the false belief that thinness and weight loss are great, while body fat and weight gain are horrible or indicate laziness, worthlessness, or immorality.

Avoid categorizing foods as "good/safe" versus "bad/dangerous." Remember, we all need to eat a balanced variety of foods.

Decide to avoid judging others and yourself on the basis of body weight or shape. Turn off the voices in your head that tell you that a person's body weight says anything about their character, personality, or value as a person.

Avoid conveying an attitude that says, "I will like you better if you lose weight, or don't eat so much, etc."

Become a critical viewer of the media and its messages about self-esteem and body image. Talk back to the television when you hear a comment or see an image that promotes thinness at all costs. Rip out (or better yet, write to the editor about) advertisements or articles in your magazines that make you feel bad about your body shape or size.

If you think someone has an eating disorder, express your concerns in a forthright, caring manner. Gently but firmly encourage the person to seek trained professional help.

Be a model of healthy self-esteem and body image. Recognize that others pay attention and learn from the way you talk about yourself and your body. Choose to talk about yourself with respect and appreciation. Choose to value yourself based on your goals, accomplishments, talents, and character. Avoid letting the way you feel about your body weight and shape determine the course of your day. Embrace the natural diversity of human bodies and celebrate your body's unique shape and size.

Support local and national nonprofit eating disorders organizations—like the National Eating Disorders Association—by volunteering your time or giving a tax deductible donation.

Section 45.2

Ten Things Parents Can Do to Help Prevent Eating Disorders

"Ten Things Parents Can Do to Help Prevent Eating Disorders" © 2005 National Eating Disorders Association. For more information, visit www .NationalEatingDisorders.org. Reviewed by David A. Cooke, M.D., FACP, October 2010.

1. Consider your thoughts, attitudes, and behaviors toward your own body and the way that these beliefs have been shaped by the forces of weightism and sexism. Then educate your children about (a) the genetic basis for the natural diversity of human body shapes and sizes and (b) the nature and ugliness of prejudice. Make an effort to maintain positive attitudes and healthy behaviors. Children learn from the things you say and do!

2. Examine closely your dreams and goals for your children and other loved ones. Are you overemphasizing beauty and body shape, particularly for girls? Avoid conveying an attitude which says, in effect, "I will like you more if you lose weight, don't eat so much, look more like the slender models in ads, fit into smaller clothes, etc." Decide what you can do and what you can stop doing to reduce the teasing, criticism, blaming, staring, etc. that reinforce the idea that larger or fatter is "bad" and smaller or thinner is "good."

3. Learn about and discuss with your sons and daughters (a) the dangers of trying to alter one's body shape through dieting, (b) the value of moderate exercise for health, and (c) the

importance of eating a variety of foods in well-balanced meals consumed at least three times a day. Avoid categorizing and labeling foods (e.g. good/bad or safe/dangerous). All foods can be eaten in moderation. Be a good role model in regard to sensible eating, exercise, and self-acceptance.

4. Make a commitment not to avoid activities (such as swimming, sunbathing, dancing, etc.) simply because they call attention to your weight and shape. Refuse to wear clothes that are uncomfortable or that you don't like but wear simply because they divert attention from your weight or shape.

5. Make a commitment to exercise for the joy of feeling your body move and grow stronger, not to purge fat from your body or to compensate for calories, power, excitement, popularity, or perfection.

6. Practice taking people seriously for what they say, feel, and do, not for how slender or "well put together" they appear.

7. Help children appreciate and resist the ways in which television, magazines, and other media distort the true diversity of human body types and imply that a slender body means power, excitement, popularity, or perfection.

8. Educate boys and girls about various forms of prejudice, including weightism, and help them understand their responsibilities for preventing them.

9. Encourage your children to be active and to enjoy what their bodies can do and feel like. Do not limit their caloric intake unless a physician requests that you do this because of a medical problem.

10. Do whatever you can to promote the self-esteem and self-respect of all of your children in intellectual, athletic, and social endeavors. Give boys and girls the same opportunities and encouragement. Be careful not to suggest that females are less important than males, e.g., by exempting males from housework or childcare. A well rounded sense of self and solid self-esteem are perhaps the best antidotes to dieting and disordered eating.

Chapter 46

Promoting Positive Self-Esteem

Chapter Contents

Section 46.1

What Is Self-Esteem?

What is self-esteem?

Self-esteem relates to how much you like yourself, and how you recognize or appreciate your individual character, qualities, skills, and accomplishments. Like body image, self-esteem can also be based on how you think other people look at you as a person. People who have low self-esteem may not always feel confident about themselves or how they look. It is often hard for them to see that they are an important and capable person. People with good self-esteem often have a positive and confident attitude about their body and mind, and can recognize their strengths as well as personal value and worth.

Why is good self-esteem important?

Good self-esteem is important for everyone because it helps you keep a positive outlook on life and makes you feel proud of the person you are, both inside and out. Most teens with good self-esteem find life much more enjoyable. They tend to have better relationships with peers and adults, find it easier to deal with mistakes or disappointments, and are more likely to stick with a task until they succeed.

Good self-esteem gives you the:

- courage to try new things;
- power to believe in yourself;
- confidence to make healthy choices for your mind and body now and throughout your life.

Treating yourself with respect and realizing that every part of you is worth caring for and protecting will help you keep a healthy attitude toward yourself. Building good self-esteem can take a long time and is not always easy, but knowing that you can improve your self-esteem is the first step.

Is there anything I can do if my self-esteem is low?

Yes! If you feel frustrated or too annoyed or upset to talk, try going for a walk or a run, listen to music, or do a favorite activity with someone you enjoy being with. Sometimes expressing how you feel can actually be more helpful than keeping feelings to yourself. Talk with a close friend or relative who you trust and who can offer encouragement and support. It can also be comforting to talk with other teens that may be going through similar experiences. Remember, everyone has had the experience of feeling badly about something!

If you are feeling very sad and discouraged most of the time, and can't seem to find ways to feel better about yourself, it is important to contact your healthcare provider or counselor. They can help you to find ways to cope.

What can I do to build self-confidence in the way I look?

There are many ways to help boost self-confidence such as finding a flattering outfit to wear, getting a new hairstyle, or simply eating nutritious foods and exercising. One of the best ways to feel good about your body is to work on having a healthy one! You may not always have control over your appearance, but you do have the power to keep a positive attitude toward yourself.

What are some ways to keep a positive attitude?

A positive attitude can come by defining an identity for yourself that is not based on looks or negative things other people may say.

You can develop good self-esteem and keep a positive attitude by:

- **Focusing on the good things you do and spending time concentrating on your unique qualities.**

- **Focusing on your education:** Learning gives you the power to make a difference in your life and in the lives of others.

- **Participating in a variety of sports or activities:** This can be a great way to stay healthy and fit, which adds to a positive body image.

- **Taking up a new hobby or learning to play an instrument:** Have you ever wanted to play the guitar? Maybe you want to learn how to play chess. Take time to find your hidden talents!

- **Setting and reaching new goals:** Having something to look forward to can give you a sense of pride and help you work through different challenges throughout your life.

- **Being an inspiration to others:** If you thought of your own ways to cope with social situations and find confidence, you may find it rewarding to share advice and offer encouragement to others.

Building a healthy body image and good self-esteem can be hard work because it takes time to become confident. As you work to improve your body image, you will experience self-acceptance and learn to recognize the qualities, skills, and talents that make you special.

Section 46.2

Building Self-Esteem: A Self-Help Guide

Excerpted from "Things You Can Do Right Away—Every Day—to Raise Your Self-Esteem," "Changing Negative Thoughts About Yourself to Positive Ones," and "Activities That Will Help You Feel Good About Yourself," from *Building Self-Esteem: A Self-Help Guide*, National Mental Health Information Center, Substance Abuse and Mental Health Services Administration, 2002. Revised by David A. Cooke, M.D., FACP, October 2010.

Things You Can Do Right Away—Every Day—to Raise Your Self-Esteem

Pay attention to your own needs and wants. Listen to what your body, your mind, and your heart are telling you. For instance, if your body is telling you that you have been sitting down too long, stand up and stretch. If your heart is longing to spend more time with a special friend, do it. If your mind is telling you to clean up your basement, listen to your favorite music, or stop thinking bad thoughts about yourself, take those thoughts seriously.

Take very good care of yourself. As you were growing up you may not have learned how to take good care of yourself. In fact, much of your attention may have been on taking care of others, on just getting by, or on "behaving well." Begin today to take good care of yourself.

Treat yourself as a wonderful parent would treat a small child or as one very best friend might treat another. If you work at taking good care of yourself, you will find that you feel better about yourself. Here are some ways to take good care of yourself:

- **Follow a healthy diet.** Eat healthy foods and avoid junk foods (foods containing a lot of sugar, salt, or fat). A healthy daily diet usually includes five or six servings of vegetables and fruit; six servings of whole-grain foods like bread, pasta, cereal, and rice; and two servings of protein foods like beef, chicken, fish, cheese, cottage cheese, or yogurt.

- **Exercise.** Moving your body helps you to feel better and improves your self-esteem. Arrange a time every day or as often as possible when you can get some exercise, preferably outdoors. You can do many different things. Taking a walk is the most common. You could run, ride a bicycle, play a sport, climb up and down stairs several times, put on a tape, or play the radio and dance to the music—anything that feels good to you. If you have a health problem that may restrict your ability to exercise, check with your doctor before beginning or changing your exercise habits.

- **Take time to do things you enjoy.** You may be so busy, or feel so badly about yourself, that you spend little or no time doing things you enjoy—things like playing a musical instrument, doing a craft project, flying a kite, or going fishing. Make a list of things you enjoy doing. Then do something from that list every day. Add to the list anything new that you discover you enjoy doing.

- **Get something done that you have been putting off.** Clean out that drawer. Wash that window. Write that letter. Pay that bill.

- **Do things that make use of your own special talents and abilities.** For instance, if you are good with your hands, then make things for yourself, family, and friends. If you like animals, consider having a pet or at least playing with friends' pets.

- **Dress in clothes that make you feel good about yourself.** If you have little money to spend on new clothes, check out thrift stores in your area.

- **Give yourself rewards—you are a great person.** Listen to some music.

- **Spend time with people who make you feel good about yourself—people who treat you well.** Avoid people who treat you badly.

- **Make your living space a place that honors the person you are.** Whether you live in a single room, a small apartment, or a large home, make that space comfortable and attractive for you. If you share your living space with others, have some space that is just for you—a place where you can keep your things and know that they will not be disturbed and that you can decorate any way you choose.

- **Make your meals a special time.** Turn off the television, radio, and stereo. Set the table, even if you are eating alone. Light a candle or put some flowers or an attractive object in the center of the table. Arrange your food in an attractive way on your plate. If you eat with others, encourage discussion of pleasant topics. Avoid discussing difficult issues at meals.

- **Keep learning.** Take advantage of opportunities to learn something new or improve your skills. Take a class or go to a seminar. Many adult education programs are free or very inexpensive. For those that are more costly, ask about a possible scholarship or fee reduction.

- **Begin doing those things that you know will make you feel better about yourself.** Go on a diet, begin an exercise program, or clean your living space.

- **Do something nice for another person.** Smile at someone who looks sad. Say a few kind words to the checkout cashier. Help your spouse with an unpleasant chore. Take a meal to a friend who is sick. Send a card to an acquaintance. Volunteer for a worthy organization.

- **Make it a point to treat yourself well every day.** Before you go to bed each night, write about how you treated yourself well during the day.

You may be doing some of these things now. There will be others you need to work on. You will find that you will continue to learn new and better ways to take care of yourself. As you incorporate these changes into your life, your self-esteem will continue to improve.

Changing Negative Thoughts about Yourself to Positive Ones

You may be giving yourself negative messages about yourself. Many people do. These are messages that you learned when you were young.

You learned from many different sources including other children, your teachers, family members, caregivers, even from the media, and from prejudice and stigma in our society.

Once you have learned them, you may have repeated these negative messages over and over to yourself, especially when you were not feeling well or when you were having a hard time. You may have come to believe them. You may have even worsened the problem by making up some negative messages or thoughts of your own. These negative thoughts or messages make you feel bad about yourself and lower your self-esteem.

Some examples of common negative messages that people repeat over and over to themselves include: "I am a jerk," "I am a loser," "I never do anything right," "No one would ever like me," "I am a klutz." Most people believe these messages, no matter how untrue or unreal they are. They come up immediately in the right circumstance—for instance, if you get a wrong answer you think "I am so stupid." They may include words like should, ought, or must. The messages tend to imagine the worst in everything, especially you, and they are hard to turn off or unlearn.

You may think these thoughts or give yourself these negative messages so often that you are hardly aware of them. Pay attention to them. Carry a small pad with you as you go about your daily routine for several days and jot down negative thoughts about yourself whenever you notice them. Some people say they notice more negative thinking when they are tired, sick, or dealing with a lot of stress. As you become aware of your negative thoughts, you may notice more and more of them.

It helps to take a closer look at your negative thought patterns to check out whether or not they are true. You may want a close friend or counselor to help you with this. When you are in a good mood and when you have a positive attitude about yourself, ask yourself the following questions about each negative thought you have noticed:

- Is this message really true?

- Would a person say this to another person? If not, why am I saying it to myself?

- What do I get out of thinking this thought? If it makes me feel badly about myself, why not stop thinking it?

You could also ask someone else—someone who likes you and who you trust—if you should believe this thought about yourself. Often, just looking at a thought or situation in a new light helps.

441

The next step in this process is to develop positive statements you can say to yourself to replace these negative thoughts whenever you notice yourself thinking them. You can't think two thoughts at the same time. When you are thinking a positive thought about yourself, you can't be thinking a negative one. In developing these thoughts, use positive words like happy, peaceful, loving, enthusiastic, warm.

Avoid using negative words such as worried, frightened, upset, tired, bored, not, never, can't. Don't make a statement like "I am not going to worry anymore." Instead say "I focus on the positive" or whatever feels right to you. Substitute "it would be nice if" for "should." Always use the present tense, e.g., "I am healthy, I am well, I am happy, I have a good job," as if the condition already exists. Use I, me, or your own name.

You can do this by folding a piece of paper in half the long way to make two columns. In one column write your negative thought and in the other column write a positive thought that contradicts the negative thought as shown in Table 46.1.

Table 46.1. Negative and Positive Thoughts

Negative Thought	Positive Thought
I am not worth anything.	I am a valuable person.
I have never accomplished anything.	I have accomplished many things.
I always make mistakes.	I do many things well.
I am a jerk.	I am a great person.
I don't deserve a good life.	I deserve to be happy and healthy.
I am stupid.	I am smart.

You can work on changing your negative thoughts to positive ones by doing the following things:

- Replacing the negative thought with the positive one every time you realize you are thinking the negative thought.

- Repeating your positive thought over and over to yourself, out loud whenever you get a chance and even sharing them with another person, if possible.

- Writing them over and over.

- Making signs that say the positive thought, hanging them in places where you will see them often—like on your refrigerator door or on the mirror in your bathroom—and repeating the thought to yourself several times when you see it.

It helps to reinforce the positive thought if you repeat it over and over to yourself when you are deeply relaxed, like when you are doing a deep-breathing or relaxation exercise, or when you are just falling asleep or waking up.

Changing the negative thoughts you have about yourself to positive ones takes time and persistence. If you use these techniques consistently for four to six weeks, you will notice that you don't think these negative thoughts about yourself as much. If they recur at some other time, you can repeat these activities. Don't give up. You deserve to think good thoughts about yourself.

Activities That Will Help You Feel Good About Yourself

Any of the following activities will help you feel better about yourself and reinforce your self-esteem over the long term. Read through them. Do those that seem most comfortable to you. You may want to do some of the other activities at another time. You may find it helpful to repeat some of these activities again and again.

Make Affirming Lists

Making lists, rereading them often, and rewriting them from time to time will help you to feel better about yourself. If you have a journal, you can write your lists there. If you don't, any piece of paper will do.

Make a list of the following things:

- At least five of your strengths—for example, persistence, courage, friendliness, creativity

- At least five things you admire about yourself—for example the way you have raised your children, your good relationship with your brother, or your spirituality

- The five greatest achievements in your life so far, like recovering from a serious illness, graduating from high school, or learning to use a computer

- At least twenty accomplishments—they can be as simple as learning to tie your shoes, to getting an advanced college degree

- Ten ways you can "treat" or reward yourself that don't include food and that don't cost anything, such as walking in the woods, window-shopping, watching children playing on a playground, gazing at a baby's face or at a beautiful flower, or chatting with a friend

- Ten things you can do to make yourself laugh
- Ten things you could do to help someone else
- Ten things that you do that make you feel good about yourself

Reinforcing a Positive Self-Image

To do this exercise you will need a piece of paper, a pencil or pen, and a timer or clock. Any kind of paper will do, but if you have paper and pen you really like, that will be even better.

Set a timer for ten minutes or note the time on your watch or a clock. Write your name across the top of the paper. Then write everything positive and good you can think of about yourself. Include special attributes, talents, and achievements. You can use single words or sentences, whichever you prefer. You can write the same things over and over if you want to emphasize them. Don't worry about spelling or grammar. Your ideas don't have to be organized. Write down whatever comes to mind. You are the only one who will see this paper. Avoid making any negative statements or using any negative words—only positive ones. When the ten minutes are up, read the paper over to yourself. You may feel sad when you read it over because it is a new, different, and positive way of thinking about yourself—a way that contradicts some of the negative thoughts you may have had about yourself. Those feelings will diminish as your reread this paper. Read the paper over again several times. Put it in a convenient place—your pocket, purse, wallet, or the table beside your bed. Read it over to yourself at least several times a day to keep reminding yourself of how great you are! Find a private space and read it aloud. If you can, read it to a good friend or family member who is supportive.

Developing Positive Affirmations

Affirmations are positive statements that you can make about yourself that make you feel better about yourself. They describe ways you would like to feel about yourself all the time. They may not, however, describe how you feel about yourself right now. The following examples of affirmations will help you in making your own list of affirmations:

- I feel good about myself.
- I take good care of myself. I eat right, get plenty of exercise, do things I enjoy, get good healthcare, and attend to my personal hygiene needs.
- I spend my time with people who are nice to me and make me feel good about myself.

- I am a good person.
- I deserve to be alive.
- Many people like me.

Make a list of your own affirmations. Keep this list in a handy place, like your pocket or purse. You may want to make copies of your list so you can have them in several different places of easy access. Read the affirmations over and over to yourself—aloud whenever you can. Share them with others when you feel like it. Write them down from time to time. As you do this, the affirmations tend to gradually become true for you.

You gradually come to feel better and better about yourself.

Appreciation Exercise

At the top of a sheet of paper write "I like _____ (your name) because:" Have friends, acquaintances, family members, and so on write an appreciative statement about you on it. When you read it, don't deny it or argue with what has been written, just accept it! Read this paper over and over. Keep it in a place where you will see it often.

Self-Esteem Calendar

Get a calendar with large blank spaces for each day. Schedule into each day some small thing you would enjoy doing, such as "go into a flower shop and smell the flowers," "call my sister," "draw a sketch of my cat," "buy new music," "tell my daughter I love her," "bake brownies," "lie in the sun for twenty minutes," "wear my favorite scent," and so on. Now make a commitment to check your "enjoy life" calendar every day and do whatever you have scheduled for yourself.

Mutual Complimenting Exercise

Get together for ten minutes with a person you like and trust. Set a timer for five minutes or note the time on a watch or clock. One of you begins by complimenting the other person—saying everything positive about the other person—for the first five minutes. Then the other person does the same thing to that person for the next five minutes. Notice how you feel about yourself before and after this exercise. Repeat it often.

Self-Esteem Resources

Go to your library. Look up books on self-esteem. Read one or several of them. Try some of the suggested activities.

Section 46.3

Developing Your Child's Self-Esteem

Healthy self-esteem is a child's armor against the challenges of the world. Kids who feel good about themselves seem to have an easier time handling conflicts and resisting negative pressures. They tend to smile more readily and enjoy life. These kids are realistic and generally optimistic.

In contrast, kids with low self-esteem can find challenges to be sources of major anxiety and frustration. Those who think poorly of themselves have a hard time finding solutions to problems. If given to self-critical thoughts such as "I'm no good" or "I can't do anything right," they may become passive, withdrawn, or depressed. Faced with a new challenge, their immediate response is "I can't."

Here's how you can play important role in promoting healthy self-esteem in your child.

What Is Self-Esteem?

Self-esteem is the collection of beliefs or feelings we have about ourselves, our "self-perceptions." How we define ourselves influences our motivations, attitudes, and behaviors and affects our emotional adjustment.

Patterns of self-esteem start very early in life. For example, a toddler who reaches a milestone experiences a sense of accomplishment that bolsters self-esteem. Learning to roll over after dozens of unsuccessful attempts teaches a baby a "can-do" attitude.

The concept of success following persistence starts early. As kids try, fail, try again, fail again, and then finally succeed, they develop ideas about their own capabilities. At the same time, they're creating a self-concept based on interactions with other people. This is why parental involvement is key to helping kids form accurate, healthy self-perceptions.

446

Self-esteem also can be defined as feelings of capability combined with feelings of being loved. A child who is happy with an achievement but does not feel loved may eventually experience low self-esteem. Likewise, a child who feels loved but is hesitant about his or her own abilities can also end up with low self-esteem. Healthy self-esteem comes when the right balance is reached.

Signs of Unhealthy and Healthy Self-Esteem

Self-esteem fluctuates as kids grow. It's frequently changed and fine-tuned, because it is affected by a child's experiences and new perceptions. So it helps to be aware of the signs of both healthy and unhealthy self-esteem.

Kids with low self-esteem may not want to try new things, and may frequently speak negatively about themselves: "I'm stupid," "I'll never learn how to do this," or "What's the point? Nobody cares about me anyway." They may exhibit a low tolerance for frustration, giving up easily or waiting for somebody else to take over. They tend to be overly critical of and easily disappointed in themselves. Kids with low self-esteem see temporary setbacks as permanent, intolerable conditions, and a sense of pessimism predominates.

Kids with healthy self-esteem tend to enjoy interacting with others. They're comfortable in social settings and enjoy group activities as well as independent pursuits. When challenges arise, they can work toward finding solutions and voice discontent without belittling themselves or others. For example, rather than saying, "I'm an idiot," a child with healthy self-esteem says, "I don't understand this." They know their strengths and weaknesses, and accept them. A sense of optimism prevails.

How Parents Can Help

How can a parent help to foster healthy self-esteem in a child? These tips can make a big difference:

- Watch what you say. Kids are very sensitive to parents' words. Remember to praise your child not only for a job well done, but also for effort. But be truthful. For example, if your child doesn't make the soccer team, avoid saying something like, "Well, next time you'll work harder and make it." Instead, try "Well, you didn't make the team, but I'm really proud of the effort you put into it." Reward effort and completion instead of outcome.

- Be a positive role model. If you're excessively harsh on yourself, pessimistic, or unrealistic about your abilities and limitations, your child may eventually mirror you. Nurture your own self-esteem, and your child will have a great role model.

- Identify and redirect your child's inaccurate beliefs. It's important for parents to identify kids' irrational beliefs about themselves, whether they're about perfection, attractiveness, ability, or anything else. Helping kids set more accurate standards and be more realistic in evaluating themselves will help them have a healthy self-concept. Inaccurate perceptions of self can take root and become reality to kids. For example, a child who does very well in school but struggles with math may say, "I can't do math. I'm a bad student." Not only is this a false generalization, it's also a belief that will set the child up for failure. Encourage kids to see a situation in its true light. A helpful response might be: "You are a good student. You do great in school. Math is just a subject that you need to spend more time on. We'll work on it together."

- Be spontaneous and affectionate. Your love will go a long way to boost your child's self-esteem. Give hugs and tell kids you're proud of them. Pop a note in your child's lunchbox that reads, "I think you're terrific!" Give praise frequently and honestly, without overdoing it. Kids can tell whether something comes from the heart.

- Give positive, accurate feedback. Comments like "You always work yourself up into such a frenzy!" will make kids feel like they have no control over their outbursts. A better statement is, "You were really mad at your brother. But I appreciate that you didn't yell at him or hit him." This acknowledges a child's feelings, rewards the choice made, and encourages the child to make the right choice again next time.

- Create a safe, loving home environment. Kids who don't feel safe or are abused at home will suffer immensely from low self-esteem. A child who is exposed to parents who fight and argue repeatedly may become depressed and withdrawn. Also watch for signs of abuse by others, problems in school, trouble with peers, and other factors that may affect kids' self-esteem. Deal with these issues sensitively but swiftly. And always remember to respect your kids.

- Help kids become involved in constructive experiences. Activities that encourage cooperation rather than competition are especially helpful in fostering self-esteem. For example, mentoring programs in which an older child helps a younger one learn to read can do wonders for both kids.

Finding Professional Help

If you suspect your child has low self-esteem, consider professional help. Family and child counselors can work to uncover underlying issues that prevent a child from feeling good about himself or herself.

Therapy can help kids learn to view themselves and the world positively. When kids see themselves in a more realistic light, they can accept who they truly are.

With a little help, every child can develop healthy self-esteem for a happier, more fulfilling life.

Chapter 47

Promoting a Healthy Body Image

Chapter Contents

Section 47.1

What Is Body Image?

"Body Image," © 2005 National Eating Disorders Association.
For more information, visit www.NationalEatingDisorders.org.
Reviewed by David A. Cooke, M.D., FACP, October 2010.

Body Image Is . . .

- How you see yourself when you look in the mirror or when you picture yourself in your mind.

- What you believe about your own appearance (including your memories, assumptions, and generalizations).

- How you feel about your body, including your height, shape, and weight.

- How you sense and control your body as you move. How you feel in your body, not just about your body.

Negative Body Image Is . . .

- A distorted perception of your shape—you perceive parts of your body unlike they really are.

- You are convinced that only other people are attractive and that your body size or shape is a sign of personal failure.

- You feel ashamed, self-conscious, and anxious about your body.

- You feel uncomfortable and awkward in your body.

Positive Body Image Is . . .

- A clear, true perception of your shape—you see the various parts of your body as they really are.

- You celebrate and appreciate your natural body shape and you understand that a person's physical appearance sys very little about their character and value as a person.

- You feel proud and accepting of your unique body and refuse to spend an unreasonable amount of time worrying about food, weight, and calories.

- You feel comfortable and confident in your body.

People with negative body image have a greater likelihood of developing an eating disorder and are more likely to suffer from feelings of depression, isolation, low self-esteem, and obsessions with weight loss.

We all may have our days when we feel awkward or uncomfortable in our bodies, but the key to developing positive body image is to recognize and respect our natural shape and learn to overpower those negative thoughts and feelings with positive, affirming, and accepting ones.

Accept yourself—Accept your body.

Celebrate yourself—Celebrate your body.

Section 47.2

Ten Steps to Positive Body Image

"Ten Steps to Positive Body Image" © 2005 National Eating Disorders Association. For more information, visit www.NationalEatingDisorders .org. Reviewed by David A. Cooke, M.D., FACP, October 2010.

One list cannot automatically tell you how to turn negative body thoughts into positive body image, but it can help you think about new ways of looking more healthfully and happily at yourself and your body. The more you do that, the more likely you are to feel good about who you are and the body you naturally have.

1. Appreciate all that your body can do. Every day your body carries you closer to your dreams. Celebrate all of the amazing things your body does for you—running, dancing, breathing, laughing, dreaming, etc.

2. Keep a top-ten list of things you like about yourself—things that aren't related to how much you weigh or what you look like. Read your list often. Add to it as you become aware of more things to like about you.

3. Remind yourself that "true beauty" is not simply skin-deep. When you feel good about yourself and who you are, you carry yourself with a sense of confidence, self-acceptance, and openness that makes you beautiful regardless of whether you physically look like a supermodel. Beauty is a state of mind, not a state of your body.

4. Look at yourself as a whole person. When you see yourself in a mirror or in your mind, choose not to focus on specific body parts. See yourself as you want others to see you—as a whole person.

5. Surround yourself with positive people. It is easier to feel good about yourself and your body when you are around others who are supportive and who recognize the importance of liking yourself just as you naturally are.

6. Shut down those voices in your head that tell you your body is not "right" or that you are a "bad" person. You can overpower those negative thoughts with positive ones. The next time you start to tear yourself down, build yourself back up with a few quick affirmations that work for you.

7. Wear clothes that are comfortable and that make you feel good about your body. Work with your body, not against it.

8. Become a critical viewer of social and media messages. Pay attention to images, slogans, or attitudes that make you feel bad about yourself or your body. Protest these messages: write a letter to the advertiser or talk back to the image or message.

9. Do something nice for yourself—something that lets your body know you appreciate it. Take a bubble bath, make time for a nap, find a peaceful place outside to relax.

10. Use the time and energy that you might have spent worrying about food, calories, and your weight to do something to help others. Sometimes reaching out to other people can help you feel better about yourself and can make a positive change in our world.

Section 47.3

Promoting Positive Body Image in Children: A Guide for Parents

"How to Raise a Healthy Child in Body and Mind: Prevention Tips for Parents," © Rebecca Manley, M.S., Multi-service Eating Disorder Association (MEDA), 1996. Reprinted with permission. For additional information, contact MEDA at 866-343-6332, or www.medainc.org. Reviewed by David A. Cooke, M.D., FACP, October 2010.

Most parents have an incredible influence on their children's lives. Many studies show that parents are often identified as role models and the people children trust most to help them define their moral standards. Therefore, it is vitally important for parents to talk with their children about developing a healthy lifestyle.

Be a positive role model. Children learn more through the actions of others than through words. Therefore, if you do not engage in unhealthy eating and exercise patterns, it is less likely your child will develop unhealthy eating and exercise habits.

Accept your child's body size. Every child is born with a different genetic makeup, which means that every child is meant to look different. Do not try to change your child's body because you have expectations of how your child should look. Try not to compare your child's size to that of another sibling or his or her friends.

Make your home environment a safe place to communicate. If your child feels he or she will be criticized for expressing feelings, he or she will be less likely to talk to you. Show that you are interested in what your child says by taking the time to stop what you are doing to really focus on your child.

Talk with your child about the media and advertising. It is amazing how many children are unaware of the techniques, such as computer graphics, to alter a picture in a magazine. Educate your child about the tricks in the modeling and advertising industries. Use television programs to talk about unrealistic body sizes and lifestyles.

Make clear rules in your home about "body teasing." "Body teasing" is mocking someone because of the way he or she looks or feels. Often teasing starts out as a fun activity but it rarely ends up that way. If every household enforced a no teasing rule there would be a lot less of this activity in schools.

Monitor your child's conversations with friends. If you find that you hear a lot of diet talk or body put downs, talk to your child about why this is happening and how this can spiral into lowered self-esteem and body image. Teach your child to be assertive and speak up when his/her friends start unhealthy talk. When your child's friends start talking badly about their bodies advise him or her to take action with words: (e.g., "Let's talk about something else," or "We spend a lot of time talking about this. Let's find other things to talk about.")

Tell your child how you felt about your body growing up. Let them know how you dealt with the thinness craze. Talk about the importance of building a strong mind and body. It is hard to have one without the other.

Section 47.4

The Link between Parents' and Kids' Body Image

"Body Image and Your Kids: Your Body Image Plays a Role in Theirs," National Women's Health Information Center, September 22, 2009.

"On a diet, you can't eat." This is what one five year-old girl had to say in a study on girls' ideas about dieting. This and other research has shown that daughters are more likely to have ideas about dieting when their mothers diet. Children pick up on comments about dieting concepts that may seem harmless, such as limiting high-fat foods or eating less. Yet, as girls enter their teen years, having ideas about dieting can lead to problems. Many things can spark weight concerns for girls and impact their eating habits in potentially unhealthy ways:

- Having mothers concerned about their own weight

- Having mothers who are overly concerned about their daughters' weight and looks

- Natural weight gain and other body changes during puberty

- Peer pressure to look a certain way

- Struggles with self-esteem

- Media images showing the ideal female body as thin

Many teenage girls of average weight think they are overweight and are not satisfied with their bodies. Having extreme weight concerns— and acting on those concerns—can harm girls' social, physical, and emotional growth. Actions such as skipping meals or taking diet pills can lead to poor nutrition and difficulty learning. For some, extreme efforts to lose weight can lead to eating disorders such as anorexia or bulimia. For others, the pressure to be thin can actually lead to binge eating disorder: overeating that is followed by extreme guilt. What's more, girls are more likely to further risk their health by trying to lose weight in unhealthy ways, such as smoking.

While not as common, boys are also at risk of developing unhealthy eating habits and eating disorders. Body image becomes an important issue for teenage boys as they struggle with body changes and pay more attention to media images of the "ideal" muscular male.

What You Can Do

Your children pay attention to what you say and do—even if it doesn't seem like it sometimes. If you are always complaining about your weight or feel pressure to change your body shape, your children may learn that these are important concerns. If you are attracted to new "miracle" diets, they may learn that restrictive dieting is better than making healthy lifestyle choices. If you tell your daughter that she would be prettier if she lost weight, she will learn that the goals of weight loss are to be attractive and accepted by others.

Parents are role models and should try to follow the healthy eating and physical activity patterns that you would like your children to follow—for your health and theirs. Extreme weight concerns and eating disorders, as well as obesity, are hard to treat. Yet, you can play an important role in preventing these problems for your children.

Follow these steps to help your child develop a positive body image and relate to food in a healthy way:

- Make sure your child understands that weight gain is a normal part of development, especially during puberty.

- Avoid negative statements about food, weight, and body size and shape.

- Allow your child to make decisions about food, while making sure that plenty of healthy and nutritious meals and snacks are available.

- Compliment your child on her or his efforts, talents, accomplishments, and personal values.

- Restrict television viewing, and watch television with your child and discuss the media images you see.

- Encourage your school to enact policies against size and sexual discrimination, harassment, teasing, and name-calling; support the elimination of public weigh-ins and fat measurements.

- Keep the communication lines with your child open.

Section 47.5

Body Image during Pregnancy: Loving Your Body at All Stages

According to Ann Douglas, author of *The Unofficial Guide to Having a Baby*, "A woman who feels good about herself will celebrate the changes that her body experiences during pregnancy, look forward to the challenge of giving birth, and willingly accept the physical and emotional changes of the postpartum period."

Loving Your Body Even Before You Are Pregnant

Loving your body before pregnancy can help you get through the physical and emotional changes during pregnancy. Having a positive body image of yourself is not about what you look like, but how you feel about yourself. This is crucial in pregnancy since there will be body changes that you cannot control. It is also helpful to understand why your body is going through these changes.

Loving Your Body When You Are Pregnant

Knowing that your body's changes are essential to your developing baby is reason enough to embrace these changes and *smile!*

Understanding What Your Body Is Doing For Your Baby

As soon as your egg is fertilized and implanted in your uterus, your body begins to go through changes. These changes are a result of your baby's growth and development. Your baby has a fetal life-support system that consists of the placenta, umbilical cord, and amniotic sac. The placenta produces hormones that are necessary to support a healthy pregnancy and baby. These hormones help prepare your breasts for lactation and are responsible for many changes in your body.

You will have an increase in blood circulation that is needed to supply the placenta. This increase in blood is responsible for that wonderful "pregnancy glow" that you may have.

Your metabolism will increase, so you may have food cravings and the desire to eat more. Your body is requiring more nutrients to feed both you and your baby.

Your uterus will enlarge and the amniotic sac (your baby's home) will be filled with amniotic fluid. The amniotic fluid is there to protect your baby from any bumps or falls.

Here are a few things you can do to love your body during pregnancy.

Exercise. Exercise during pregnancy can help you feel fit, strong, and sexy. According to the American College of Obstetricians and Gynecologists, pregnant women are encouraged to exercise at least thirty minutes a day throughout pregnancy, unless your healthcare provider instructs differently.

Before starting any exercise program *always* check with your healthcare provider.

Pamper yourself. Treat yourself to a body massage or a makeover. Go shopping! What better excuse to go shopping? There are cute and even sophisticated maternity clothes to buy. This is your time to shine. Make the most of these wonderful nine months.

Have a good support network. It is a good idea to surround yourself with positive people. During your pregnancy you can be more vulnerable to negative self-talk and it can affect you in a negative way. If you are feeling that you are not getting the support you need, share that with those around you.

Loving Your Body After Pregnancy

After your baby is born your body has to adjust and return to a nonpregnant body. Your uterus will need time to shrink, so don't expect a flat belly after your delivery. Remember, your body has been through a lot in giving birth and needs time to recuperate. Give yourself some time to rest and catch up on some sleep. It's ok to ask your family and friends for help with the baby so you can catch some zzzz's.

Exercise can also help you get your pre-pregnancy body back. Join a gym that offers childcare or load up your stroller and walk through the neighborhood. This will also help get you out of the house so you can feel refreshed.

Chapter 48

Determining a Healthy Weight

Chapter Contents

Section 48.1

How to Assess Your Weight

Excerpted from "Assessing Your Weight," November 10, 2009,
and "About BMI for Children and Teens," January 27, 2009,
Centers for Disease Control and Prevention.

Assessing Your Weight

If you've been thinking about your current weight, it may be because
you've noticed a change in how your clothes fit. Or maybe you've been
told by a healthcare professional that you have high blood pressure
or high cholesterol and that excessive weight could be a contributing
factor. The first step is to assess whether or not your current weight
is healthy.

Adult Body Mass Index or BMI

One way to begin to determine whether your weight is a healthy
one is to calculate your "body mass index" (BMI). For most people, BMI
is a reliable indicator of body fatness. It is calculated based on your
height and weight.

To calculate your BMI, use the formula in Figure 48.1. Or determine
your BMI by finding your height and weight in Figure 48.2.

$$BMI = \frac{weight \ (pounds) \ x \ 703}{height \ squared \ (inches^2)}$$

Figure 48.1. *How to calculate body mass index*

Understanding Your BMI

- If your BMI is less than 18.5, it falls within the "underweight"
  range.

- If your BMI is 18.5 to 24.9, it falls within the "normal" or healthy
  weight range.

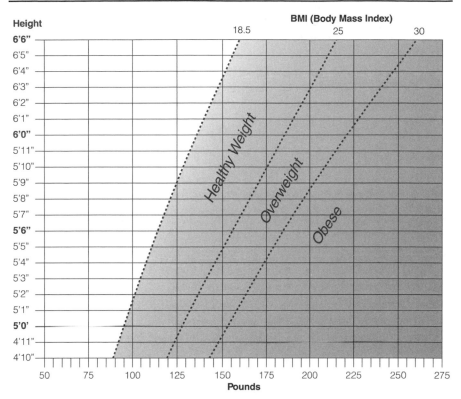

Find your weight on the bottom of the graph. Go straight up from that point until you come to the line that matches your height. Then look to find your weight group. The higher your BMI is over 25, the greater chance you may have of developing health problems.

Figure 48.2. Body mass index chart (Height is figured without shoes and weight is figured without clothes.)

- If your BMI is 25.0 to 29.9, it falls within the "overweight" range.
- If your BMI is 30.0 or higher, it falls within the "obese" range.

"Underweight," "normal," "overweight," and "obese" are all labels for ranges of weight. Obese and overweight describe ranges of weight that are greater than what is considered healthy for a given height, while underweight describes a weight that is lower than what is considered healthy. If your BMI falls outside of the "normal" or healthy weight range, you may want to talk to your doctor or healthcare provider about how you might achieve a healthier body weight. Obesity and overweight have been shown to increase the likelihood of certain diseases and other health problems.

463

At an individual level, BMI can be used as a screening tool but is not diagnostic of the body fatness or health of an individual. A trained healthcare provider should perform appropriate health assessments in order to evaluate an individual's health status and risks.

Waist Circumference

Another way to assess your weight is to measure your waist size. Your waistline may be telling you that you have a higher risk of developing obesity-related conditions if you are:

- a man whose waist circumference is more than forty inches;
- a non-pregnant woman whose waist circumference is more than thirty-five inches.

Excessive abdominal fat is serious because it places you at greater risk for developing obesity-related conditions, such as type 2 diabetes, high blood cholesterol, high triglycerides, high blood pressure, and coronary artery disease. Individuals who have excessive abdominal fat should consult with their physicians or other healthcare providers to develop a plan for losing weight.

How to Measure Your Waist Size[1]

To measure your waist size (circumference), place a tape measure around your bare abdomen just above your hip bone. Be sure that the tape is snug, but does not compress your skin, and is parallel to the floor. Relax, exhale, and measure your waist.

About BMI for Children and Teens

What is BMI?

Body Mass Index (BMI) is a number calculated from a child's weight and height. BMI is a reliable indicator of body fatness for most children and teens. BMI does not measure body fat directly, but research has shown that BMI correlates to direct measures of body fat, such as underwater weighing and dual energy x-ray absorptiometry (DXA).[2] BMI can be considered an alternative for direct measures of body fat. Additionally, BMI is an inexpensive and easy-to-perform method of screening for weight categories that may lead to health problems.

For children and teens, BMI is age- and sex-specific and is often referred to as BMI-for-age.

What Is a BMI Percentile

After BMI is calculated for children and teens, the BMI number is plotted on the Centers for Disease Control and Prevention (CDC) BMI-for-age growth charts (for either girls or boys) to obtain a percentile ranking. Percentiles are the most commonly used indicator to assess the size and growth patterns of individual children in the United States. The percentile indicates the relative position of the child's BMI number among children of the same sex and age. The growth charts show the weight status categories used with children and teens (underweight, healthy weight, overweight, and obese).

BMI-for-age weight status categories and the corresponding percentiles are shown in Table 48.1.

Table 48.1. BMI-for-Age Weight Status Categories and Percentiles

Weight Status Category	Percentile Range
Underweight	Less than the fifth percentile
Healthy weight	Fifth percentile to less than the eighty-fifth percentile
Overweight	Eighty-fifth to less than the ninety-fifth percentile
Obese	Equal to or greater than the ninety-fifth percentile

How Is BMI Used with Children and Teens?

BMI is used as a screening tool to identify possible weight problems for children. CDC and the American Academy of Pediatrics (AAP) recommend the use of BMI to screen for overweight and obesity in children beginning at two years old.

For children, BMI is used to screen for obesity, overweight, healthy weight, or underweight. However, BMI is not a diagnostic tool. For example, a child may have a high BMI for age and sex, but to determine if excess fat is a problem, a healthcare provider would need to perform further assessments. These assessments might include skinfold thickness measurements, evaluations of diet, physical activity, family history, and other appropriate health screenings.

465

How Is BMI Calculated and Interpreted for Children and Teens?

Calculating and interpreting BMI using the BMI percentile calculator involves the following steps:

1. Before calculating BMI, obtain accurate height and weight measurements.

2. Calculate the BMI and percentile using Figure 48.1, Figure 48.3, and Figure 48.4.

3. Review the calculated BMI-for-age percentile and results. The BMI-for-age percentile is used to interpret the BMI number because BMI is both age- and sex-specific for children and teens. These criteria are different from those used to interpret BMI for adults—which do not take into account age or sex. Age and sex are considered for children and teens for two reasons:

    *   The amount of body fat changes with age. (BMI for children and teens is often referred to as BMI-for-age.)

    *   The amount of body fat differs between girls and boys.

        The CDC BMI-for-age growth charts for girls and boys take into account these differences and allow translation of a BMI number into a percentile for a child's or teen's sex and age.

4. Find the weight status category for the calculated BMI-for-age percentile as shown in the Table 48.1. These categories are based on expert committee recommendations.

Why Can't Healthy Weight Ranges Be Provided for Children and Teens?

Healthy weight ranges cannot be provided for children and teens for the following reasons:

*   Healthy weight ranges change with each month of age for each sex.
*   Healthy weight ranges change as height increases.

Can I Determine If My Child or Teen Is Obese by Using an Adult BMI Calculator?

No. The adult calculator provides only the BMI number and not the BMI age- and sex-specific percentile that is used to interpret BMI and determine the weight category for children and teens. It is not appropriate to use the BMI categories for adults to interpret BMI numbers for children and teens.

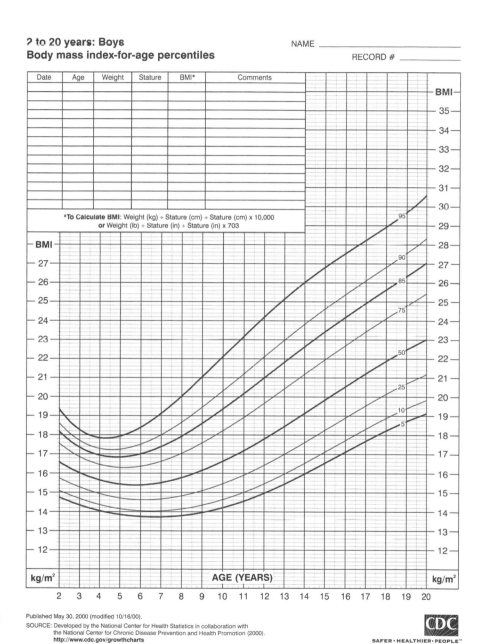

2 to 20 years: Boys
Body mass index-for-age percentiles

NAME _____

RECORD # _____

Date	Age	Weight	Stature	BMI*	Comments

*To Calculate BMI: Weight (kg) ÷ Stature (cm) ÷ Stature (cm) x 10,000
or Weight (lb) ÷ Stature (in) ÷ Stature (in) x 703

AGE (YEARS)

kg/m²   kg/m²

2 3 4 5 6 7 8 9 10 11 12 13 14 15 16 17 18 19 20

Published May 30, 2000 (modified 10/16/00).
SOURCE: Developed by the National Center for Health Statistics in collaboration with
the National Center for Chronic Disease Prevention and Health Promotion (2000).
http://www.cdc.gov/growthcharts

CDC
SAFER·HEALTHIER·PEOPLE™

Figure 48.3. *Body Mass Index-for-Age Percentiles, Boys, 2 to 20 Years*

467

2 to 20 years: Girls
Body mass index-for-age percentiles

NAME _____

RECORD # _____

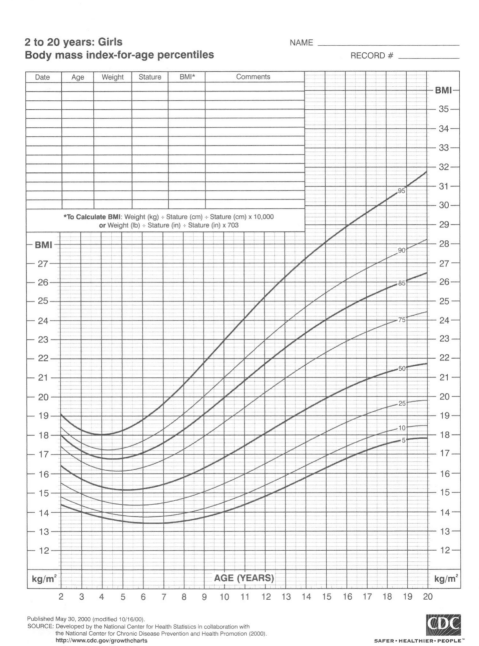

Published May 30, 2000 (modified 10/16/00).
SOURCE: Developed by the National Center for Health Statistics in collaboration with
the National Center for Chronic Disease Prevention and Health Promotion (2000).
http://www.cdc.gov/growthcharts

Figure 48.4. *Body Mass Index-for-Age Percentiles, Girls, 2 to 20 Years*

468

References

1. U.S. Department of Health and Human Services, A Healthier You, page 14. Available online: http://www.health.gov/dietaryguidelines/dga2005/healthieryou.

2. Mei Z, Grummer-Strawn LM, Pietrobelli A, Goulding A, Goran MI, Dietz WH. Validity of body mass index compared with other body-composition screening indexes for the assessment of body fatness in children and adolescents. *American Journal of Clinical Nutrition* 2002;7597–985.

3. Freedman DS, Dietz WH, Srinivasan SR, Berenson GS. The relation of overweight to cardiovascular risk factors among children and adolescents: The Bogalusa Heart Study. *Pediatrics* 1999;103:1175–82.

4. Must A and Anderson SE. Effects of obesity on morbidity in children and adolescents. *Nutrition in Clinical Care* 2003;6(1):4–12.

5. Whitaker RC, Wright JA, Pepe MS, Seidel KD, Dietz WH. Predicting obesity in young adulthood from childhood and parental obesity. *New England Journal of Medicine* 1997;37(13):869–73.

6. Ferraro KF, Thorpe RJ Jr, Wilkinson JA. The life course of severe obesity: does childhood overweight matter? *Journal of Gerontology: Social Sciences* 2003;58B(2):S110–19.

Section 48.2

Should I Gain Weight?

"I want to play hockey, like I did in middle school, but now that I'm in high school, the other guys have bulked up and I haven't. What can I do?"

"All of my friends have broad shoulders and look like they lift weights. No matter what I do, I just look scrawny. What can I do?"

"It's not like I want to gain a lot of weight, but I'd like to look like I have some curves, like the girls I see on TV. What can I do?"

A lot of teens think that they're too skinny, and wonder if they should do something about it.

Why Do People Want to Gain Weight?

Some of the reasons people give for wanting to gain weight are:

- **I'm worried that there's something wrong with me:** If you want to gain weight because you think you have a medical problem, talk to your doctor. Although certain health conditions can cause a person to be underweight, most of them have symptoms other than skinniness, like stomach pain or diarrhea. So it's likely that if some kind of medical problem is making you skinny, you probably wouldn't feel well.

- **I'm worried because all of my friends have filled out and I haven't:** Many guys and girls are skinny until they start to go through puberty. The changes that come with puberty include weight gain and, in guys, broader shoulders and increased muscle mass. Because everyone is on a different schedule, some of your friends may have started to fill out when they were as young as eight (if they're girls) or ten (if they're guys). But for some normal kids, puberty may not start until twelve or later for girls and fourteen or later for guys. And whenever you start puberty, it may take three or four years for you to fully develop and gain all of the weight and muscle mass you will have as an adult. Some people experience what's called delayed puberty. If you are one of these "late bloomers," you may find that some relatives of yours developed late, too. Most teens who have delayed puberty don't need to do anything; they'll eventually develop normally—and that includes gaining weight and muscle. If you are concerned about delayed puberty, though, talk to your doctor.

- **I've always wanted to play a certain sport; now I don't know if I can:** Lots of people come to love a sport in grade school or middle school—and then find themselves on the bench when their teammates develop faster. If you've always envisioned yourself playing football, it can be tough when your body doesn't seem to want to measure up. You may need to wait until your body goes through puberty before you can play football on the varsity squad. Another option to consider is switching your ambitions to another sport. If you were the fastest defensive player on your middle school football team but now it seems that your body type is long and lean, maybe track and field is for you. Many adults find that the sports they love the most are those that fit their body types the best.

- **I just hate the way I look:** Developing can be tough enough without the pressure to be perfect. Your body changes (or doesn't change), your friends' bodies change (or don't), and you all spend a lot of time noticing. It's easy to judge both yourself and others based on appearances. Sometimes, it can feel like life is some kind of beauty contest! Your body is your own, and as frustrating as it may seem to begin with, there are certain things you can't speed up or change. But there is one thing you can do to help: Work to keep your body healthy so that you can grow and develop properly. Self-esteem can play a part here, too. People who learn to love their bodies and accept them for what they are carry themselves well and project a type of self-confidence that helps them look attractive. If you're having trouble with your body image, talk about how you feel with someone you like and trust who's been through it—maybe a parent, doctor, counselor, coach, or teacher.

It's the Growth, Not the Gain

No matter what your reason is for wanting to gain weight, here's a simple fact: The majority of teens have no reason—medical or otherwise—to try to gain weight. An effort like this will at best simply not work and at worst increase your body fat, putting you at risk for health problems.

So focus on growing strong, not gaining weight. Keeping your body healthy and fit so that it grows well is an important part of your job as a teen. Here are some things you can do to help this happen.

Make Nutrition Your Mission

Your friends who want to slim down are eating more salads and fruit. Here's a surprise: So should you. You can do more for your body by eating a variety of healthier foods instead of trying to pack on weight by forcing yourself to eat a lot of unhealthy high-fat, high-sugar foods. Chances are, trying to force-feed yourself won't help you gain weight anyway, and if you do, you'll mostly just be gaining excess body fat.

Eating a variety of healthy foods, making time for regular meals and snacks, and eating only until you are full will give your body its best chance to stay healthy as it gets the fuel and nutrients it needs.

Good nutrition doesn't have to be complicated. Here are some simple tips:

- Eat lots of vegetables and fruits.
- Choose whole grains.
- Eat breakfast every day.
- Eat healthy snacks.
- Limit less nutritious foods, like chips and soda.

Eating well at this point in your life is important for lots of reasons. Good nutrition is a key part of normal growth and development. It's also wise to learn good eating habits now—they'll become second nature, which will help you stay healthy and fit without even thinking about it.

Keep on Moving

Another way to keep your body healthy is to incorporate exercise into your routine. This can include walking to school, playing Frisbee with your friends, or helping out with some household chores. Or you might choose to work out at a gym or with a sports team. A good rule of thumb for exercise amounts during the teen years: Try to get at least sixty minutes of moderate to vigorous physical activity every day.

Strength training, when done safely, is a healthy way to exercise, but it won't necessarily bulk you up. Guys especially get more muscular during puberty, but puberty is no guarantee that you'll turn into a cover model for *Muscle & Fitness* in a couple of years—some people just don't have the kind of body type for this to happen. Our genes play an important role in determining our body type. Adult bodies come in all different shapes and sizes, and some people stay lean their entire lives, no matter what they do.

If you've hit puberty, the right amount of strength training will help your muscles become stronger and have more endurance. And, once a boy has reached puberty, proper weight training can help him bulk up, if that's the goal. Girls can benefit from strength training, too, but they won't bulk up like boys. Be sure to work with a certified trainer, who can show you how to do it without injuring yourself.

Get the Skinny on Supplements

Thinking about drinking something from a can or taking a pill to turn you buff overnight? Guess what: Supplements or pills that make promises like this are at best a waste of money and at worst potentially harmful to your health.

The best way to get the fuel you need to build muscle is by eating well. Before you take any kind of supplement at all, even if it's just a vitamin pill, talk to your doctor.

Sleep Your Way to Stunning

Sleep is an important component of normal growth and development. If you get enough, you'll have the energy to fuel your growth. Your body is at work while it sleeps—oxygen moves to the brain, growth hormones are released, and your bones keep on developing, even while you're resting.

Focus on feeling good. It can help to know that your body is likely to change in the months and years ahead. Few of us look like we did at fifteen when we're twenty-five. But it's also important to realize that feeling good about yourself can make you more attractive to others, too.

Section 48.3

Are You Overweight?

"Are You Overweight?" by Abigail H. Natenshon, MA, LCSW, GCFP. © 2010. Reprinted with permission. Abigail H. Natenshon has been a psychotherapist specializing in eating disorders for four decades. As the director of Eating Disorder Specialists of Illinois: A Clinic Without Walls, she has authored two books, *When Your Child Has an Eating Disorder: A Step-by-Step Workbook for Parents and Caregivers* and *Doing What Works: An Integrative System for the Treatment of Eating Disorders from Diagnosis to Recovery*. Natenshon, who is also a Guild Certified Feldenkrais Practitioner, hosts three informative websites, including www.empoweredparents.com, www .empoweredkidz.com, and www.treatingeatingdisorders.com.

Are You Overweight?

This is a tough question. Sometimes people believe that if they do not look as thin as Heather Locklear or Kate Moss they must be overweight. This is certainly not the case; only a very small percentage of people are born with an ectomorph body type that would allow them to look this thin and still be healthy. Misconceptions about being overweight abound; people assume that overweight people do not care about their appearance, that they are lazy, undisciplined, and irresponsible about themselves and their appearance. Some believe that if they do weigh more than they should or they want to, then that makes them physically unfit, unattractive, and unacceptable to their peers. Few people understand that obesity is a factor that is largely determined by natural factors such as genetics, and the maternal environment provided the fetus while in utero. Nor are various forms of weight measurements such as body mass index (BMI) accurate indicators of overweight in children and teens because healthy weight ranges change with each month of age for each sex, and because healthy weight ranges change as height increases.

Clearly, the most destructive of all misconceptions about being overweight is that dieting is the best and only way to lose weight. In fact, the opposite is true. In fact, studies show that:

- dieting is the worst way to lose weight;
- young people who restrict food or diet early in life have a much greater chance of becoming obese adults;

- ninety-five percent of dieters gain back all of their weight, and more, within five years;

- dieters lose weight in muscle tissue and gain it back in fat.
  Here are some facts that you need to know:

- Certain people who are large in size or who might appear to be overweight are not unhealthy. Some people are born with naturally larger bones and an endomorph body type, which is rounder and softer and gains weight more easily. Size and shape acceptance becomes critical in such instances.

- Aside from genetic factors, people may become the size and shape they are because of the nature and quality of their eating and exercise lifestyle. People who eat well and exercise regularly have the capacity to remain physically fit, strong, and healthy, despite their genetically determined body type and shape.

- It is only when a person is overweight as a result of eating too much of the wrong kinds of foods in erratic eating patterns, and/ or from a lack of exercise, that overweight can become a health hazard. Be aware that when mesomorph body types become overweight, they may look like endomorph body types.

Do You Have a Healthy Relationship with Food?

The important question to ask yourself is not whether you are too fat. It is whether or not you have a healthy "relationship" with food:

- Do you envision food as fuel and as nourishment, as tasting good and being an enjoyable and regular part of your life?

- Do you see food as a life-giving substance that allows your brain to function optimally, and your muscles and bones to grow healthfully?

- Do you see eating as pleasurable and satisfying and at the center of sociability with family and friends?

Hopefully, you were able to answer these questions affirmatively. If not, why not? Does food and eating frighten and worry you? Are you preoccupied with counting calories and feeling concerned that every bite you put in your mouth will appear on your body, that food is fattening, and in some ways, feels to you like an enemy? If so, you may be experiencing the early signs of a clinical eating disorder or at the very least, disordered eating and you may want to seek some help.

If you believe that you are overweight and are aware that you do not eat regular, healthy meals; if instead of eating nutritious foods to sustain your growing body, you turn to easily accessible "junk" foods (foods without nutritional value); and if you would like to lose weight in order to become more physically fit and to look better, it is important for you to begin thinking about eating differently, not less. Does this come as a surprise to you?

What does it mean to become a healthy eater? Healthy eating is the ability to eat regularly, freely, and pleasurably without fear of becoming overweight. Did you know that when you eat regular meals, you enhance the functioning of your body's metabolism and insure that once your body reaches its set point weight, its "happy weight," or the weight it needs and wants to be in order to function at its best, you will stop gaining weight naturally, without trying? Did you know that healthy eating in the form of nutritious, balanced, and varied meals also offers the best way to lose weight in a healthy way, and for the long term, should that ever become a necessity.

How Should You Eat to Allow Your Body to Reach Its Set Point Weight?

- Always eat three square meals a day. If you skip meals, you will damage the function of your metabolism and will no longer be able to burn fat effectively.

- Never substitute a protein bar for a meal.

- Be sure to eat protein, carbohydrates, and fat at each meal. Protein makes your mind alert and gives you a feeling of being full. Carbohydrates give you energy, and fat makes you feel satisfied, contributes to your neurological and reproductive development, and carries vitamins throughout your body.

- Recognize that eating fat doesn't make you fat.

- If you decide to limit your fat intake, consider limiting the saturated fats only.

- Never miss breakfast. People who eat less in the early part of the day eat 40 percent more during the latter part of the day.

- Limit the amount of soda pop that you drink. Drink water instead. It is better for you. Beware of diet drinks that are loaded with chemicals that make you feel hungry for sugar.

- When you snack, treat your body to something that will help you to grow up and to grow strong. Cheese and crackers, peanut butter on bread, yogurt, and fruit are all great alternatives to cookies and cakes.

- Remember that cookies and cakes aren't bad—as long as you eat them in moderation! Remember, there are no bad foods. Excess is bad; food is not.

- The more a person deprives himself of a certain kind of food, the more apt (s)he is to binge and gorge on that food when (s)he succumbs. A healthy eater is a person who can eat all kinds of foods, in moderation, and without fear.

- Make sure you get regular exercise. Walk to school when you can, take the dog out for a walk, enjoy and rake leaves in the fall, play in and shovel snow in the winter, plant and enjoy the flowers in the spring.

First Things First

In your effort to learn to eat differently, it is essential first to become aware of your eating habits and exercise lifestyle. Then, decide if you would like to make some changes and if so, what changes. Consider the following:

- Make a journal of what you eat during every day. You will begin to learn a great deal about yourself, your eating habits, and what you might like to change.

- Do not eat anywhere other than the kitchen or dining room table, sitting down, with a plate in front of you.

- Don't eat in front of the television. The less television watching you do, the more exercise you are likely to get.

- Ask your parents to fill the house with "nutritionally dense" foods, or foods that are good for you. Offer to go food shopping with them so you can show them what you like to eat. They can help you find the most healthful foods for you.

- Cook meals with your parents. It's great fun and a wonderful skill to have.

- Be sure to include your parents in your hopes, plans, and efforts. They will want to know how they can help and support you.

477

- Always eat moderately and wisely and you will find you will be able to eat fearlessly and to trust your body to be healthy and not get fat.

Food should be enjoyed. It is one of the greatest gifts we as humans have. Your relationship with food is something that is clearly within your power to change if you are not happy with it at the moment. Learning to eat healthfully will improve how you feel about each day, as well as how you feel about yourself.

Eating healthfully is the route to living healthfully, and living healthfully is the prerequisite to becoming the adult that you would like to be one day.

Section 48.4

Weight Cycling: An Unhealthy Pattern

"Weight Cycling," Weight-Control Information Network,
National Institute of Diabetes and Digestive and Kidney Diseases,
National Institutes of Health, NIH Publication No. 01-3901, May 2008.

What is weight cycling?

Weight cycling is the repeated loss and regain of body weight. This sometimes happens to people who go on weight-loss diets. A small cycle may include loss and regain of five to ten pounds. In a large cycle, weight can change by fifty pounds or more.

Is weight cycling harmful to my health?

Experts are not sure if weight cycling leads to health problems. However, some studies suggest a link to high blood pressure, high cholesterol, gallbladder disease, and other problems. One study showed other problems may be linked to weight cycling as well. The study showed that women who weight cycle gain more weight over time than women who do not weight cycle. Binge eating (when a person eats a lot of food while feeling out of control) was also linked to women who weight cycle. The same study showed that women who weight cycle were also less likely to use physical activity to control their weight.

Weight cycling may affect your mental health too. People who weight cycle may feel depressed about their weight. However, weight cycling should not be a reason to "feel like a failure." If you feel down, try to focus on making changes in your eating and physical activity habits. Keeping a good attitude will help you stay focused. In addition, talk with a healthcare professional about your weight and ways you can manage it. Doing so may help you determine why you weight cycle. Understanding the cause of your weight cycling may help you in the process of lifelong weight management.

How can I manage weight and avoid weight cycling?

Experts recommend different strategies for different people. The goal for everyone is to achieve a healthy weight. This can help prevent the health problems linked to weight cycling.

People who are not overweight or obese, and have no health problems related to weight, should maintain a stable weight.

People who are overweight or obese should try to achieve and maintain a modest weight loss. An initial goal of losing 10 percent of your body weight can help in your efforts to improve overall health.

If you need to lose weight, be ready to make lifelong changes. Healthy eating and physical activity are the keys to your efforts. Focus on making healthful food choices, such as eating more high-fiber foods like fruits and vegetables and cutting down on foods that are high in saturated or trans fats. And make room for physical activity. Studies show that many people who weight cycle do not participate in regular physical activity. Walking, jogging, or other activities can help keep you active and feeling good.

If I weight cycle after a diet, will I gain more weight than I had before the diet? Will I have less muscle?

Studies do not show that fat tissue increases after a weight cycle. Study results do not support decreases in muscle either. Many people simply regain the weight they lost while on the diet—they have the same amount of fat and muscle as they did before the weight cycle.

Some people worry that weight cycling can put more fat around their stomach area. This is important since people who carry extra body weight around this area are more likely to develop type 2 diabetes. Studies show that people do not have more fat around their stomach after a weight cycle. However, other studies suggest that women who are overweight and have a history of weight cycling have thicker layers of fat around their stomach, compared to women who do not weight cycle. It is not clear how this relates to weight cycling.

If I regain lost weight, will it be even harder to lose it again?

Losing weight after a weight cycle should not be harder. Studies show weight cycling does not affect how fast you burn food energy, which is called your "metabolic rate." This rate slows as we get older, but healthy eating and regular physical activity can still help you achieve a healthy weight.

Is staying overweight healthier than weight cycling?

This is a hard question to answer since experts are not sure whether weight cycling causes health problems. However, experts are sure that if you are overweight, losing weight is a good thing. Being overweight or obese is associated with the following health problems:

- High blood pressure
- Heart disease
- Stroke
- Gallbladder disease
- Fatty liver disease
- Type 2 diabetes
- Certain types of cancer
- Arthritis
- Breathing problems, such as sleep apnea (when breathing stops for short periods during sleep)

Not everyone who is overweight or obese has the same risk for these problems. Risk is affected by several factors: your gender, family history of disease, the amount of extra weight you have, and where fat is located on your body. You can improve your health with a modest weight loss. Losing just 10 percent of your body weight over six months will help.

Experts need to learn more about weight cycling. Knowing if it is a cause or effect of poor physical and mental health is important. In the meantime, you can help yourself if you are overweight or obese. Try to eat a healthy diet and get plenty of physical activity. If you go through a weight cycle, do not feel like a failure. Just keep trying your best.

Chapter 49

Maintaining Your Weight

Chapter Contents

Section 49.1

Maintaining a Healthy Weight: Balancing Calories

Excerpted from "Balancing Calories," Centers for
Disease Control and Prevention, April 1, 2009.

The Caloric Balance Equation

When it comes to maintaining a healthy weight for a lifetime, the bottom line is—calories count! Weight management is all about balance—balancing the number of calories you consume with the number of calories your body uses or "burns off."

A calorie is defined as a unit of energy supplied by food. A calorie is a calorie regardless of its source. Whether you're eating carbohydrates, fats, sugars, or proteins, all of them contain calories.

Caloric balance is like a scale. To remain in balance and maintain your body weight, the calories consumed (from foods) must be balanced by the calories used (in normal body functions, daily activities, and exercise):

- If you are maintaining your weight you are "in balance." You are eating roughly the same number of calories that your body is using. Your weight will remain stable.

- If you are gaining weight you are "in caloric excess." You are eating more calories than your body is using. You will store these extra calories as fat and you'll gain weight.

- If you are losing weight you are "in caloric deficit." You are eating fewer calories than you are using. Your body is pulling from its fat storage cells for energy, so your weight is decreasing.

Am I in Caloric Balance?

If you are maintaining your current body weight, you are in caloric balance. If you need to gain weight or to lose weight, you'll need to tip the balance scale in one direction or another to achieve your goal.

If you need to tip the balance scale in the direction of losing weight, keep in mind that it takes approximately 3,500 calories below your calorie needs to lose a pound of body fat.[1] To lose about one to two pounds per week, you'll need to reduce your caloric intake by 500 to 1000 calories per day.[2]

Physical activities (both daily activities and exercise) help tip the balance scale by increasing the calories you expend each day.

Recommended Physical Activity Levels

- Two and a half hours (150 minut.es) of moderate-intensity aerobic activity (i.e., brisk walking) every week and muscle-strengthening activities on two or more days a week that work all major muscle groups (legs, hips, back, abdomen, chest, shoulders, and arms).

- Increasing the intensity or the amount of time that you are physically active can have even greater health benefits and may be needed to control body weight.

- Encourage children and teenagers to be physically active for at least sixty minutes each day, or almost every day.

The bottom line is, each person's body is unique and may have different caloric needs. A healthy lifestyle requires balance, in the foods you eat, in the beverages you consume, in the way you carry out your daily activities, and in the amount of physical activity or exercise you include in your daily routine. While counting calories is not necessary, it may help you in the beginning to gain an awareness of your eating habits as you strive to achieve energy balance. The ultimate test of balance is whether or not you are gaining, maintaining, or losing weight.

Questions and Answers about Calories

Are fat-free and low-fat foods low in calories? Not always. Some fat-free and low-fat foods have extra sugars, which push the calorie amount right back up. Just because a product is fat-free, it doesn't mean that it is "calorie-free," and calories do count! Always read the Nutrition Facts food label to find out the calorie content. Remember, this is the calorie content for one serving of the food item, so be sure and check the serving size. If you eat more than one serving, you'll be eating more calories than is listed on the food label.

If I eat late at night, will these calories automatically turn into body fat? The time of day isn't what affects how your body uses calories. It's the overall number of calories you eat and the calories you burn over the course of twenty-four hours that affects your weight.

I've heard it is more important to worry about carbohydrates than calories. Is this true? By focusing only on carbohydrates, you can still eat too many calories. Also, if you drastically reduce the variety of foods in your diet, you could end up sacrificing vital nutrients and not be able to sustain the diet over time.

Does it matter how many calories I eat as long as I'm maintaining an active lifestyle? While physical activity is a vital part of weight control, so is controlling the number of calories you eat. If you consume more calories than you use through normal daily activities and physical activity, you will still gain weight.

References

1. DHHS, A Healthier You, page 19. Available online: http://www .health.gov/dietaryguidelines/dga2005/healthieryou/html/ chapter5.html

2. DHHS, AIM for a Healthy Weight, page 5. Available online: http://www.nhlbi.nih.gov/health/public/heart/obesity/aim _hwt.pdf (PDF-2.17Mb)

Section 49.2

Helping Children Maintain a Healthy Weight

Excerpted from "Tips for Parents: Ideas to
Help Children Maintain a Healthy Weight," Centers for
Disease Control and Prevention, May 19, 2009.

You've probably read about it in newspapers and seen it on the news: in the United States, the number of obese children and teens has continued to rise over the past two decades.1 You may wonder: Why are doctors and scientists troubled by this trend? And as parents or other concerned adults, you may also ask: What steps can we take to help prevent obesity in our children? This section provides answers to some of the questions you may have and provides you with resources to help you keep your family healthy.

Why Is Childhood Obesity Considered a Health Problem?

Doctors and scientists are concerned about the rise of obesity in children and youth because obesity may lead to the following health problems:

- Heart disease, caused by high cholesterol and/or high blood pressure

- Type 2 diabetes

- Asthma

- Sleep apnea

- Social discrimination

Childhood obesity is associated with various health-related consequences. Obese children and adolescents may experience immediate health consequences and may be at risk for weight-related health problems in adulthood.

Psychosocial Risks

Some consequences of childhood and adolescent overweight are psychosocial. Obese children and adolescents are targets of early and systematic social discrimination.2 The psychological stress of social stigmatization can cause low self-esteem which, in turn, can hinder academic and social functioning, and persist into adulthood.3

Cardiovascular Disease Risks

Obese children and teens have been found to have risk factors for cardiovascular disease (CVD), including high cholesterol levels, high blood pressure, and abnormal glucose tolerance. In a population-based sample of five- to seventeen-year-olds, almost 60 percent of overweight children had at least one CVD risk factor while 25 percent of overweight children had two or more CVD risk factors.2

Additional Health Risks

Less common health conditions associated with increased weight include asthma, hepatic steatosis, sleep apnea, and type 2 diabetes:

- Asthma is a disease of the lungs in which the airways become blocked or narrowed, causing breathing difficulty. Studies have identified an association between childhood overweight and asthma.4,5

- Hepatic steatosis is the fatty degeneration of the liver caused by a high concentration of liver enzymes. Weight reduction causes liver enzymes to normalize.2

- Sleep apnea is a less common complication of overweight for children and adolescents. Sleep apnea is a sleep-associated breathing disorder defined as the cessation of breathing during sleep that lasts for at least ten seconds. Sleep apnea is characterized by loud snoring and labored breathing. During sleep apnea, oxygen levels in the blood can fall dramatically. One study estimated that sleep apnea occurs in about 7 percent of overweight children.6

- Type 2 diabetes is increasingly being reported among children and adolescents who are overweight.[7] Onset of diabetes in children and adolescents can result in advanced complications such as CVD and kidney failure.[8]

In addition, studies have shown that obese children and teens are more likely to become obese as adults.[9,10]

What Can I Do As a Parent or Guardian to Help Prevent Childhood Overweight and Obesity?

To help your child maintain a healthy weight, balance the calories your child consumes from foods and beverages with the calories your child uses through physical activity and normal growth.

Remember that the goal for overweight and obese children and teens is to reduce the rate of weight gain while allowing normal growth and development. Children and teens should *not* be placed on a weight reduction diet without the consultation of a healthcare provider.

Encourage Healthy Eating Habits

There's no great secret to healthy eating. To help your children and family develop healthy eating habits, try the following things:

- Provide plenty of vegetables, fruits, and whole-grain products.
- Include low-fat or non-fat milk or dairy products.
- Choose lean meats, poultry, fish, lentils, and beans for protein.
- Serve reasonably sized portions.
- Encourage your family to drink lots of water.
- Limit sugar-sweetened beverages.
- Limit consumption of sugar and saturated fat.

Remember that small changes every day can lead to a recipe for success!

Make Favorite Dishes Healthier

The recipes that you may prepare regularly, and that your family enjoys, with just a few changes can be healthier and just as satisfying.

Remove Calorie-Rich Temptations

Although everything can be enjoyed in moderation, reducing the calorie-rich temptations of high-fat and high-sugar, or salty snacks can also help your children develop healthy eating habits. Instead allow your children to eat them only occasionally, so that they truly will be treats! Here are examples of easy-to-prepare, low-fat and low-sugar treats that contain one hundred calories or fewer:

- A medium-size apple
- A medium-size banana
- 1 cup blueberries
- 1 cup grapes
- 1 cup carrots, broccoli, or bell peppers with 2 tbsp. hummus

Help Kids Stay Active

Children and teens should participate in at least sixty minutes of moderate-intensity physical activity most days of the week, preferably daily.[11] Remember that children imitate adults. Start adding physical activity to your own daily routine and encourage your child to join you.

Some examples of moderate intensity physical activity include the following:

- Brisk walking
- Playing tag
- Jumping rope
- Playing soccer
- Swimming
- Dancing

Reduce Sedentary Time

In addition to encouraging physical activity, help children avoid too much sedentary time. Although quiet time for reading and homework is fine, limit the time your children watch television, play video games, or surf the web to no more than two hours per day. Additionally, the American Academy of Pediatrics (AAP) does not recommend television viewing for children age two or younger.[12] Instead, encourage your children to find fun activities to do with family members or on their own that simply involve more activity.

References

1. Ogden CL, Carroll MD, Curtin LR, McDowell MA, Tabak CJ, Flegal KM. Prevalence of overweight and obesity in the United States, 1999–2004. *JAMA* 2006;295(13):1549–55.

2. Dietz W. Health consequences of obesity in youth: Childhood predictors of adult disease. *Pediatrics* 1998;101:518–25.

3. Swartz MB and Puhl R. Childhood obesity: a societal problem to solve. *Obesity Reviews* 2003; 4(1):57–71.

4. Rodriguez MA, Winkleby MA, Ahn D, Sundquist J, Kraemer HC. Identification of populations subgroups of children and adolescents with high asthma prevalence: findings from the Third National Health and Nutrition Examination Survey. *Arch Pediatr Adolesc Med* 2002;156:269–75.

5. Luder E, Melnik TA, Dimaio M. Association of being over-weight with greater asthma symptoms in inner city black and Hispanic children. *J Pediatr* 1998;132:699–703.

6. Mallory GB, Fiser DH, Jackson R. Sleep-associated breathing disorders in morbidly obese children and adolescents. *J Pediatr* 1989;115:892–97.

7. Fagot-Campagna A, Narayan KMV, Imperatore G. Type 2 diabetes in children: exemplifies the growing problem of chronic diseases [Editorial]. *BMJ* 2001;322:377–78.

8. Must A, Anderson SE. Effects of obesity on morbidity in children and adolescents. *Nutr Clin Care* 2003;6:1;4–11.

9. Whitaker RC, Wright JA, Pepe MS, Seidel KD, Dietz WH. Predicting obesity in young adulthood from childhood and parental obesity. *N Engl J Med* 1997; 37(13):869–73.

10. Serdula MK, Ivery D, Coates RJ, Freedman DS. Williamson DF. Byers T. Do obese children become obese adults? A review of the literature. *Prev Med* 1993;22:167–77.

11. http://www.aap.org/family/tv1.htm,* accessed 12/18/06.

12. This physical activity recommendation is from the Dietary Guidelines for Americans 2005: http://www.health.gov/dietaryguidelines/dga2005/document/html/chapter4.htm

Chapter 50

Weight Gain Guidelines

Chapter Contents

Section 50.1

Restoring Normal Weight

"Eating Disorders," © 2010 A.D.A.M., Inc.
Reprinted with permission.

Nutrition rehabilitation and psychotherapy are the cornerstones of anorexia nervosa treatment. Patients may also require treatment of medical problems related to the condition, such as bone loss and imbalances in important electrolytes.

Restoring Normal Weight and Nutritional Intervention

Nutritional intervention is essential. Weight gain is associated with fewer symptoms of anorexia and with improvements in both physical and mental function. Restoring good nutrition can help reduce bone loss, and raising the level of energy available to the body by balancing food intake and exercise can normalize hormonal function. Restoring weight is also essential before the patient can fully benefit from additional psychotherapeutic treatments.

Goals for Weight Gain and Good Nutrition

A weight-gain goal of two to three pounds a week for hospitalized patients, and one-half to one pound a week for outpatients, is strongly encouraged. Patients typically begin with a calorie count as low as 1,000 to 1,600 calories a day, which is then gradually increased to 2,000 to 3,500 calories a day. Patients may initially experience intensified anxiety and depressive symptoms, as well as fluid retention, in response to weight gain. These symptoms decrease as the weight is maintained.

Tubal Feedings

Feeding tubes that pass through the nose to the stomach are not commonly used, since they may discourage a return to normal eating habits and because many patients interpret their use as punishing forced feeding. However, for patients who are at significant risk or for those who refuse to eat, tube feeding through the nose or through a tube inserted through the abdomen into the stomach can help with weight gain and improve the nutritional status of the patient.

Intravenous Feedings

Intravenous feedings may be needed in life-threatening situations. This involves inserting a needle into the vein and infusing fluids containing nutrients directly into the bloodstream. Intravenous feedings must be administered carefully. When given at home, no more than the prescribed amount should be used. Overzealous administration of glucose solutions can cause phosphate levels to drop severely and trigger a condition called hypophosphatemia. Emergency symptoms include irritability, muscle weakness, bleeding from the mouth, disturbed heart rhythms, seizures, and coma.

Section 50.2

Weight Gain Tips for Athletes

To gain weight, athletes need to consume more calories than they use. This weight gain will include water, fat, and protein in muscle. To limit the amount of fat gain and increase muscle gains, athletes need to use effective exercise training and nutrition programs.

A common misconception among athletes is that the best way to build muscle or "bulk up" is to eat a high-protein diet. Adequate protein intake is essential when you are increasing muscle mass, but most of the energy needed to fuel muscle growth comes from an adequate calorie intake from carbohydrates and fats.

Weight gainer supplements are marketed to athletes with claims that these supplements will aid in the gain of muscle mass. Although these supplements may help increase daily calorie and protein intake, they have no benefits over food choices that provide the same amount of calories and protein.

Tips for a Healthy Weight Gain

1. Increasing calorie intake by 500 to 1,000 calories per day can help supply the extra calories needed to gain lean weight.

2. It takes time to increase muscle weight. Most athletes can successfully gain one-half to one pound of muscle weight per week if they eat enough food to meet their additional calorie and protein needs for weight gain or and train properly.

3. Choose higher-calorie foods. For example, choose juices over whole fruits and low-fat milk over skim milk or water.

4. Eat larger food portions. Don't skip meals. Increasing the amounts of food that you eat at one time will help supply the calories needed to gain muscle weight.

5.   Eat five or more meals a day. Eat plenty of high-calorie snacks plus meals throughout the day.

6.   Drink plenty of fluids that supply calories like juice, milk, milkshakes, and sports beverages. For example, drinking 1.5 quarts of grape or cranberry juice supplies 1,000 calories; 1.5 quarts of 2 percent milk supplies 720 calories.

7.   Set realistic goals. Genetic factors can play a large role in physique. You are not going to look like Arnold if your parents look like Pee Wee Herman.

8.   Get regular, restful sleep—seven to eight hours per night. Growth hormone peaks in deep sleep. Adequate rest is essential for your body to build new lean body mass.

9.   Be aware of the calories from all the food and drinks you swallow. Nibbling on food throughout the day, even if it is just a bite here or there, can contribute substantially to your total calorie intake. Beverages, like regular soda, slushes, fruit punches, lattes and other coffees with flavoring and milk, beer, cocktails and other beverages with alcohol, and sports drinks, can add up to a lot of extra calorie consumption. Limit high intakes of these high-calorie drinks.

Nutritional Strategies for Weight Gain

Eating additional calories from a well-balanced diet of a variety of performance foods is essential for healthy weight gain. Choose your foods wisely, and eat more servings of wholesome foods from each food group instead of just increasing fat or protein intake. Eating this way and proper exercise will help maximize your lean weight gain and minimize unwanted fat weight gain.

High-Calorie Snack Ideas

Snacking is a great way to increase calories. Be careful of snacks that help increase your calorie intake but are loaded with fat.

Eat high-calorie, nutrient-dense snacks:

- Soft pretzels with peanut butter
- Low-fat milkshakes
- Dried fruits
- Bean and cheese burritos
- Bagels and peanut butter
- Baked potatoes with chili
- Granola and yogurt
- Yogurt, fruit, and nuts

495

- Peanut butter and jelly sandwiches

- Low-fat cheese and crackers

- Fruit smoothies

- High-calorie granola bars or energy bars

- Apple, cranberry, and grape juices

- Almonds, walnuts, peanuts

- Instant breakfast drinks

- Canned Liquid meals

Table 50.1. Weight Gain Plan Following the Sports Food Swap© Guidelines

Meal	Swaps	Calories
Breakfast	1 cup 2 percent milk	120
	3 eggs, scrambled	300
	1 wheat English muffin	160
	1 large banana	130
	2 tablespoons jam	96
Snack	1 apple	60
	15 wheat crackers (thin)	130
	1 string cheese	75
Lunch	12 ounces 2 percent milk	180
	4 slices roasted turkey breast, lettuce, tomato, pickle	150
	2 slices wheat bread	160
	1 cup baby carrots	60
	1 pear	60
Snack	1 cup low-fat vanilla yogurt	200
	1/2 cup blueberries	60
	1/4 cup low-fat granola	90
Dinner	12 ounces 2 percent Milk	180
	5 ounces grilled chicken breast	335
	1 cup wild rice	165
	1 cup sliced peaches	110
	2 cups broccoli with melted cheddar cheese	190
Snack	1 cup orange juice	170
	1 soft pretzel	190
	2 tablespoons peanut butter	186
		Total: 3,557 calories

Chapter 51

Healthy Weight Loss Guidelines

Chapter Contents

Section 51.1

Why Do People Diet?

"The Deal with Diets," August 2009, reprinted with permission from www
.KidsHealth.org. Copyright © 2009 The Nemours Foundation. This information
was provided by KidsHealth, one of the largest resources online for medically
reviewed health information written for parents, kids, and teens. For more
articles like this one, visit www.KidsHealth.org, or www.TeensHealth.org.

High-protein diets. Low-fat diets. All-vegetable diets. No-carb diets.
With all the focus on dieting, how do you figure out what's healthy and
what isn't?

Lots of people feel pressured to lose weight and try different types
of diets. But if you really need to lose weight, improving your eating
habits and exercising will help you more than any diet.

Why Do People Diet?

People diet for many reasons. Some are at an unhealthy weight and
need to pay closer attention to their eating and exercise habits. Some
play sports and want to be in top physical condition. Others may think
they would look and feel better if they lost a few pounds.

Some people may diet because they think they are supposed to look
a certain way. Actors and actresses are thin, and most fashions are
shown off by very thin models. But this look is unrealistic for most
people—not to mention physically damaging to the models and stars
who struggle to maintain it.

By the time they turn twelve or thirteen, most teen girls start to
go through body changes that are natural and necessary: Their hips
broaden, their breasts develop, and suddenly the way they look may
not match girls on TV or in magazine ads. Guys develop at different
rates, too. Those guys with washboard abs you see in clothing ads are
usually in their twenties.

Can Diets Be Unhealthy?

Any diet on which you eat fewer calories than you need to get
through the day—like an 800-calorie-per-day diet, for instance—can

be dangerous. Diets that don't allow any fat also can be bad for you. Everyone needs a certain amount of fat in their diet—up to 30 percent of total calories—so no one should eat a completely fat-free diet.

Don't fall for diets that restrict certain food groups, either. A diet that requires you to say no to bread or pasta or allows you to eat only fruit is unhealthy. You won't get the vitamins and minerals you need. And although you may lose weight, you'll probably gain it back as soon as you start eating normally again.

Some people start dieting because they think all the problems in their lives are because of weight. Others have an area of their lives that they can't control, like an alcoholic parent, so they focus excessively on something they can control—their exercise and food intake.

People who diet may get lots of praise and compliments from friends and family when they start losing pounds, which makes them feel good. But eventually a person reaches a weight plateau—and doesn't lose as much weight as before because the body is trying to maintain a healthy weight. People in these situations eventually discover that, even if they do lose weight, they aren't any happier.

Some people may find it hard to control their eating, so they stick with an extreme diet for a little while, but then eat tons of food. Feeling guilty about the binge, they vomit or use laxatives. Eating too little to maintain a healthy weight (anorexia) or eating only to throw up the calories (bulimia) are both eating disorders, which are harmful to a person's health. Someone with an eating disorder needs medical treatment right away.

So How Can I Lose Weight Safely?

When you're a teen, dieting can be dangerous because you may not get the right kinds and amounts of nutrients, which can lead to poor growth and other health problems. But eating healthy meals and snacks combined with reasonable amounts of exercise can help you lose weight and develop properly at the same time. For a lot of people, just being more active might help them lose weight without even changing what they eat. Regular exercise also helps them feel healthier and better about themselves.

The best way to diet is to eat a wide variety of enough food to meet your body's needs. Aim to eat more fruits and veggies, cut back on meats high in fat (like burgers and hot dogs), greasy fried foods, and sweets, and drink more water instead of sugary drinks like sports drinks or sodas.

If you are concerned about your body's size or think you need to lose weight, talk with your doctor or a registered dietitian, who may reassure you that you are at a healthy weight. Or if you are overweight, he or she can sit down with you and determine the best way for you to reach a healthy weight.

Great Ways to Find Good Health

If you want to change your health habits, here are some tried-and-true tips:

- Exercise! Find a sport you like, walk to school, or ride a bike a few times per week.

- Drink milk, including fat-free or low-fat milk. (Many teens mistakenly think that milk has more calories than other drinks like soda. But a cup of skim milk has only 80 calories as well as protein and calcium. A can of soda has 150 calories of sugar and no other nutrients at all.)

- Eat a variety of foods, including plenty—at least five servings a day—of fruits and veggies. (And no, unfortunately, potato chips don't count as veggies!)

- Drink plenty of water (at least four to six eight-ounce glasses a day).

- Eat lean, high-protein foods, like lean meat, chicken, fish, or beans.

- Eat whole grains (like whole-wheat bread or pasta), which provide fiber, B vitamins, and iron.

- Eat breakfast. Studies show that people who eat breakfast do better in school, tend to eat less throughout the day, and are less likely to be overweight.

- Choose smaller portions at fast-food restaurants. Avoid super-sizing even if it feels like better value.

- Stay away from fad diets—you might lose a few pounds temporarily, but if you don't focus on changing your habits, you'll probably just gain it back when you go back to your usual way of eating.

- Don't take diet pills, even ones you get over the counter.

- Avoid seeing foods as "good" or "bad" or eliminating entire groups of foods, like dairy. If you eliminate entire food groups, you may miss out on important nutrients, like calcium.

- If you choose to become a vegetarian, talk to your doctor or dietitian about how to make nutritious vegetarian choices.

Dieting Danger Signs

How do you know if your diet is out of control? Warning signs include:

- continuing to diet, even if not overweight;
- physical changes, such as weakness, headaches, or dizziness;
- withdrawal from family and friends;
- poor school performance;
- eating in secret;
- thinking about food all the time;
- restricting activities because of food or compulsive exercise;
- fear of food;
- wearing baggy clothes as a way to hide thinness;
- vomiting after meals or using laxatives.

If you, or someone you know, shows any of these signs, talk to a trusted adult or doctor.

Dieting and weight control can consume your life. By accepting your body and making healthy choices, you can keep your weight under control and enjoy life at the same time.

Section 51.2

Why Diets Don't Work

Weight-loss and fad diets involve restricting food intake to levels which often leave a person constantly hungry and in some cases, lacking the necessary nutrients they need to maintain physical health and energy levels. The restrictive nature of dieting does not work, as fad diets do not provide a sustainable meal plan for the long term. Ninety-five percent of people who diet regain the weight and more within two years. Aside from the dangers of dieting, there are a number of physical and emotional reasons why diets do not work:

- **Famine response:** When food intake is reduced, bodies respond as if they are in famine or starvation situation. As a survival instinct, the body can adjust its metabolism or the amount of energy it uses to maintain bodily functions. Although it is very difficult to increase the body's metabolism (increase the rate we burn energy), the body attempts to protect itself against famine by reducing the metabolic rate, which can happen within forty-eight hours of restricting either the type or the amount of food, and can decrease by as much as 40 percent.

- **Leptin:** Leptin is a hormone produced by the fat cells in our bodies. It exists in the body in proportionate amounts to our weight. When body fat decreases, so do leptin levels. Bodies want to compensate for this loss in leptin and respond by increasing hunger urges and decreasing metabolism, which reduces the rate at which energy is burned.

- **Rising obesity rates coinciding with growth of weight-loss industry:** The past few decades have seen a marked increase in the size and profitability of the weight-loss industry, with a boom in the number and sales of countless diet plans. However over this time, we have also seen a significant increase in obesity rates across first-world countries. While there is no hard evidence of this correlation, it seems the more preoccupied and diet-obsessed we as a society become, the more we see these weight-loss efforts fail as evident in rising obesity rates.

- **Food in social settings:** Food is often associated with many social occasions and family gatherings, such as going out to dinner or a barbecue. People who are dieting often avoid social situations and family mealtimes, leading to feelings of isolation and a loss of support.

- **Abstinence leads to bingeing:** When food intake is restricted, a person experiences physical and emotional deprivation. This compels a person to eat, which commonly leads to overeating or bingeing. As a result, a person is likely to feel sensations of guilt and failure. This often becomes a cycle which is difficult to break and has devastating effects on a person's self esteem.

Section 51.3

Weight Management Myths

"Don't Eat After 7 and Six Other Weight Management Myths," by
Michelle May, M.D. © 2010 Eating Disorder Hope (www.eating
disorderhope.com). Reprinted with permission.

Diets are filled with dogma about when, what, and how much to eat. Certainly "the rules" are usually based on observations that make sense, but unless you understand why you do certain things, you'll break the rules as soon as the temptation is greater than your motivation. Let's examine some of these myths, where they come from, and how to make long-term changes that will work for you.

Myth: Don't Eat After 7 p.m.

Your metabolism doesn't shut off at 7:01 p.m., so why is this rule so common? It is based on the observation that a lot of people who struggle with their weight overeat in the evening. Most people have already eaten dinner so they aren't snacking because they're hungry. They snack because of boredom, television, loneliness, and other triggers.

Rather than creating a rule to address those habits, ask yourself "Am I hungry?" whenever you feel like eating in the evenings. If you truly are, eat, keeping in mind that your day is winding down so you won't need a huge meal. If you aren't, consider why you feel like eating and come up with a better way to address that need. Ken, a man in one of my workshops, realized he was just bored so he started doing stained glass in the evenings to entertain himself. Whatever works!

Myth: Eat Small Meals Every Three Hours

This rule is based on the fact that many thin people tend to eat frequent small meals. However, most of the thin people I know don't check their watch to tell them it's time to eat—they eat when their body tells them to. They eat when they're hungry and stop when they're satisfied. Since that tends to be a small meal, they get hungry again in a few hours.

Instead of watching the clock, begin to tune in to the physical symptoms of hunger to tell you when to eat. And remember, your stomach is only about the size of your fist so it only holds a handful of food comfortably. By learning to listen to your body's signals, you are likely to follow a frequent small meal pattern naturally.

Myth: Don't Let Yourself Get Hungry

This one is based on the belief that overweight people are incapable of controlling themselves when they are hungry. In my experience with hundreds of workshop participants, once they learn to tell the difference between physical hunger and head hunger, the opposite is true.

Think about it. When you're hungry, food tastes better and is more satisfying. My grandmother used to say, "Hunger is the best seasoning." Besides, if you aren't hungry when you start eating, what's going to tell you to stop? Of course, you also need to learn to recognize hunger and make time to eat before you are too hungry since it's harder to make great choices when you are starving!

Myth: Exercise More When You Cheat

I *hate* this one because it has caused millions of people to equate physical activity with punishment for eating. As a result, many people either hate to exercise or use exercise to earn the right to eat.

While it's true that your weight is determined by your overall calories in versus your calories out, exercise is only part of the equation and has so many other important benefits. Instead of using exercise to pay penance, focus on how great you feel, how much more energy you have, how much better you sleep, and how much healthier you are becoming. In the long run, you are more likely to do something because it feels good than because you are forced to.

Myth: Follow Your Diet Six Days a Week Then You Can Have a Cheat Day

This is absurd! What if you were a harsh, overly strict parent six days a week then completely ignored your kids every Saturday? How would this approach work for your marriage or managing your employees?

It just doesn't make sense to try to be perfect (whatever that is) Sunday through Friday while obsessing about everything you're going to eat on your day off. Then on Saturday you overeat just because you're allowed to so you end up feeling miserable all day. Huh? Personally, I would rather enjoy eating the foods I love every day mindfully and in moderation. I call this being "in charge" instead of going back and forth between being in control and out of control.

Myth: Eat X Number of Calories (or X Number of Points) Every Day

Does it make sense that you would need exactly the same amount of fuel every day? Aren't there just days when you are hungrier than others, maybe because of your activity levels or hormonal cycles?

Rather than setting yourself up to "cheat" on those hungry days and forcing yourself to eat more food than you want on your less hungry days, allow yourself the flexibility to adjust your intake based on your actual needs rather than an arbitrary number. Important: for this to work long term, you also need to learn to tell the difference between physical hunger and head hunger.

Myth: Carbs Are Bad (or Fat Is Bad)

This "good food–bad food" thinking makes certain foods special. As a result, you may feel deprived and think about them even more than you did before. Worse yet, healthy foods become a four-letter word.

The truth is all foods fit into a healthy diet. Since different foods have various nutritional qualities and calorie content, you can use the principles of balance, variety, and moderation to guide you without trying to restrict an entire food group.

Truth: You Are In Charge

I assume the rule-makers are well intentioned and don't realize that they've created a tight rope that most people will fall off of sooner or later. If your head hadn't already told you that all these rules are crazy, wasn't your heart saying there had to be a better way?

It's time to give yourself a wider path that you can stay on forever by allowing yourself the flexibility to make decisions that both nourish and nurture you.

Section 51.4

Tips for Losing Weight Safely

"How Can I Lose Weight Safely?" February 2009, reprinted with permission from www.KidsHealth.org. Copyright © 2009 The Nemours Foundation. This information was provided by KidsHealth, one of the largest resources online for medically reviewed health information for parents, kids, and teens. For more articles like this one, visit www.KidsHealth.org, or www.TeensHealth.org.

Finding a Healthy Weight

Weight loss is a tricky topic. Lots of people are unhappy with their present weight, but most aren't sure how to change it—and many would be better off staying where they are. You may want to look like the models or actors in magazines and on TV, but those goals might not be healthy or realistic for you. Besides, no magical diet or pill will make you look like someone else.

So what should you do about weight control?

Being healthy is really about being at a weight that is right for you. The best way to find out if you are at a healthy weight or if you need to lose or gain weight is to talk to a doctor or dietitian, who can compare your weight with healthy norms to help you set realistic goals. If it turns out that you can benefit from weight loss, then you can follow a few of the simple suggestions listed below to get started.

Weight management is about long-term success. People who lose weight quickly by crash dieting or other extreme measures usually gain back all (and often more) of the pounds they lost because they haven't permanently changed their habits.

Tips for Success

Therefore, the best weight-management strategies are those that you can maintain for a lifetime. That's a long time, so we'll try to keep these suggestions as easy as possible!

Make it a family affair. Ask your family to lend help and support and to make dietary or lifestyle changes that will benefit the whole family, if possible. People who have the support of their families tend to have better results with their weight-management programs. But remember, you should all work together in a friendly and helpful way—making weight loss into a competition is a recipe for disaster!

Watch your drinks. It's amazing how many extra calories can be lurking in the sodas, juices, and other drinks that you take in every day. Simply cutting out a can of soda or one sports drink can save you 150 calories or more each day. Drink water or other sugar-free drinks to quench your thirst and stay away from sugary juices and sodas. Switching from whole to nonfat or low-fat milk is also a good idea.

Start small. Small changes are a lot easier to stick with than drastic ones. Try reducing the size of the portions you eat and giving up regular soda for a week. Once you have that down, start gradually introducing healthier foods and exercise into your life.

Stop eating when you're full. Lots of people eat when they're bored, lonely, or stressed, or keep eating long after they're full out of habit. Try to pay attention as you eat and stop when you're full. Slowing down can help because it takes about twenty minutes for your brain to recognize how much is in your stomach. Sometimes taking a break before going for seconds can keep you from eating another serving.

Avoid eating when you feel upset or bored—try to find something else to do instead (a walk around the block or a trip to the gym are good alternatives). Many people find it's helpful to keep a diary of what they eat and when. Reviewing the diary later can help them identify the emotions they have when they overeat or whether they have unhealthy habits. Your doctor or a registered dietitian can give you pointers on how to do this.

Eat less more often. Many people find that eating a couple of small snacks throughout the day helps them to make healthy choices at meals. Stick a couple of healthy snacks (carrot sticks, whole-grain pretzels, or a piece of fruit) in your backpack so that you can have one or two snacks during the day. Adding healthy snacks to your three squares and eating smaller portions when you sit down to dinner can help you to cut calories without feeling deprived.

Five a day keep the pounds away. Ditch the junk food and dig out the fruits and veggies! Five servings of fruits and veggies aren't just a good idea to help you lose weight—they'll help keep your heart and the rest of your body healthy. Other suggestions for eating well: replace white bread with whole wheat, trade your sugary sodas for water and low-fat milk, and make sure you eat a healthy breakfast.

Having low-sugar, whole-grain cereal and low-fat milk with a piece of fruit is a much better idea than inhaling a donut as you run to the bus stop or eating no breakfast at all! A registered dietitian can give you lots of other snack and menu ideas.

More Tips

Avoid fad diets. It's never a good idea to trade meals for shakes or to give up a food group in the hope that you'll lose weight—we all need a variety of foods to stay healthy. Stay away from fad diets because you're still growing and need to make sure you get proper nutrients. Avoid diet pills (even the over-the-counter or herbal variety). They can be dangerous to your health; besides, there's no evidence that they help keep weight off over the long term.

Don't banish certain foods. Don't tell yourself you'll never again eat your absolutely favorite peanut butter chocolate ice cream or a bag of chips from the vending machine. Making these foods forbidden is sure to make you want them even more. Also, don't go fat free: You need to have some fat in your diet to stay healthy, so giving up all fatty foods all the time isn't a good idea. The key to long-term success is making healthy choices most of the time. If you want a piece of cake at a party, go for it! But munch on the carrots rather than the chips to balance it out.

Get moving. You may find that you don't need to cut calories as much as you need to get off your behind. Don't get stuck in the rut of thinking you have to play a team sport or take an aerobics class to get exercise. Try a variety of activities from hiking to cycling to dancing until you find ones you like.

Not a jock? Find other ways to fit activity into your day: walk to school or work, jog up and down the stairs a couple of times before your morning shower, turn off the tube and work in the garden, or take a stroll around the neighborhood—anything that gets you moving. Your goal should be to work up to sixty minutes of exercise every day. But everyone has to begin somewhere. It's fine to start out by simply taking a few turns around the block and building up your levels of fitness gradually.

Build muscle. Muscle burns more calories than fat. So adding strength training to your exercise routine can help you reach your weight loss goals as well as give you a toned bod. And weights are not the only way to go: Try resistance bands, Pilates, or push-ups to get strong. A good, well-balanced fitness routine includes aerobic workouts, strength training, and flexibility exercises.

Forgive yourself. So you were going to have one cracker with spray cheese on it and the next thing you know the can's pumping air and the box is empty? Drink some water, brush your teeth, and move on. Everyone who's ever tried to lose weight has found it challenging. When you slip up, the best idea is to get right back on track and don't look back. Avoid telling yourself that you'll get back on track tomorrow or next week or after New Year's. Start now.

Try to remember that losing weight isn't going to make you a better person—and it won't magically change your life. It's a good idea to maintain a healthy weight because it's just that: healthy.

Section 51.5

Choosing a Safe and Successful Weight-Loss Program

Reprinted from the Weight-control Information Network, National
Institute of Diabetes and Digestive and Kidney Diseases, National
Institutes of Health, NIH Publication No. 08-3700, April 2008.

Choosing a weight-loss program may be a difficult task. You may
not know what to look for in a weight-loss program or what questions
to ask. This section can help you talk to your healthcare professional
about weight loss and get the best information before choosing a
program.

Talk With Your Healthcare Professional

You may want to talk with your doctor or other healthcare professional about controlling your weight before you decide on a weight-loss
program. Doctors do not always address issues such as healthy eating,
physical activity, and weight management during general office visits.
It is important for you to start the discussion in order to get the information you need. Even if you feel uncomfortable talking about your
weight with your doctor, remember that he or she is there to help you
improve your health. Here are some tips:

- Tell your healthcare professional that you would like to talk
  about your weight. Share your concerns about any medical conditions you have or medicines you are taking.

- Write down your questions in advance.

- Bring pen and paper to take notes.

- Bring a friend or family member along for support if this will
  make you feel more comfortable.

- Make sure you understand what your healthcare provider is saying. Do not be afraid to ask questions if there is something you
  do not understand.

- Ask for other sources of information like brochures or websites.

- If you want more support, ask for a referral to a registered dietitian, a support group, or a commercial weight-loss program.

- Call your healthcare professional after your visit if you have more questions or need help.

Ask Questions

Find out as much as you can about your health needs before joining a weight-loss program. Here are some questions you might want to ask your healthcare professional.

About Your Weight

- Do I need to lose weight? Or should I just avoid gaining more?

- Is my weight affecting my health?

- Could my extra weight be caused by a health problem such as hypothyroidism or by a medicine I am taking? (Hypothyroidism is when your thyroid gland does not produce enough thyroid hormone, a condition that can slow your metabolism—how your body creates and uses energy.)

About Weight Loss

- What should my weight-loss goal be?

- How will losing weight help me?

About Nutrition and Physical Activity

- How should I change my eating habits?

- What kinds of physical activity can I do?

- How much physical activity do I need?

About Treatment

- Should I take weight-loss drugs?

- What about weight-loss surgery?

- What are the risks of weight-loss drugs or surgery?

- Could a weight-loss program help me?

A Responsible and Safe Weight-Loss Program

If your healthcare provider tells you that you should lose weight and you want to find a weight-loss program to help you, look for one that is based on regular physical activity and an eating plan that is balanced, healthy, and easy to follow. Weight-loss programs should encourage healthy behaviors that help you lose weight and that you can stick with every day. Safe and effective weight-loss programs should include the following:

- Healthy eating plans that reduce calories but do not forbid specific foods or food groups.

- Tips to increase moderate-intensity physical activity.

- Tips on healthy habits that also keep your cultural needs in mind, such as lower-fat versions of your favorite foods.

- Slow and steady weight loss. Depending on your starting weight, experts recommend losing weight at a rate of one-half to two pounds per week. Weight loss may be faster at the start of a program.

- Medical care if you are planning to lose weight by following a special formula diet, such as a very low-calorie diet (a program that requires careful monitoring from a doctor).

- A plan to keep the weight off after you have lost it.

Get Familiar with the Program

Gather as much information as you can before deciding to join a program. Professionals working for weight-loss programs should be able to answer the questions listed below.

What does the weight-loss program consist of?

- Does the program offer one-on-one counseling or group classes?

- Do you have to follow a specific meal plan or keep food records?

- Do you have to purchase special food, drugs, or supplements?

- If the program requires special foods, can you make changes based on your likes and dislikes and food allergies?

- Does the program help you be more physically active, follow a specific physical activity plan, or provide exercise instruction?

- Does the program teach you to make positive and healthy behavior changes?

- Is the program sensitive to your lifestyle and cultural needs?
- Does the program provide ways to keep the weight off? Will the program provide ways to deal with such issues as what to eat at social or holiday gatherings, changes to work schedules, lack of motivation, and injury or illness?

What are the staff qualifications?

- Who supervises the program?
- What type of weight management training, experience, education, and certifications do the staff have?

Does the product or program carry any risks?

- Could the program hurt you?
- Could the recommended drugs or supplements harm your health?
- Do participants talk with a doctor?
- Does a doctor run the program?
- Will the program's doctors work with your personal doctor if you have a medical condition such as high blood pressure or are taking prescribed drugs?
- Is there ongoing input and follow-up from a healthcare professional to ensure your safety while you participate in the program?

How much does the program cost?

- What is the total cost of the program?
- Are there other costs, such as weekly attendance fees, food and supplement purchases, etc.?
- Are there fees for a follow-up program after you lose weight?
- Are there other fees for medical tests?

What results do participants typically have?

- How much weight does an average participant lose and how long does he or she keep the weight off?
- Does the program offer publications or materials that describe what results participants typically have?

If you are interested in finding a weight-loss program near you, ask your healthcare provider for a referral or contact your local hospital.

Section 51.6

When Dieting Becomes Dangerous

Reprinted from "Dieting," "Dangers of Dieting," and "Competitive Dieting," © 2009 Eating Disorders Foundation of Victoria. Reprinted with permission. For additional information and resources, visit www.eatingdisorders.org.au.

Dieting

Many dieting behaviors can be damaging to physical and psychological health. Fluctuating weight is common for most people who diet frequently, as most people regain all the weight they have lost after a diet. Weight loss or weight gain may lead to long-term physical side effects. As well as the physical effects, dieting can be damaging to people's emotional and psychological health, for example, people who diet frequently are more likely to experience depression.

Dieting is the number one risk factor in the development of an eating disorder. Research shows that women who diet severely are eighteen times more likely to develop an eating disorder. Women who diet moderately are five times more likely to develop an eating disorder.

Dangers of Dieting

- Dieting is the greatest risk factor for the development of an eating disorder. Sixty-eight percent of fifteen-year-old females are on a diet, of these, 8 percent are severely dieting. Adolescent girls who diet only moderately are five times more likely to develop an eating disorder than those who don't diet, and those who diet severely are eighteen times more likely to develop an eating disorder.

- Recurrent dieting can eventually lead to weight gain. Ninety-five percent of people who go on weight loss diets regain everything they have lost plus more within two years.

- Most weight-loss diets are highly restrictive and leave dieters feeling constantly hungry. Dieters can often ignore this hunger for a short time but such deprivation eventually leads to powerful food cravings and over-compensatory behavior in the form of bingeing. This results in feelings of guilt, blame, and failure which take a major toll on self-esteem. This cycle can continue throughout a person's lifetime and is a major risk factor in the development of an eating disorder.

- Dieting can reduce the body's metabolism (the rate it burns energy). Healthy metabolism usually returns with normal eating.

- Bad breath, fatigue, overeating, headaches and muscle cramps, constipation, sleep disturbance, and loss of bone density are just some of the effects dieting can have on our bodies.

- The unconscious activity of the body (the energy our bodies require to keep our nervous system, heart function, breathing, etc) requires roughly two-thirds of our daily energy intake.

- Diets disconnect people from their natural bodily responses through imposed meal plans which may overlook hunger, physical activity, and a person's individual nutritional requirements.

Competitive Dieting

Competitive dieting is a dangerous phenomenon which, when taken to extreme levels, can lead to food and weight obsession, as well as disordered eating behaviors. Television shows such as *The Biggest Loser* have seen a marked trend in competitive dieting programs across many workplaces and gyms, whereby people are encouraged to participate individually or as teams to lose the most amount of weight in a specified time period, often for a prize or some form of reward.

Another common and dangerous instance where competitive dieting is common is among high school girls. Many full-blown eating disorders can stem from a seemingly innocent experimentation with dieting whereby a group of friends decide to start a diet together. It is common in competitive dieting circumstances for somebody to start a diet with friends and become obsessed with losing the most weight, which can lead to unhealthy and dangerous behaviors regarding food intake and/ or physical activity levels. In males, it is more common to see competitive situations surrounding physical activity, e.g., in sports. This may be equally dangerous for the development of disordered eating or lifestyle behaviors if the competition is taken to extreme levels.

Regardless of the context, competitive dieting is a dangerous and unhealthy trend. While participating in competitive dieting will not amount to an eating disorder in every instance, if a person possesses certain personality traits, brain chemistry, and/or external factors they are placing themselves at considerable risk of developing an eating disorder.

Section 51.7

Is Dieting OK for Kids?

Everyone has been on a diet. Does that sound strange? Well, it's
true. A diet is simply the collection of the foods you regularly eat. But
the word "diet" also can mean an attempt to lose weight by limiting
calories or types of food.

You may know some adults and kids who worry about their weight
and say they're going on a diet. You might wonder if you should be on
a diet, too. But the majority of kids do not need to—and should not—
diet this way. Why? Let's find out.

Dieting to Lose Weight

All foods and many drinks contains calories, a kind of energy. When
someone diets to lose weight, the person is trying to eat fewer calories
than the body uses. By doing this, the person may lose body fat and
decrease his or her weight. Likewise, if a person eats more calories
than the body uses, the person may gain weight.

Kids usually do not need to diet in this way. Unlike adults, kids are still
growing and developing. During this time, kids need a variety of healthy
foods to keep their bodies growing properly. Some kids are overweight,
but even overweight kids often can improve their health simply by eating
nutritious foods and being more active. Being overweight can cause health
problems, but kids may hurt their health even more by doing something
drastic, like skipping meals or deciding to eat only lettuce.

Who Needs to Diet?

Though some people may feel they weigh too much or too little, there is
no perfect body shape. Some people have larger frames (bigger bones) and
will always look bigger and heavier than people with smaller frames.

Talk to your doctor if you have questions about your weight. Your doctor can examine you and check your body mass index (BMI). That's a way of estimating how much body fat you have. If the doctor is concerned about your weight, he or she can recommend a couple of goals:

- For you to gain weight at a slower pace
- For you to maintain your current weight

For some kids, the doctor may recommend losing some weight, but this should be done with the doctor's help. Kids who need to lose weight may visit with a dietitian who can explain how to reduce calories safely while still getting all the necessary nutrients.

Dangerous Diets

Diets that don't include a variety of nutritious foods, or have too few calories, can be dangerous for kids. Some types of dangerous diets are called "fad diets," because a fad means something that's popular for a short while. Fad diets usually promise quick weight loss and require the person to follow a strict set of guidelines.

Some dangerous diets cut out entire categories of foods or require the person to eat just one thing, such as cabbage soup—yuck! The truth is there is no quick fix when it comes to weight loss. So pills, special drinks, all-liquid diets, and other gimmicks are poor choices, especially for kids. If someone offers you a diet pill or suggests you start having a magic milkshake that can make you thinner, tell them no! These diets can make people sick. They also usually end with the person regaining any weight that was lost.

Someone who is willing to take extreme steps to be thinner could have an eating disorder. These include anorexia nervosa (starving oneself) or bulimia nervosa (eating and then deliberately throwing up). They are serious conditions that need a doctor's attention.

Help for a Dangerous Dieter

If you know a friend or sibling who's following a dangerous diet, you need to tell an adult. You could turn to a parent, a teacher, or another adult you trust. You could also tell the person yourself that their eating habits are unhealthy, but you probably will need to get an adult involved, too.

It's not unusual for kids—or adults—to wish they were taller, or thinner, or that they could change something about their appearance. If you feel this way, talk to a parent or an adult you trust. You may

518

need someone to help you understand these feelings and get a handle on whether your weight is a health concern.

The body changes that happen to kids during puberty include weight gain. This is normal, but it's a good idea to talk with your doctor about it if you or your parents have questions.

What Kids Can Do

So if kids don't need to diet, how can they stay at a healthy weight? All kids can benefit from eating a balanced diet and getting plenty of physical activity.

Kids have a lot of choices when it comes to activity and exercise. Some like to play on sports teams or dance in troupes. Others may prefer to be more casual, riding their bikes or shooting hoops at the park. Just helping your parents rake leaves or clean the house is a kind of physical activity, though not as much fun as something like swimming! And it's a good idea to cut down on pastimes that aren't very active—such as watching TV or playing computer games.

Kids can also try to eat a variety of healthy foods. A balanced diet means that you don't eat the same thing every day and that you eat a mix of foods from different food groups. These include:

- fruits and vegetables;

- milk and dairy products;

- meat, nuts, and other protein-rich foods;

- grains, especially whole-grain foods, such as whole-grain breads and cereals.

This kind of diet helps your body by giving it the right nutrients. For instance, protein helps build your muscles and other body structures. Calcium helps your growing bones. And you need vitamins and other nutrients to keep your body working as it should. Fiber prevents constipation and carbohydrates give you energy, just to name a few.

Now that you understand more about diets, you can tell people you're on a very special one—a balanced, healthy diet just right for a kid!

519

Chapter 52

Guidelines for Healthy Eating

Chapter Contents

Section 52.1

Components of a Balanced Diet: What Teens and Families Need

Excerpted from "Body Basics," U.S. Department of Health and Human Services Office on Women's Health, January 2009.

A healthy, balanced diet for children, teens, and adults includes a mix of different foods. Here's what a healthy eating plan looks like.

Fruits

Try to eat 2 cups (4 portions) of fruit each day.
Choose whole fruits (fresh, frozen, or canned) more often than fruit juice.

Vegetables

Eat 2½ cups (5 portions) of vegetables each day.
Aim for a variety of vegetables each week, including dark green vegetables, like spinach and broccoli; orange vegetables, like carrots; dry beans, such as lentils, white beans, and kidney beans; starchy vegetables such as corn and sweet potatoes; and other vegetables.

Milk and Milk Products

Adults and children nine years of age and older should try to eat or drink 3 cups (3 portions) of milk and milk products each day. (One portion is 1½ ounces of natural cheese or 2 ounces processed cheese.)
Milk and milk products include fat-free or low-fat milk, low-fat yogurt, and low-fat cheeses.

Whole Grains

Try to eat 6 ounces of grains (at least half as whole grains) each day.
Examples of whole grains include whole wheat, brown rice, oats or oatmeal, whole rye, corn, whole-grain barley, and popcorn. Remember,

the whole grain should be first on the ingredients list. Wheat flour, enriched flour, and de-germinated cornmeal are not whole grains.

Meat and Beans

Aim for 5½ ounces (2 portions) of meat and beans each day.

Try different types of protein-rich foods. Examples include lean meats, poultry, fish (grilled, baked, broiled), nuts, eggs, beans, peas, and peanut butter.

Fats, Salts, Sugars

Limit your intake of fats, salts, and sugars each day.

Read the Nutrition Facts labels to find foods low in saturated fats, trans fats, cholesterol, and sugars.

Section 52.2

How Much Food Should I Eat?
A Guide to Portion Size

Portion Distortion

Cookies as big as Frisbees. Muffins the size of flowerpots. Bowls of pasta so deep, your fork can barely find the bottom. One reason people's waistlines have expanded over the past few decades is because food portions have too.

People today eat way more than they used to—and way more than they need to. This means that they're constantly taking in more calories than their bodies can burn. Unfortunately, lots of us don't realize that we're eating too much because we've become so used to seeing (and eating!) large portions.

Portion sizes began to increase in the 1980s and have been ballooning ever since. Take bagels, for example: twenty years ago, the average bagel had a three-inch diameter and 140 calories. Today, bagels have a six-inch diameter and 350 calories. One bagel that size actually contains half a person's recommended number of grain servings for an entire day!

The price of such overabundance is high. It's common knowledge that people who consistently overeat are likely to become overweight. But they also risk getting a number of medical problems, including high blood pressure, high cholesterol, type 2 diabetes, bone and joint problems, breathing and sleeping problems, and even depression. Later in life, people who overeat are at greater risk for heart disease, heart failure, and stroke.

It's easy to understand why the food industry tends to serve way more food than is necessary: Customers love to feel like they're getting the best value for their money! But the value meal is no deal when it triples our calories and sets the stage for health problems.

So what can you do to take back control? A good place to start is knowing about two things that can help you eat smart: serving sizes and recommended amounts of different foods.

Help Yourself: The Truth about Serving Sizes

Look at the label on any product package and you'll see a nutrition information section that gives a serving size for that food. Contrary to popular belief, this serving size is not telling you the amount you should be eating. It's simply a guide to help you see how many calories and nutrients—as well as how much fat, sugar, and salt—you get from eating a specific quantity of that food.

Sometimes the serving size on a package will be a lot less than you are used to eating. In some cases, it's perfectly OK (and even a good idea) to eat more than the serving size listed on the package. For example, if you're cooking frozen vegetables and see the serving size is one cup, it's no problem to eat more because most vegetables are low in calories and fat yet high in nutrition.

But when it comes to foods that are high in calories, sugar, or fat, the serving size can alert you that you may be getting more than is healthy. If you buy a twenty-ounce bottle of soda and drink it all at once, the amount you consumed is twenty ounces. But if the label shows the serving size is eight ounces, not only did you have 2½ servings, you also had 2½ times the listed calories as well as 2½ times the sugar.

Eat Smart: What's Recommended

Serving sizes tell you how much nutrition you're getting from a particular food but they don't tell you which foods you need to stay healthy—and how much of those foods you should eat. That's where the U.S. Department of Agriculture's MyPyramid comes in.

MyPyramid divides foods into six groups:

1. Grains

2. Vegetables

3. Fruits

4. Oils

5. Dairy

6. Meat and beans

MyPyramid then offers guidelines to help people figure out how much of these foods they should eat based on age, gender, and activity level.

Once we know the types of foods and quantities we should be eating, it's easier to figure out how much of that heaping plate of food our bodies actually need as opposed to how much they want. Instead of going along with what your school cafeteria or favorite restaurant puts on your plate, you can take control by eating only the amount you need.

The Divided Plate and Other Portion Tips

Serving sizes on food labels and recommended amounts on My-Pyramid are usually given in grams, ounces, or cups. Of course, most of us don't carry around food scales and measuring cups. So how can we translate those amounts into quantities we can relate to? That's where the following visual cues come in. (Just be warned: Some might seem small, especially to recovering super-sizers!)

One easy way to size up portions if you don't have any measurements is to take a look at your hand. A clenched fist is about a cup—and a cup is the amount experts recommend for a portion of pasta, rice, cereal, vegetables, and fruit. A meat portion should be about as big as your palm. And limit the amount of added fats (like butter, mayo, or salad dressing) to the size of the top of your thumb.

Another great way to visualize appropriate portions is to use the concept of the "divided plate." Think of your plate as divided into four equal sections. Use one of the top quarters for protein. Use the other top quarter for starch, preferably a whole grain. Then fill the bottom half with veggies. None of the foods should overlap—or be piled high! Not only will dividing your plate like this help you keep portions under control, it can also help you to balance your meals.

Portion-Control Tips

Being aware of realistic portion sizes and visualizing portions or using the "divided plate" concept will help you avoid overeating. But sometimes these visual cues can be hard—especially when foods are difficult to measure, like a sandwich, or they're foods like chips and cookies that we tend to eat right out of the bag.

More tips for portion control:

- Eat your meals on a smaller plate so your meal looks larger. A sandwich on a dinner-size plate looks lost; on an appetizer plate it looks downright hefty.

- Avoid taking an entire bag of chips or a container of ice cream to the couch. You're far less likely to overdo it if you serve yourself a portion in the kitchen first.

- Try single-serving size foods (like those cute little eight-ounce cans of soda!) to help your body learn what an appropriate portion size is. These days all kinds of snacks and beverages are available in "100-calorie" portions. Of course, the key is to eat just one!

- Eat three well-rounded meals (with vegetables, proteins, and carbs) and one or two healthy snacks at regular times throughout the day. Skipping meals or waiting too long between them can make you more likely to overdo it at the next meal.

- Add more salads and fruit to your diet, especially at the start of a meal. This can help control hunger and give a sense of fullness while controlling calorie intake.

- Try not to rush through your meals. Eat slowly and chew well—giving yourself a chance to feel full before you take more. If you do want seconds, go for more salad or veggies.

- Be aware that most restaurant portions are three or four times the right serving size. Try sharing meals with friends, ordering an appetizer as a main dish, or packing up the extra to take home before you begin to eat.

- Don't be tempted to go for the giant value meal or the jumbo drink just because they're only a few cents more than the regular size.

Most important, make it a habit to let your stomach rather than your eyes tell you when you're done with a meal. The key to maintaining a healthy weight is to listen to your body's natural signals about when it's hungry and when it's full. Sometimes these signals can be confused by constant overeating or constant dieting, which is why it pays to watch portion sizes and make smart food choices.

Section 52.3

How to Read Food Labels

Excerpted from "Food Labels and More," National Women's
Health Information Center, June 17, 2008.

The Nutrition Facts Label

You've probably seen the Nutrition Facts label on many food packages.
The label states how many calories and how much saturated fat, trans fat,
cholesterol, dietary fiber, and other nutrients are in each serving.

Here are the key steps for using the Nutrition Facts label:

- Check the serving size and number of servings. The serving size for
  a food is based on the amount of that food that people usually eat
  at one time. Serving sizes are standardized for similar kinds of food
  so that you can compare the nutritional value of these foods. So, for
  instance, all cans of peaches should have the same serving size.

- Pay attention to the number of calories. On the label, you'll find
  the number of calories per serving and the number of calories
  from fat in each serving.

- The Nutrition Facts label shows the % (percentage) Daily Value
  (% DV) of certain nutrients contained in one serving of the food.
  The % DVs are based on a daily diet of two thousand calories.
  You may need more or less than two thousand calories per day.
  Still, the % DVs gives you a general idea of whether a food is low
  or high in a certain nutrient. Five percent or less is low; 20 per-
  cent or more is high.

- Look for foods that are low in total fat, saturated fat, trans fat,
  cholesterol, and sodium. Trans fat doesn't have a % DV, but you
  should eat as little of it as possible.

- Look for foods that are high in dietary fiber.

- Look for foods that are high in potassium, vitamins A and C,
  calcium, and iron. Some food labels also show % DVs for other
  vitamins and minerals. You'll want to choose foods that are high
  in those nutrients as well.

- When choosing a food for its protein content (such as red meat, poultry, dry beans, milk, and milk products), choose those that are lean, low-fat, or fat free.

Pay Attention to Food Ingredients

Besides the Nutrition Facts label, most food packages also have an ingredients list. Ingredients are listed in order by weight:

- If you're trying to avoid foods with a lot of added sugar, limit foods that list added sugars as the first few ingredients.

- If you're trying to increase your fiber intake, choose foods with a whole grain, such as whole wheat, listed as the first ingredient. Other whole grains are whole oats, oatmeal, whole-grain corn, popcorn, brown rice, wild rice, whole rye, whole-grain barley, buckwheat, triticale, bulgur (cracked wheat), millet, quinoa, and sorghum.

Other Labels on Foods You Eat

Some foods have labels such as "fat-free," "reduced calorie," or "light." Below are some useful definitions for you.

Calorie terms:

- Low-calorie: Forty calories or fewer per serving

- Reduced-calorie: At least 25 percent fewer calories per serving when compared with a similar food

- Light or lite: One-third fewer calories; if more than half the calories are from fat, fat content must be reduced by 50 percent or more

Sugar terms:

- Sugar-free: Less than one-half gram sugar per serving

- Reduced sugar: At least 25 percent less sugar per serving when compared with a similar food

Fat terms:

- Fat-free or 100 percent fat free: Less than one-half gram fat per serving

- Low-fat: Three grams or less fat per serving

- Reduced-fat: At least 25 percent less fat when compared with a similar food

It's important to remember that fat-free doesn't mean calorie free. People tend to think they can eat as much as they want of fat-free foods. Even if you cut fat from your diet but consume more calories than you use, you will gain weight. Also, fat-free or low-fat foods may contain high amounts of added sugars or sodium to make up for the loss of flavor when fat is removed. For example, a fat-free muffin may be just as high in calories as a regular muffin. So, remember, it is important to read your food labels and compare products.

Section 52.4

Benefits of Healthy Eating

"Nutrition and the Health of Young People," Centers
for Disease Control and Prevention, October 20, 2008.

Healthy eating contributes to overall healthy growth and development, including healthy bones, skin, and energy levels, and a lowered risk of dental caries, eating disorders, constipation, malnutrition, and iron-deficiency anemia.[1]

Diet and Disease

Early indicators of atherosclerosis, the most common cause of heart disease, begin as early as childhood and adolescence. Atherosclerosis is related to high blood cholesterol levels, which are associated with poor dietary habits.[2]

Osteoporosis, a disease where bones become fragile and can break easily, is associated with inadequate intake of calcium.[3]

Type 2 diabetes, formerly known as adult-onset diabetes, has become increasingly prevalent among children and adolescents as rates of overweight and obesity rise.[4] A Centers for Disease Control and Prevention (CDC) study estimated that one in three American children born in 2000 will develop diabetes in their lifetime.[5]

Overweight and obesity, influenced by poor diet and inactivity, are significantly associated with an increased risk of diabetes, high blood pressure, high cholesterol, asthma, joint problems, and poor health status.[6]

Obesity Among Youth

The prevalence of overweight among children aged six to eleven years has more than doubled in the past twenty years and among adolescents aged twelve to nineteen has more than tripled.[7,8]

Overweight children and adolescents are more likely to become overweight or obese adults;[9] one study showed that children who became obese by age eight were more severely obese as adults.[10]

Eating Behaviors of Young People

Less than 40 percent of children and adolescents in the United States meet the U.S. dietary guidelines for saturated fat.[11]

In 2007, only 21.4 percent of high school students reported eating fruits and vegetables five or more times daily (when fried potatoes and potato chips are excluded) during the past seven days.[12]

Only 39 percent of children ages two to seventeen meet the USDA's dietary recommendation for fiber (found primarily in dried beans and peas, fruits, vegetables, and whole grains).[13]

Eighty-five percent of adolescent females do not consume enough calcium.[3] During the last twenty-five years, consumption of milk, the largest source of calcium, has decreased 36 percent among adolescent females.[14] Additionally, from 1978 to 1998, average daily soft drink consumption almost doubled among adolescent females, increasing from six ounces to eleven ounces, and almost tripled among adolescent males, from seven ounces to nineteen ounces.[11,15]

A large number of high school students use unhealthy methods to lose or maintain weight. A nationwide survey found that during the thirty days preceding the survey, 12.3 percent of students went without eating for twenty-four hours or more; 4.5 percent had vomited or taken laxatives in order to lose weight; and 6.3 percent had taken diet pills, powders, or liquids without a doctor's advice.[12]

Diet and Academic Performance

Research suggests that not having breakfast can affect children's intellectual performance.[16]

The percentage of young people who eat breakfast decreases with age: while 92 percent of children ages six to eleven eat breakfast, only 77 percent of adolescents ages twelve to nineteen eat breakfast.[11]

Hunger and food insufficiency in children are associated with poor behavioral and academic functioning.[17,18]

References

1. U.S. Department of Health and Human Services and U.S. Department of Agriculture. *Dietary Guidelines for Americans, 6th Edition*, 2005. Washington, DC, U.S. Government Printing Office.

2. Kavey RW, Daniels SR, Lauer RM, Atkins DL, Hayman LL, Taubert K. American Heart Association guidelines for primary prevention of atherosclerotic cardiovascular disease beginning in childhood. *Journal of Pediatrics* 2003;142(4):368–72.

3. U.S. Department of Health and Human Services. *Bone Health and Osteoporosis: A Report of the Surgeon General*. Rockville, MD: Department of Health and Humans Services, Office of the Surgeon General, 2004.

4. Rosenbloom AL, Joe JR, Young RS, Winter WE. Emerging epidemic of type 2 diabetes in youth. *Diabetes Care* 1999;22(2): 345–54.

5. Venkat Narayan KM, Boyle JP, Thompson TJ, Sorensen SW, Williamson DF. Lifetime risk for diabetes mellitus in the United States. *Journal of the American Medical Association* 2003;290(14):1884–90.

6. Mokdad AH, Ford ES, Bowman BA, et al. Prevalence of obesity, diabetes, and obesity-related health risk factors, 2001. *Journal of the American Medical Association* 2003;289(1):76–79.

7. Ogden CL, Flegal KM, Carroll MD, Johnson CL. Prevalence and trends in overweight among US children and adolescents, 1999–2000. *Journal of the American Medical Association* 2002;288:1728–32.

8. Ogden CL, Carroll MD, Curtin LR, McDowell MA, Tabak CJ, Flegal KM. Prevalence of overweight and obesity in the United States,1999–2004. *Journal of the American Medical Association* 2006;295:1549–55.

9. Ferraro KF, Thorpe RJ Jr, Wilkinson JA. The life course of severe obesity: Does childhood overweight matter? *Journal of Gerontology* 2003;58B(2):S110–19.

10. Freedman DS, Khan LK, Dietz WH, Srinivasan SR, Berenson GS. Relationship of childhood obesity to coronary heart disease risk factors in adulthood: the Bogalusa Heart Study. *Pediatrics* 2001;108(3):712–18.

11. U.S. Department of Agriculture. *Continuing Survey of Food Intakes by Individuals 1994–96*, 1998.

12. Centers for Disease Control and Prevention. Youth Risk Behavior Surveillance—United States, 2007. *Morbidity & Mortality Weekly Report* 2008;57(SS-05):1–131.

13. Lin BH, Guthrie J, Frazao E. American children's diets not making the grade. *Food Review* 2001;24(2):8–17.

14. Cavadini C, Siega-Riz AM, Popkin BM. US adolescent food intake trends from 1965 to 1996. *Archives of Disease in Childhood* 2000;83(1):18–24.

15. U.S. Department of Agriculture. *Continuing Survey of Food Intakes by Individuals, 1987–88*, Appendix A.

16. Pollitt E, Matthews R. Breakfast and cognition: an integrative summary. *American Journal of Clinical Nutrition* 1998;67(suppl): 804S–13S.

17. Alaimo K, Olson CM, and Frongillo EA. "Food Insufficiency and American School-Aged Children's Cognitive, Academic and Psychosocial Developments." *Pediatrics* 108.1 (2001):44–53.

18. Kleinman, R. E., et al. "Hunger in children in the United States: Potential behavioral and emotional correlates." *Pediatrics* 101 (1998):1–6.

Section 52.5

Winning Nutrition for Athletes

Excerpted from "Winning Nutrition for Athletes,"
© 2010 The President's Council on Physical Fitness and Sports.

What diet is best for athletes?

All athletes need a diet that provides enough energy in the form of carbohydrates and fats as well as essential protein, vitamins, and minerals. This means a diet containing 55 to 60 percent of calories from carbohydrates (10 to 15 percent from sugars and the rest from starches), no more than 30 percent of calories from fat, and the remaining (about 10 to15 percent) from protein.

That translates into eating a variety of foods every day—grains, vegetables, fruits, beans, lean meats, and low-fat dairy products. The base of the diet should come from carbohydrates in the form of starches and sugars. Fluids, especially water, are also important to the winning combination. Dehydration can stop even the finest athlete from playing his or her best game.

Are carbohydrates important for athletes?

When starches or sugars are eaten, the body changes them all to glucose, the only form of carbohydrate used directly by muscles for energy. Whether carbohydrates are in the form of starches (in vegetables and grains), sucrose (table sugar), fructose (found in fruits and juices), or lactose (milk sugar), carbohydrates are digested and ultimately changed to glucose.

The body uses this glucose in the blood for energy. Most glucose is stored as glycogen in the liver and muscles. During exercise glycogen is broken down in the muscles and provides energy. Usually there is enough glycogen in muscles to provide fuel for 90 to 120 minutes of exercise.

Most exercise and sport games do not use up glycogen stores so eating carbohydrates during the activity usually isn't needed. But for some athletes, eating or drinking carbohydrates during exercise helps maintain their blood glucose and energy levels.

Most athletes need not be concerned with "carbohydrate loading," the special technique of eating a lot of carbohydrates for several days before an endurance event. Instead, focus on getting enough carbohydrates every day. The best way to ensure plenty of energy for exercise is to eat a nutritious, balanced diet that is high in carbohydrates and low in fat with lots of different foods.

Do athletes need extra protein or protein supplements to build muscles?

No. Muscles develop from training and exercise. A certain amount of protein is needed to help build the muscles but a nutritious, balanced diet that includes two or three servings from the meat/bean/egg group (six to seven ounces total) and two to three servings of dairy daily will supply all of the protein that the muscles need.

Extra servings of protein in foods or protein supplements do not assist in muscle development. Unlike carbohydrates, protein cannot be stored in the body and any excess will be burned for energy or stored as body fat.

What should an athlete eat before, during, and after exercise?

The most important thing is to concentrate on eating a nutritious, balanced diet every day. This provides plenty of energy to grow and exercise. Here are a few tips about eating before, during and after exercise.

Before:

- Have some high-carbohydrate foods like bananas, bagels, or fruit juices. These foods are broken down quickly and provide glucose to the muscles.

- The timing of this meal depends on athletes' preference for eating before exercise, but researchers have found that eating something from one to four hours before exercise helps keep plenty of blood glucose available for working muscles.

- It is also critical to drink plenty of cool water before exercise to keep muscles hydrated.

During:

- Perspiration and exertion deplete the body of fluids necessary for an optimal performance and lead to dehydration. It is important to drink plenty of cool water, at least a half a cup of water every twenty minutes of exercise. Adding a teaspoon of sugar, a little fruit juice, or a small amount of powdered drink mix flavors plain water and may encourage fluid intake.

- Usually there is no need to worry about replacing carbohydrates unless the exercise lasts more than ninety minutes and is hard and continuous. When this happens, drinking a sports drink or other beverage with some sugar in it will provide fuel and water to the muscles being exercised.

- Make a homemade sports drink by mixing no more than 4 teaspoons of sugars, ¼ teaspoon of salt, and some flavoring (like a teaspoon of lemon juice) in eight ounces of water.

After:

- If the exercise was strenuous and lasted a long time, glycogen stores may need refueling. Consuming foods and beverages high in carbohydrates right after exercise will replenish glycogen stores if they are low after exercising.

- No matter the intensity of the exercise, it's important to drink plenty of water and eat a nutritious, balanced meal that has lots of carbohydrate-rich foods such as grains, pastas, potatoes, vegetables, and fruits. A teaspoon of sugar, at only 15 calories per teaspoon, adds flavor to these foods and may increase taste appeal. (Like all carbohydrates, sugar has four calories per gram, and there are four grams to a teaspoon. The FDA's 1993 food labeling regulations require rounding to fifteen calories on consumer packages.)

Section 52.6

The Importance of Family Meals

"The Top Ten Reasons to Have Family Meals," © Rebecca Manley, MS, Multi-service Eating Disorder Association (MEDA), 2007. Reprinted with permission. For additional information, contact MEDA at 866-343-6332, or www.medainc.org.

1. Meals reassure children that they will be fed. Children of all ages feel better with structure. Knowing what to expect helps them to feel safe in the world and decreases anxiety. By providing meals at approximately the same time every day, you are letting your child know that you will take care of his/her hunger needs.

2. Meals are a great way to connect about the day. The world is such a busy place. By taking thirty minutes out of your day to talk to your child about his/her day, you will be creating a safe space to share thoughts about school, work, and friendships.

3. Meals are great venues for introducing new foods. This does not mean that meals need to be complicated events; it just means that you are providing a scheduled routine where children can experiment with new things. By adding a new fruit, vegetable, or protein dish to the table, you are giving children the opportunity to explore a variety of new foods.

4. Meals teach responsibility. Children of all ages can be a major part of the mealtime process. Toddlers can help fold napkins, preschoolers can set the table, kindergarteners can help with mixing dips, elementary school children can cut vegetables or do simple recipes, middle school and high school children can put together entire meals (with supervision). Let children pick out foods at the store to prepare in a recipe later. By giving children responsibilities involving meal time, you are not only teaching them how to make healthy meals, you are increasing their self-esteem by showing them they can accomplish something.

5. Meals make eating important. Sports, play-dates, work, school functions, everything seems to come before a family meal. By scheduling mealtimes you are modeling to your child that sitting and eating is important. Sitting and eating a healthy meal should be as important as going to bed each night.

6. Meals teach manners. Teaching a child about table manners will help your child feel more comfortable when going out to eat or to a friend's house for dinner, and in turn, help your child feel more confident.

7. Meals teach kids how to connect to their hunger. By taking the time to sit and eat, you are teaching kids how to slow down and listen to their body's hunger. When you eat on the run, in the car, in front of the television, you can't listen properly to what your body is telling you, am I full? Am I still hungry? Am I thirsty? Model verbal cues while having a family meal: "I think I am done eating. My body feels full."

8. Meals teach the importance of connection. Research shows that people who are more connected with others are less likely to be depressed. By taking the time to bring your family together, and by making mealtimes a pleasurable experience, you are setting the stage for great connections. You are reinforcing the importance of talking to others and sharing your feeling and thoughts.

9. Meals teach kids about customs. Everyone has at least one family tradition from their childhood. Turkey on Thanksgiving or special bread on Christmas or Chanukah. Use mealtimes to teach your child about past and current customs regarding food. Talk about the customs of others.

10. Meals help families grow physically, emotionally, and socially. By providing a meal of healthy food, good conversation, and your undivided attention, you are giving your child the opportunity to grow and develop the body confidence he/she needs for life.

Chapter 53

Guidelines for Healthy Exercise

Chapter Contents

Section 53.1

Physical Activity for a Healthy Weight

Centers for Disease Control and Prevention, January 27, 2009.

Why is physical activity important?

Regular physical activity is important for good health, and it's especially important if you're trying to lose weight or to maintain a healthy weight:

- When losing weight, more physical activity increases the number of calories your body uses for energy or "burns off." The burning of calories through physical activity, combined with reducing the number of calories you eat, creates a "calorie deficit" that results in weight loss.

- Most weight loss occurs because of decreased caloric intake. However, evidence shows the only way to maintain weight loss is to be engaged in regular physical activity.

- Most importantly, physical activity reduces risks of cardiovascular disease and diabetes beyond that produced by weight reduction alone.

Physical activity also helps to do the following:

- Maintain weight
- Reduce high blood pressure
- Reduce risk for type 2 diabetes, heart attack, stroke, and several forms of cancer
- Reduce arthritis pain and associated disability
- Reduce risk for osteoporosis and falls
- Reduce symptoms of depression and anxiety

How much physical activity do I need?

When it comes to weight management, people vary greatly in how much physical activity they need. Here are some guidelines to follow.

To maintain your weight: Work your way up to 150 minutes of moderate-intensity aerobic activity, 75 minutes of vigorous-intensity aerobic activity, or an equivalent mix of the two each week. Strong scientific evidence shows that physical activity can help you maintain your weight over time. However, the exact amount of physical activity needed to do this is not clear since it varies greatly from person to person. It's possible that you may need to do more than the equivalent of 150 minutes of moderate-intensity activity a week to maintain your weight.

To lose weight and keep it off: You will need a high amount of physical activity unless you also adjust your diet and reduce the number of calories you're eating and drinking. Getting to and staying at a healthy weight requires both regular physical activity and a healthy eating plan.

What do moderate- and vigorous-intensity mean?

Moderate. While performing the physical activity, if your breathing and heart rate are noticeably faster but you can still carry on a conversation, it's probably moderately intense.
Examples include the following:

- Walking briskly (a fifteen-minute mile)
- Light yard work (raking/bagging leaves or using a lawn mower)
- Light snow shoveling
- Actively playing with children
- Biking at a casual pace

Vigorous. If your heart rate is increased substantially and you are breathing too hard and fast to have a conversation, it's probably vigorously intense.
Examples include the following:

- Jogging/running
- Swimming laps
- Rollerblading/inline skating at a brisk pace
- Cross-country skiing
- Most competitive sports (football, basketball, or soccer)
- Jumping rope

How many calories are used in typical activities?

Table 53.1 shows calories used in common physical activities at both moderate and vigorous levels.

Table 53.1. Calories Used per Hour in Common Physical Activities

Moderate Physical Activity	Approximate Calories/30 Minutes for a 154 lb Person[1]	Approximate Calories/Hr for a 154 lb Person[1]
Hiking	185	370
Light gardening/yard work	165	330
Dancing	165	330
Golf (walking and carrying clubs)	165	330
Bicycling (<10 mph)	145	290
Walking (3.5 mph)	140	280
Weightlifting (general light workout)	110	220
Stretching	90	180

Vigorous Physical Activity	Approximate Calories/30 Minutes for a 154 lb Person[1]	Approximate Calories/Hr for a 154 lb Person[1]
Running/jogging (5 mph)	295	590
Bicycling (>10 mph)	295	590
Swimming (slow freestyle laps)	255	510
Aerobics	240	480
Walking (4.5 mph)	230	460
Heavy yard work (chopping wood)	220	440
Weightlifting (vigorous effort)	220	440
Basketball (vigorous)	220	440

Note: [1]Calories burned per hour will be higher for persons who weigh more than 154 lbs (70 kg) and lower for persons who weigh less.

Source: Adapted from Dietary Guidelines for Americans 2005, page 16, Table 4.

Section 53.2

Benefits of Exercise

You've probably heard countless times how exercise is "good for you." But did you know that it can actually help you feel good, too? Getting the right amount of exercise can rev up your energy levels and even help improve your mood.

Rewards and Benefits

Experts recommend that teens get sixty minutes or more of moderate to vigorous physical activity each day. Here are some of the reasons:

- **Exercise benefits every part of the body, including the mind:** Exercising causes the body to produce endorphins, chemicals that can help a person to feel more peaceful and happy. Exercise can help some people sleep better. It can also help some people who have mild depression and low self-esteem. Plus, exercise can give people a real sense of accomplishment and pride at having achieved a certain goal—like beating an old time in the hundred-meter dash.

- **Exercising can help you look better:** People who exercise burn more calories and look more toned than those who don't. In fact, exercise is one of the most important parts of keeping your body at a healthy weight.

- **Exercise helps people lose weight and lower the risk of some diseases:** Exercising to maintain a healthy weight decreases a person's risk of developing certain diseases, including type 2 diabetes and high blood pressure. These diseases, which used to be found mostly in adults, are becoming more common in teens.

- **Exercise can help a person age well:** This may not seem important now, but your body will thank you later. Women are especially prone to a condition called osteoporosis (a weakening of the bones) as they get older. Studies have found that weight-bearing exercise, like jumping, running, or brisk walking, can help girls (and guys!) keep their bones strong.

The three components to a well-balanced exercise routine are: aerobic exercise, strength training, and flexibility training.

Aerobic Exercise

Like other muscles, the heart enjoys a good workout. You can provide it with one in the form of aerobic exercise. Aerobic exercise is any type of exercise that gets the heart pumping and quickens your breathing. When you give your heart this kind of workout regularly, it will get stronger and more efficient in delivering oxygen (in the form of oxygen-carrying blood cells) to all parts of your body.

If you play team sports, you're probably meeting the recommendation for sixty minutes or more of moderate to vigorous activity on practice days. Some team sports that give you a great aerobic workout are swimming, basketball, soccer, lacrosse, hockey, and rowing.

But if you don't play team sports, don't worry—there are plenty of ways to get aerobic exercise on your own or with friends. These include biking, running, swimming, dancing, in-line skating, tennis, cross-country skiing, hiking, and walking quickly. In fact, the types of exercise that you do on your own are easier to continue when you leave high school and go on to work or college, making it easier to stay fit later in life as well.

Strength Training

The heart isn't the only muscle to benefit from regular exercise. Most of the other muscles in your body enjoy exercise, too. When you use your muscles and they become stronger, it allows you to be active for longer periods of time without getting worn out.

Strong muscles are also a plus because they actually help protect you when you exercise by supporting your joints and helping to prevent injuries. Muscle also burns more energy when a person's at rest than fat does, so building your muscles will help you burn more calories and maintain a healthy weight.

Different types of exercise strengthen different muscle groups, for example:

- For arms, try rowing or cross-country skiing. Pull-ups and push-ups, those old gym class standbys, are also good for building arm muscles.

- For strong legs, try running, biking, rowing, or skating. Squats and leg raises also work the legs.

- For shapely abs, you can't beat rowing, yoga or Pilates, and crunches.

Flexibility Training

Strengthening the heart and other muscles isn't the only important goal of exercise. Exercise also helps the body stay flexible, meaning that your muscles and joints stretch and bend easily. People who are flexible can worry less about strained muscles and sprains.

Being flexible may also help improve a person's sports performance. Some activities, like dance or martial arts, obviously require great flexibility, but increased flexibility can also help people perform better at other sports, such as soccer or lacrosse.

Sports and activities that encourage flexibility are easy to find. Martial arts like karate also help a person stay flexible. Ballet, gymnastics, Pilates, and yoga are other good choices. Stretching after your workout will also help you improve your flexibility.

What's Right for Me?

One of the biggest reasons people drop an exercise program is lack of interest: If what you're doing isn't fun, it's hard to keep it up. The good news is that there are tons of different sports and activities that you can try out to see which one inspires you.

When picking the right type of exercise, it can help to consider your workout personality. For example, do you like to work out alone and on your own schedule? If so, solo sports like biking or snowboarding may be for you. Or do you like the shared motivation and companionship that comes from being part of a team?

You also need to plan around practical considerations, such as whether your chosen activity is affordable and available to you. (Activities like horseback riding may be harder for people who live in cities, for example.) You'll also want to think about how much time you can set aside for your sport.

It's a good idea to talk to someone who understands the exercise, like a coach or fitness expert at a gym. He or she can get you started on a program that's right for you and your level of fitness.

Another thing to consider is whether any health conditions may affect how—and how much—you exercise. Doctors know that most people benefit from regular exercise, even those with disabilities or conditions like asthma. But if you have a health problem or other considerations (like being overweight or very out of shape), talk to your doctor before beginning an exercise plan. That way you can get information on which exercise programs are best and which to avoid.

Too Much of a Good Thing

As with all good things, it's possible to overdo exercise. Although exercising is a great way to maintain a healthy weight, exercising too much to lose weight isn't healthy. The body needs enough calories to function properly. This is especially true for teens, who are still growing.

Exercising too much in an effort to burn calories and lose weight (also called compulsive exercise) can be a sign of an eating disorder. If you ever get the feeling that your exercise is in charge of you rather than the other way around, talk with your doctor, a parent, or another adult you trust.

It's also possible to overtrain—something high school athletes need to watch out for. If you participate in one sport, experts recommend that you limit that activity to a maximum of five days a week, with at least two to three months off per year. You can still train more than that as long as it's cross-training in a different sport (such as swimming or biking if you play football).

Participating in more than one activity or sport can help athletes use different skills and avoid injury. Also, never exercise through pain. And, if you have an injury, make sure you give yourself enough time to heal. Your body—and your performance—will thank you.

Considering the benefits to the heart, muscles, joints, and mind, it's easy to see why exercise is wise. And the great thing about exercise is that it's never too late to start. Even small things can count as exercise when you're starting out—like taking a short bike ride, walking the dog, or raking leaves.

If you're already getting regular exercise now, keep it up. Staying fit is often one of the biggest challenges for people as they get busy with college and careers.

Section 53.3

How to Know When a Young Athlete's Exercise Is a Problem

"How to Know When a Young Athlete's Exercise Is a Problem," by Roberta Sherman, Ph.D., *Eating Disorders Recovery Today*, Fall 2007, Volume 5, Number 4. © 2007 Gürze Books. Reprinted with permission.

Sport participation can be very helpful to a young athlete in terms of developing self-esteem, self-efficacy, and sportsmanship. Unfortunately, it can also be a mechanism for the development of an eating disorder. Although unhealthy eating behaviors can sometimes be difficult to identify in the sport environment, recognizing unhealthy exercise can be even more complicated. In part, the difficulty results from the emphasis on rigorous training. Most coaches at the collegiate and elite levels believe that training is the single most important factor in enhancing athletic performance, and many believe that "more is better" regarding the frequency, duration, and intensity of training. Right or wrong, many of the current trends in sport, including those related to training, tend to filter down from the collegiate and elite levels to high school, middle school, and even younger levels of competition.

Sports at higher levels (i.e., collegiate and elite) usually have the most knowledgeable and well-trained medical and training personnel looking out for the athletes' welfare. Unfortunately, sports at lower levels tend not only to have less experienced and less informed coaches, but also tend to have minimal medical and training staffs. Thus, young athletes could be at significant risk.

In this section, I will provide suggestions regarding not only how to identify possible exercise or training problems with your young athlete, but also how you might take a more active role in making sport participation safer and more enjoyable for him or her.

Detecting Possible Problems

Part of the difficulty in identifying "excessive" exercise in athletes is that exercise or, more specifically, training, is so valued in the sport environment. Often people who train harder and/or more intensely are viewed as being "good" athletes. One way to detect a possible problem is to look at your child or adolescent's training compared to her teammates. Is she doing significantly more? If so, this may be indicative of a problem. Additionally, is she exercising more than the coach is requiring or recommending? If so, it may be suggestive of a problem.

However, this approach to identification is not always straightforward. Coaches are often looking for the athlete who will train harder than her teammates. It is difficult for a coach (and sometimes a parent) to view an athlete who works harder and longer than the others as having a problem. On the contrary, these athletes are more often valued because of their "work ethic." Their extra training may be rewarded and reinforced. It is difficult to know if the athlete is simply a good, hard-working competitor, or a person with a problem. Nonetheless, this is a good place to start the identification process.

Because sports differ with respect to their physical requirements (i.e., cross country vs. softball, tennis vs. swimming, etc.), training demands will differ. But when attempting to determine if training is safe and healthy, it is often more helpful to look at additional factors. The obvious ones involve physical/medical symptoms. These might include menstrual abnormalities, stress fractures, recurrent injuries, and injuries due to overuse. Interestingly, many athletes who train intensely experience frequent colds and upper respiratory infections that are believed to result from decreased immunity related to their strenuous training. Many of these physical symptoms result from psychological issues related to exercise. Things to look for might include exercising against medical advice, exercising despite injury or illness, an inability to change an exercise routine, or exercise that interferes with everyday activities such as school, work, or relationships.

One final way to assess the appropriateness of an athlete's training relates to decreased athletic performance. A decrement in performance is a cardinal symptom of what has been termed "overtraining syndrome" or "staleness." Other overtraining symptoms include appetite disturbance, depression, and "heavy legs," a sensation that athletes report feeling when they are experiencing overtraining. The recommended treatment for overtraining is complete rest. Ironically, many athletes increase their training when performance declines.

Parents can play an important role in making sport participation safer and more enjoyable. Since youth sport athletes are probably at greater risk than those who compete at higher levels, parents should take a more active role in monitoring the sport activities of their children to ensure their health and safety. A good place to start is to become knowledgeable regarding unhealthy exercise and weight loss methods often practiced by athletes, and how these can affect a child's health. Use reputable and well-documented sources of information regarding healthy sport training and competition. Additionally, parents should not assume that their child is healthy simply because she is performing well athletically. You know your child better than anyone. Be assertive with coaches when you are concerned, and don't hesitate to withhold sport participation until your concerns have been alleviated through proper assessment and treatment.

One last important point regarding the appropriateness of sport participation for children and adolescents is warranted. These issues related to training should not be misconstrued to mean that young people should avoid sport participation. What should be avoided are the unhealthy attitudes and behaviors that are often associated with exercise, both inside and outside of sports.

Chapter 54

Coping with Holidays and Food-Related Challenges

Navigating through the holiday season can be a mixed blessing. Although culturally this is known to be a positive, cheerful time, it is also undoubtedly stressful for many individuals. There are increased demands including a hectic social calendar, buying gifts, decorating, and hosting friends and family. Financial challenges are present for many people as money constraints might require some stretching to make ends meet. Holidays can be a particularly poignant time for those who have lost a loved one or those who are unable to be with the people they care about. Finally, for those of you spending time with family, it often can come with increased conflict. That discomfort with a family member that you have been ignoring all year . . . well, you will face it now—staring across from you at the dinner table!

During the holidays, there is also the inevitable focus on food. Many of the engagements that occur around this season include social eating. Meeting up with family and friends that you see infrequently can involve pressure related to body image and food consumption as well. I have worked with individuals on all ends of the weight spectrum who find body image and weight to be a challenging aspect of their lives. I have also heard that for individuals with a current issue or history of using food-related behaviors as a means to cope with stress, it can be a particularly challenging time. My clients have often related to me that they feel "under the microscope" during the holidays. Within the culture of the United States, we are inundated

"Thriving During the Holidays," by Tera Lensegrav-Benson, Ph.D. © 2010 Eating Disorder Hope (www.eatingdisorderhope.com). Reprinted with permission.

with information in the media related to looking great in that holiday dress while simultaneously being blasted with the idea that weight gain during this time of year is a given. Consequently, as in any stressful or potentially "triggering" situation, those who suffer currently or have a history of eating disorders are at higher risk for engaging in disordered eating as well as struggles with mindset/body image during the holidays.

Do you have to accept that this time of year is going to send your issues with weight and food into an utter tailspin? Is there hope to come out of the holiday season with any semblance of balance?

The short answer is yes!

It is possible to effectively negotiate this time of year. If you reconceptualize your approach, you may feel empowered by the way you are able to make decisions in line with your values.

How to Cope Effectively

Prioritize

Holidays present an opportunity to take stock of your life. A continually emerging therapy approach, acceptance and commitment therapy (ACT), uses the concept of values-based living as one of its cornerstones. This philosophy is especially salient during the holidays. Specifically, if you are making decisions that are inconsistent with your personal values it is likely to result in increased stress and life dissatisfaction.

Define your values. First, delve into what you are passionate about, defining what gives your life meaning (this is often done most effectively with a therapist if you are working with one). This is highly personal, so try not to fall into a trap of coming up with the values you think that you "should" have. For example, do you live for social engagements which could mean that relationships are a core value for you? You will know if you are hitting home with this if it you become enlivened when you think about it.

Accept new viewpoints. Then, consider how your values apply to the holiday season. Ask yourself genuinely what this time of year means to you. It is certain that during the holidays, you will have to navigate through competing interests. Do you honor a specific tradition because you always do it or because it truly impacts you in a positive way? For example, if you have a core value of relationships, do your holiday traditions revolve around this concept?

Take action. Finally, you can then prioritize options and determine what commitments and tasks are meaningful enough for you to devote your energy to. For example, you may decide to stop doing certain holiday traditions such as traveling away from home in light of the need to act more in line with your newly defined value of connecting with your immediate family.

Just Say No to Perfection

Let go . . . of the idea of a "perfect" anything: the perfectly decorated tree, the perfect gift, being the perfect hostess, the list could go on and on. Yet, I often hear from my clients that perfection (particularly as a means to cope with stress) is something they are hanging on to. This is a set-up for disappointment because being human inherently means that perfection is a very unlikely outcome. It is okay to give yourself permission to let go of the rule that the holidays will only be good if you can do things perfectly.

Balance

It can be easy with the hustle and bustle of the season to let the positive things that you have incorporated into your life (work on balanced eating, exercise, mindfulness) go. This is not the time to give up the healthy habits that you have going! If you are committed to something that you value such as recovery or eating in moderation, renew your commitment to yourself at this time. You will find that if you are able to maintain balance in your life and stay on track with the positive changes you have been working on, you will be more likely to successfully navigate the holiday season.

Get Support

Social support has been demonstrated to be a very important feature in maintaining good mental and physical health. Don't be afraid to rely on the people who are supportive of your efforts to become or stay balanced with food issues. If you aren't working with a therapist but feel that you could benefit, this is a good time to give yourself the gift of the treatment that you need.

Part Seven

Additional Help and Information

Chapter 55

Glossary of Terms Related to Eating Disorders

abuse: Misuse, wrong use, especially excessive use, of anything.[2]

adipose tissue: Fat tissue.[1]

aerobic: Fat-fueled; aerobic exercise increases basal metabolic rate, reduces appetite, firms muscles, improves cardiac and respiratory function, and burns flab.[1]

adult-onset: Occurring for the first time in those who have reached maturity.[1]

amenorrhea: The loss of the menstrual cycle. In terms of eating disorders this is usually the result of excessive weight loss and often accompanied by excessive exercise.[1]

anorectic: A name frequently used for diet medications that curb appetite.[1]

anorexia nervosa: Self-induced starvation with at least 15 percent of original body weight lost. Victims also have amenorrhea, fat phobia, and a severe distortion of body image.[1]

The terms in this glossary marked [1] were reprinted with permission from "Eating Disorders Glossary," by Nancy A. Rudd, Liz Davis, and Penny Winkle. © 2010 The Ohio State University Body Image Health Task Force. For additional information, visit http://ehe.osu.edu/cs/bitf/. The terms marked [2] were excerpted from Stedman's Electronic Medical Dictionary v.5.0, © 2000 Lippincott Williams and Wilkins.

behavior therapy: An offshoot of psychotherapy involving the use of procedures and techniques associated with research in the fields of conditioning and learning for the treatment of a variety of psychologic conditions; distinguished from psychotherapy because specific symptoms (e.g., phobia, enuresis, high blood pressure) are selected as the target for change, planned interventions or remedial steps to extinguish or modify these symptoms are then employed, and the progress of changes is continuously and quantitatively monitored.[2]

body dysmorphic disorder: A psychosomatic (somatoform) disorder characterized by preoccupation with some imagined defect in appearance in a normal-appearing person.[2]

body image: Personal conception of one's own body as distinct from one's actual anatomic body or the conception other persons have of it.[2]

body mass index: An anthropometric measure of body mass, defined as weight in kilograms divided by height in meters squared; a method of determining caloric nutritional status.[2]

bulimorexia: Binging followed by purging through laxative abuse, forced vomiting, excessive exercise, or enema abuse.[1]

bulimia nervosa: Uncontrolled eating in the presence of a strong desire to lose weight.[1]

catharsis: The emotional reenactment in thought or symbolic form of a painful experience that brings relief of the distress caused by the original experience.[1]

cognitive therapy: Any of a variety of techniques in psychotherapy that utilizes guided self-discovery, imaging, self-inspection, symbolic modeling, and related forms of explicitly elicited cognitions as the principal mode of treatment.[2]

diuretic: A chemical that stimulates the production of urine. Also known as a water pill.[1]

eating disorders: A group of mental disorders including anorexia nervosa, bulimia nervosa, pica, and rumination disorder of infancy.[2]

emetic: Relating to or causing vomiting; an agent that causes vomiting (e.g., ipecac syrup).[2]

enema: The injection of a liquid into the lower bowel through the rectum to compel elimination.[1]

etiology: Cause or origin. Specifically, all the causes of a disease or abnormal condition.[1]

family therapy: A type of group psychotherapy in which a family in conflict meets as a group with the therapist and explores its relationships and processes; focus is on the resolution of current interactions between members rather than on individual members.[2]

gastroplasty: A surgical procedure used to reduce the digestive capacity by shortening the small intestine or shrinking the effective size of he stomach.[1]

hunger: The physical urge to eat that is prompted by immediate need for energy.[1]

intervention: An action or ministration that produces an effect or that is intended to alter the course of a pathologic process.[2]

juvenile-onset: Occurring between infancy to young adulthood.[1]

ketosis: A condition characterized by the enhanced production of ketone bodies, as in diabetes mellitus or starvation.[2]

laxative: Mildly cathartic, having the action of loosening the bowels; a mild cathartic, a remedy that moves the bowels slightly without pain or violent action.[2]

malnutrition: Faulty nutrition resulting from malabsorption, poor diet, or overeating.[2]

nutrition: A function of living plants and animals, consisting in the taking in and metabolism of food material whereby tissue is built up and energy liberated.[2]

obesity: This controversial term is often used to describe individuals at least 20 percent above the weight recommended for one's height.[1]

oral expulsion syndrome (OES): The chewing but avoidance of swallowing food. OES is a diet technique in some people, but the reflection of emotional disturbance and eating disorders in most.[1]

osteoporosis: Reduction in the quantity of bone or atrophy of skeletal tissue; an age-related disorder characterized by decreased bone mass and increased susceptibility to fractures.[2]

panacea: A remedy for all ills or difficulties.[1]

pathorexia: Disordered appetite. It refers to the whole spectrum of food disorder problems.[1]

phobia: An unrealistic fear, often with obsessional characteristics.[1]

pica: A perverse appetite for substances not fit as food or of no nutritional value.[2]

postpartum depression: A depression that follows child birth in some mothers. Cases can be mild or severe enough to be labeled psychosis and require hospitalization.[1]

purgatives: A substance or method used to eliminate food before it can be digested.[1]

purging: A forced cleansing or release. In terms of eating disorders this is usually done by vomiting or laxative abuse.[1]

recovery: A getting back or regaining; recuperation.[2]

relapse: Return of the manifestations of a disease after an interval of improvement.[2]

rumination: The apparently voluntary regurgitation, chewing, and reswallowing of food.[1]

set point (theory): The weight a person or an animal maintains and returns to after dieting or overfeeding. Set point varies with age and activity levels, and may be raised if the organism is subject to chronic deprivation.[1]

starvation: Lengthy and continuous deprivation of food.[2]

steatopygia: Large buttocks and heavy upper thigh distribution of fat deposits.[1]

sublimate: The expression of an "unacceptable" impulse or urge in a positive or acceptable way. The standard of unacceptable and acceptable usually relate to societal norms.[1]

thermogenesis: The generation of heat, particularly in brown fat deposits, that provides necessary warmth, and may also be a way the body burns excess food and so avoids weight gain.[1]

Chapter 56

Directory of Eating Disorder Resources

Academy for Eating Disorders
111 Deer Lake Road, Suite 100
Deerfield, IL 60015
Phone: 847-498-4274
Fax: 847-480-9282
Website: http://www.aedweb.org
E-mail: info@aedweb.org

The Alliance for Eating Disorders Awareness
P.O. Box 13155
North Palm Beach, FL 33408
Toll-Free: 866-662-1235
Phone: 561-841-0900
Fax: 561-653-0043
Website: www.
eatingdisorderinfo.org

American Dietetic Association
120 S. Riverside Plaza
Suite 2000
Chicago, IL 60606-6995
Toll-Free: 800-877-1600
Phone: 312-899-0040
Website: http://www.eatright.org

Body Positive
P.O. Box 7801
Berkeley, CA 94707
Phone: 510-528-0101
Fax: 510-558-0979
Website:
http://www.thebodypositive.org
E-mail:
info@thebodypositive.org

Resources in this chapter were compiled from several sources deemed reliable. All contact information was verified and updated in September 2010.

Bulimia Nervosa Resource Guide

ECRI Institute
Attn: Bulimia Guide Webmaster
5200 Butler Pike
Plymouth Meeting, PA 19462
Website:
http://www.bulimiaguide.org

Caring Online

Website:
http://www.caringonline.com

Casa Palmera

14750 El Camino Real
Del Mar, California 92014
Phone: 866-768-6719 or
858-481-4411
(non-admission related
questions)
Website:
http://www.casapalmera.com

Eating Disorder Foundation

3003 East Third Avenue
Suite 110
Denver, CO 80206
Phone: 303-322-3373
Website: http://www.
eatingdisorderfoundation.org

Eating Disorder Referral and Information Center

Website:
http://www.edreferral.com

Eating Disorders Coalition

720 7th Street NW, Suite 300
Washington, DC 20001
Phone: 202-543-9570
Website: http://www
.eatingdisorderscoalition.org
E-mail: manager@
eatingdisorderscoalition.org

Eating Disorders Foundation of Victoria

1513 High Street, Glen Iris, VIC 3146
Australia
Website:
http://www.eatingdisorders.org.au
E-mail: edfv@
eatingdisorders.org.au

Eating Disorders Recovery Center

232 Vance Rd., Suite 206
St. Louis, MO 63088
Phone: 636-225-3700
Website: http://www.addictions.net

Female Athlete Triad Coalition

Website:
http://www.femaleathletetriad
.org

girlshealth.gov

8270 Willow Oaks Corporate
Drive, Suite 301
Fairfax, VA 22031
Website:
http://www.girlshealth.gov

Harris Center for Education and Advocacy in Eating Disorders

2 Longfellow Place
Suite 200
Boston, MA 02114
Phone: 617-726-8470
Website:
http://www2.massgeneral.org/
harriscenter/index.asp

Multi-Service Eating Disorders Association

92 Pearl Street
Newton, MA 02458
Toll-Free: 866-343-MEDA
Phone: 617-558-1881
Website:
http://www.medainc.org
E-mail: info@medainc.org

National Association of Anorexia Nervosa and Associated Disorders (ANAD)

P.O. Box 640
Naperville, IL 60566
Phone: 630-577-1333 (general)
or 630-577-1330 (Helpline)
Website: http://www.anad.org

National Center for Overcoming Overeating

Website:
http://www.overcoming
overeating.com
E-mail: webmaster@
overcomingovereating.com

National Eating Disorder Information Centre

ES 7-421, 200 Elizabeth Street
Toronto, Ontario M5G 2C4
Canada
Toll-free: 866-NEDIC-20
(866-633-4220)
Phone: 416-340-4156
Fax: 416-340-4736
Website:
http://www.nedic.ca/index.shtml
E-mail: nedic@uhn.on.ca

National Eating Disorders Association

Informational and Referral
Program
603 Stewart Street, Suite 803
Seattle, WA 98101
Toll-Free: 800-931-2237
Phone: 206-382-3587
Fax: 206-829-8501
Website: http://
www.nationaleatingdisorders.org

National Institute of Diabetes and Digestive and Kidney Diseases (NIDDK)

Office of Communications and
Public Liaison
NIDDK, NIH
Bldg 31, Rm 9A06
31 Center Drive, MSC 2560
Bethesda, MD 20892-2560
Phone: 301-496-3583
Website:
http://www.niddk.nih.gov

National Institute of Mental Health (NIMH)
6001 Executive Boulevard
Room 8184 MSC 9663
Bethesda, MD 20892-9663
Toll-Free:
866-615-NIMH (6464)
Phone: 301-443-4513
Fax: 301-443-4279
TTY: 301-443-8431
TTY Toll-Free: 866-415-8051
Website:
http://www.nimh.nih.gov
E-mail: nimhinfo@nih.gov

National Women's Health Information Center (NWHIC)
Toll-free: 800-994-9662
TDD: 888-220-5446
Website:
http://www.womenshealth.gov

Overeaters Anonymous
P.O. Box 44020
Rio Rancho, NM 87174-4020
Phone: 505-891-2664
Fax: 505-891-4320
Website: http://www.oa.org

Rader Programs
Toll-Free: 877-632-4293
Website:
http://www.raderprograms.com

Sheena's Place
87 Spadina Road
Toronto, Ontario
Canada M5R 2T1
Phone: 416-927-8900
Fax: 416-927-8844
Website:
http://www.sheenasplace.org
E-mail: info@sheenasplace.org

Something Fishy
Website: http://www.something
-fishy.org

Weight Control Information Network
1 WIN Way
Bethesda, MD 20892–3665
Toll-Free: 877-946-4627
Phone: 202-828–1025
Fax: 202-828-1028
Website:
http://www.win.niddk.nih.gov
E-mail: win@info.niddk.nih.gov

Index

Index

Page numbers followed by 'n' indicate a footnote. Page numbers in *italics* indicate a table or illustration.

567

Taylor, C. Barr 390–91
teenagers *see* adolescents
temporary paralysis, described 263
temporomandibular joint disorders
   (TMJ), described 267
"Ten Steps to Positive Body Image"
   (National Eating Disorders
   Association) 453n
"Ten Things Parents Can Do to
   Help Prevent Eating Disorders"
   (National Eating Disorders
   Association) 433n
tests
   anorexia nervosa 40
   bone density 277–78
   eating disorders 334, 337–39
   osteoporosis 310
   rumination disorder 78–79
text messaging, relapse
   prevention 413
therapeutic bind, described 371
therapists, overview 344–53
therapy
   anorexia nervosa 41, 45
   binge eating disorder 34
   bulimia nervosa 51–54
   eating disorders 185, 197–98
   ethnic factors, eating disorders
      168–71
   levels of care overview 358–65
   treatment resistance 354–55
   types, overview 366–72
thermogenesis, defined 560
"Things You Can Do Right Away
   - Every Day - to Raise Your Self-
   Esteem" (SAMHSA) 438n
"Thriving During the Holidays"
   (Lensegrav-Benson) 551n
throat problems, bulimia
   nervosa 293–94
thrombocytopenia, anorexia
   nervosa 280
"Tips for Coaches: Preventing
   Eating Disorders in Athletes"
   (National Eating Disorders
   Association) 155n
"Tips for Parents: Ideas to Help
   Children Maintain a Healthy
   Weight" (CDC) 485n

Topamax (topiramate)
   bulimia nervosa 385
   eating disorders 198, 395
   sleep eating 86
topiramate
   bulimia nervosa 385
   eating disorders 198, 395
   sleep eating 86
"The Top Ten Reasons to Have
   Family Meals" (Manley) 537n
treatment facilities, overview 342–44,
   352–53
treatment resistance,
   described 354–55
tube feeding, restoring
   normal weight 492–93
twins studies, anorexia nervosa
   214–15

U

"Understanding Eating Disorders"
   (NIH) 24n
underwater weighing, body fat 464
University of Arizona, weight gain
   tips publication 494n
University of California,
   sense of taste publication 211n
University of North Carolina
   publications
      heredity, anorexia 213n
University of Texas, publications
   oral health, eating
      disorders 303n
   reproductive issues 301n
University of Virginia, ADHD,
   eating disorders publication 179n

V

venlafaxine 394

W

Wack, Elizabeth 411n
waist measurement,
   described 464
warning signs overview,
   eating disorders 314–15

Health Reference Series
Complete Catalog
List price $93 per volume. School and library price $84 per volume.

Adolescent Health Sourcebook, 3rd Edition

Basic Consumer Health Information about Adolescent Growth and Development, Puberty, Sexuality, Reproductive Health, and Physical, Emotional, Social, and Mental Health Concerns of Teens and Their Parents, Including Facts about Nutrition, Physical Activity, Weight Management, Acne, Allergies, Cancer, Diabetes, Growth Disorders, Juvenile Arthritis, Infections, Substance Abuse, and More

Along with Information about Adolescent Safety Concerns, Youth Violence, a Glossary of Related Terms, and a Directory of Resources

Edited by Amy L. Sutton. 600 pages. 2010. 978-0-7808-1140-9.

Adult Health Concerns Sourcebook

Basic Consumer Health Information about Medical and Mental Concerns of Adults, Including Facts about Choosing Healthcare Providers, Navigating Insurance Options, Maintaining Wellness, Preventing Cancer, Heart Disease, Stroke, Diabetes, and Osteoporosis, and Understanding Aging-Related Health Concerns, Including Menopause, Cognitive Changes, and Changes in the Coronary and Vascular Systems

Along with Tips on Caring for Aging Parents and Dealing with Health-Related Work and Travel Issues, a Glossary, and a Directory of Resources for Additional Help and Information

Edited by Sandra J. Judd. 648 pages. 2008. 978-0-7808-0999-4.

"Provides a thorough list of topics that are important to adult health and for caregivers."
—*CHOICE, Nov '08*

"Written in easy-to-understand language... the content is well-organized and is intended to aid adults in making health care-related decisions."
—*AORN Journal, Dec '08*

AIDS Sourcebook, 4th Edition

Basic Consumer Health Information about Human Immunodeficiency Virus (HIV) and Acquired Immunodeficiency Syndrome (AIDS), Featuring Updated Statistics and Facts about Risks, Prevention, Screening, Diagnosis, Treatments, Side Effects, and Complications, and Including a Section about the Impact of HIV/AIDS on the Health of Women, Children, and Adolescents

Along with Tips on Managing Life with AIDS, Reports on Current Research Initiatives and Clinical Trials, a Glossary of Related Terms, and Resource Directories for Further Help and Information

Edited by Ivy L. Alexander. 680 pages. 2008. 978-0-7808-0997-0.

SEE ALSO *Contagious Diseases Sourcebook, 2nd Edition*

Alcoholism Sourcebook, 3rd Edition

Basic Consumer Health Information about Alcohol Use, Abuse, and Dependence, Featuring Facts about the Physical, Mental, and Social Health Effects of Alcohol Addiction, Including Alcoholic Liver Disease, Pancreatic Disease, Cardiovascular Disease, Neurological Disorders, and the Effects of Drinking during Pregnancy

Along with Information about Alcohol Treatment, Medications, and Recovery Programs, in Addition to Tips for Reducing the Prevalence of Underage Drinking, Statistics about Alcohol Use, a Glossary of Related Terms, and Directories of Resources for More Help and Information

Edited by Joyce Brennfleck Shannon. 600 pages. 2010. 978-0-7808-1141-6.

SEE ALSO *Drug Abuse Sourcebook, 3rd Edition*

Allergies Sourcebook, 3rd Edition

Basic Consumer Health Information about Allergic Disorders, Such as Anaphylaxis, Hives,

Eczema, Rhinitis, Sinusitis, and Conjunctivitis, and Their Triggers, Including Pollen, Mold, Dust Mites, Animal Dander, Insects, Chemicals, Food, Food Additives, and Medications

Along with Advice about the Diagnosis and Treatment of Allergy Symptoms, a Glossary of Related Terms, a Directory of Resources for Help and Information, and Suggestions for Additional Reading

Edited by Amy L. Sutton. 588 pages. 2007. 978-0-7808-0950-5.

SEE ALSO *Asthma Sourcebook, 2nd Edition*

Alzheimer Disease Sourcebook, 4th Edition

Basic Consumer Health Information about Alzheimer Disease, Other Dementias, and Related Disorders, Including Multi-Infarct Dementia, Dementia with Lewy Bodies, Frontotemporal Dementia (Pick Disease), Wernicke-Korsakoff Syndrome (Alcohol-Related Dementia), AIDS Dementia Complex, Huntington Disease, Creutzfeldt-Jacob Disease, and Delirium

Along with Information about Coping with Memory Loss and Forgetfulness, Maintaining Skills, and Long-Term Planning for People with Dementia, and Suggestions Addressing Common Caregiver Concerns, Updated Information about Current Research Efforts, a Glossary of Related Terms, and Directories of Sources for Additional Help and Information

Edited by Karen Bellenir. 603 pages. 2008. 978-0-7808-1001-3.

"An invaluable resource for persons who have received a diagnosis, for caregivers, and for family members dealing with this insidious disease. It is recommended for public, community college, and ready-reference sections in academic libraries."
—*American Reference Books Annual, 2009*

SEE ALSO *Brain Disorders Sourcebook, 3rd Edition*

Arthritis Sourcebook, 3rd Edition

Basic Consumer Health Information about the Risk Factors, Symptoms, Diagnosis, and Treatment of Osteoarthritis, Rheumatoid Arthritis, Juvenile Arthritis, Gout, Infectious Arthritis, and Autoimmune Disorders Associated with Arthritis

Along with Facts about Medications, Surgeries, and Self-Care Techniques to Manage Pain and Disability, Tips on Living with Arthritis, a Glossary of Related Terms, and Resources for Additional Help and Information

Edited by Amy L. Sutton. 600 pages. 2010. 978-0-7808-1077-8.

Asthma Sourcebook, 2nd Edition

Basic Consumer Health Information about the Causes, Symptoms, Diagnosis, and Treatment of Asthma in Infants, Children, Teenagers, and Adults, Including Facts about Different Types of Asthma, Common Co-Occurring Conditions, Asthma Management Plans, Triggers, Medications, and Medication Delivery Devices

Along with Asthma Statistics, Research Updates, a Glossary, a Directory of Asthma-Related Resources, and More

Edited by Karen Bellenir. 581 pages. 2006. 978-0-7808-0866-9.

SEE ALSO *Lung Disorders Sourcebook; Respiratory Disorders Sourcebook, 2nd Edition*

Attention Deficit Disorder Sourcebook

Basic Consumer Health Information about Attention Deficit/Hyperactivity Disorder in Children and Adults, Including Facts about Causes, Symptoms, Diagnostic Criteria, and Treatment Options Such as Medications, Behavior Therapy, Coaching, and Homeopathy

Along with Reports on Current Research Initiatives, Legal Issues, and Government Regulations, and Featuring a Glossary of Related Terms, Internet Resources, and a List of Additional Reading Material

Edited by Dawn D. Matthews. 447 pages. 2002. 978-0-7808-0624-5.

"Recommended reference source."
—*Booklist, Jan '03*

SEE ALSO *Learning Disabilities Sourcebook, 3rd Edition*

Autism and Pervasive Developmental Disorders Sourcebook

Basic Consumer Health Information about Autism Spectrum and Pervasive Developmental Disorders, Such as Classical Autism, Asperger Syndrome, Rett Syndrome, and Childhood Disintegrative Disorder, Including Information about Related Genetic Disorders and Medical Problems and Facts about Causes, Screening Methods, Diagnostic Criteria, Treatments and Interventions, and Family and Education Issues

Along with a Glossary of Related Terms, Tips for Evaluating the Validity of Health Claims, and a Directory of Resources for Additional Help and Information

Edited by Sandra J. Judd. 603 pages. 2007. 978-0-7808-0953-6.

"This book provides a current overview of disorders on the autism spectrum and information about various therapies, educational resources, and help for families with practical issues such as workplace adjustments, living arrangements, and estate planning. It is a useful resource for public and consumer health libraries."
—*American Reference Books Annual, 2009*

SEE ALSO *Learning Disabilities Sourcebook, 3rd Edition*

Back and Neck Disorders Sourcebook, 2nd Edition

Basic Consumer Health Information about Spinal Pain, Spinal Cord Injuries, and Related Disorders, Such as Degenerative Disk Disease, Osteoarthritis, Scoliosis, Sciatica, Spina Bifida, and Spinal Stenosis, and Featuring Facts about Maintaining Spinal Health, Self-Care, Pain Management, Rehabilitative Care, Chiropractic Care, Spinal Surgeries, and Complementary Therapies

Along with Suggestions for Preventing Back and Neck Pain, a Glossary of Related Terms, and a Directory of Resources

Edited by Amy L. Sutton. 607 pages. 2004. 978-0-7808-0738-9.

"Recommended... An easy to use, comprehensive medical reference book."
—*E-Streams, Sep '05*

"For anyone who has back or neck problems, this book is ideal. Its easy-to-understand language and variety of topics makes this sourcebook a worthwhile read. The price... is reasonable for the amount of information contained in the book"
—*Occupational Therapy in Health Care, 2007*

Blood & Circulatory Disorders Sourcebook, 3rd Edition

Basic Consumer Health Information about Blood and Circulatory System Disorders, Such as Anemia, Leukemia, Lymphoma, Rh Disease, Hemophilia, Thrombophilia, Other Bleeding and Clotting Deficiencies, and Artery, Vascular, and Venous Diseases, Including Facts about Blood Types, Blood Donation, Bone Marrow and Stem Cell Transplants, Tests and Medications, and Tips for Maintaining Circulatory Health

Along with a Glossary of Related Terms and a List of Resources for Additional Help and Information

Edited by Sandra J. Judd. 600 pages. 2010. 978-0-7808-1081-5.

SEE ALSO *Leukemia Sourcebook*

Brain Disorders Sourcebook, 3rd Edition

Basic Consumer Health Information about Acquired and Traumatic Brain Injuries, Brain Tumors, Cerebral Palsy and Other Genetic and Congenital Brain Disorders, Infections of the Brain, Epilepsy, and Degenerative Neurological Disorders Such as Dementia, Huntington Disease, and Amyotrophic Lateral Sclerosis (ALS)

Along with Information on Brain Structure and Function, Treatment and Rehabilitation Options, a Glossary of Terms Related to Brain Disorders, and a Directory of Resources for More Information

Edited by Joyce Brennfleck Shannon. 600 pages. 2010. 978-0-7808-1083-9.

SEE ALSO *Alzheimer Disease Sourcebook, 4th Edition*

Breast Cancer Sourcebook, 3rd Edition

Basic Consumer Health Information about Breast Health and Breast Cancer, Including Facts about Environmental, Genetic, and Other Risk Factors, Prevention Efforts, Screening and Diagnostic Methods, Surgical Treatment Options and Other Care Choices, Complementary and Alternative Therapies, and Post-Treatment Concerns

Along with Statistical Data, News about Research Advances, a Glossary of Related Terms, and Directories of Resources for Additional Information and Support

Edited by Karen Bellenir. 606 pages. 2009. 978-0-7808-1030-3.

"A very useful reference for people wanting to learn more about breast cancer and how to negotiate their care or the care of a loved one. The third edition is necessary as information/treatment options continue to evolve."
—*Doody's Review Service, 2009*

SEE ALSO *Cancer Sourcebook for Women, 3rd Edition, Women's Health Concerns Sourcebook, 3rd Edition*

Breastfeeding Sourcebook

Basic Consumer Health Information about the Benefits of Breastmilk, Preparing to Breastfeed, Breastfeeding as a Baby Grows, Nutrition, and More, Including Information on Special Situations and Concerns Such as Mastitis, Illness, Medications, Allergies, Multiple Births, Prematurity, Special Needs, and Adoption

Along with a Glossary and Resources for Additional Help and Information

Edited by Jenni Lynn Colson. 367 pages. 2002. 978-0-7808-0332-9.

SEE ALSO *Pregnancy and Birth Sourcebook, 3rd Edition*

Burns Sourcebook

Basic Consumer Health Information about Various Types of Burns and Scalds, Including Flame, Heat, Cold, Electrical, Chemical, and Sun Burns

Along with Information on Short-Term and Long-Term Treatments, Tissue Reconstruction, Plastic Surgery, Prevention Suggestions, and First Aid

Edited by Allan R. Cook. 604 pages. 1999. 978-0-7808-0204-9.

"This is an exceptional addition to the series and is highly recommended for all consumer health collections, hospital libraries, and academic medical centers."
—*E-Streams, Mar '00*

"This key reference guide is an invaluable addition to all health care and public libraries in confronting this ongoing health issue."
—*American Reference Books Annual, 2000*

SEE ALSO *Dermatological Disorders Sourcebook, 2nd Edition*

Cancer Sourcebook, 5th Edition

Basic Consumer Health Information about Major Forms and Stages of Cancer, Featuring Facts about Head and Neck Cancers, Lung Cancers, Gastrointestinal Cancers, Genitourinary Cancers, Lymphomas, Blood Cell Cancers, Endocrine Cancers, Skin Cancers, Bone Cancers, Metastatic Cancers, and More

Along with Facts about Cancer Treatments, Cancer Risks and Prevention, a Glossary of Related Terms, Statistical Data, and a Directory of Resources for Additional Information

Edited by Karen Bellenir. 1105 pages. 2007. 978-0-7808-0947-5.

"The 5th, updated edition of Cancer Sourcebook should be in every public and health lending library collection... An unparalleled discussion essential for any health collections considering an all-in-one basic general reference."
—*California Bookwatch, Aug '07*

SEE ALSO *Breast Cancer Sourcebook, 3rd Edition, Cancer Survivorship Sourcebook, Leukemia Sourcebook*

Cancer Sourcebook for Women, 4th Edition

Basic Consumer Health Information about Gynecologic Cancers and Other Cancers of Special Concern to Women, Including Cancers of the Breast, Cervix, Colon, Lung, Ovaries, Thyroid, and Uterus

Along with Facts about Benign Conditions of the Female Reproductive System, Cancer Risk

Factors, Diagnostic and Treatment Procedures, Side Effects of Cancer and Cancer Treatments, Women's Issues in Cancer Survivorship, a Glossary of Related Terms, and a Directory of Resources for Additional Help and Information

Edited by Karen Bellenir. 600 pages. 2010. 978-0-7808-1139-3.

SEE ALSO Breast Cancer Sourcebook, 3rd Edition, Women's Health Concerns Sourcebook, 3rd Edition

Cancer Survivorship Sourcebook

Basic Consumer Health Information about the Physical, Educational, Emotional, Social, and Financial Needs of Cancer Patients from Diagnosis, through Cancer Treatment, and Beyond, Including Facts about Researching Specific Types of Cancer and Learning about Clinical Trials and Treatment Options, and Featuring Tips for Coping with the Side Effects of Cancer Treatments and Adjusting to Life after Cancer Treatment Concludes

Along with Suggestions for Caregivers, Friends, and Family Members of Cancer Patients, a Glossary of Cancer Care Terms, and Directories of Related Resources

Edited by Karen Bellenir. 633 pages. 2007. 978-0-7808-0985-7.

"Well organized and comprehensive in coverage, the book speaks to issues encountered both during and after cancer treatment. Recommended for consumer health and public libraries."
—*Library Journal, Aug 1 '07*

"Cancer Survivorship Sourcebook will be useful to anyone who has a friend or loved one with a cancer diagnosis."
—*American Reference Books Annual, 2008*

SEE ALSO *Cancer Sourcebook, 5th Edition, Disease Management Sourcebook*

Cardiovascular Disorders Sourcebook, 4th Edition

Basic Consumer Health Information about Heart and Blood Vessel Diseases and Disorders, Such as Angina, Heart Attack, Heart Failure, Cardiomyopathy, Arrhythmias, Valve Disease, Atherosclerosis, Aneurysms, and

Congenital Heart Defects, Including Information about Cardiovascular Disease in Women, Men, Children, Adolescents, and Minorities

Along with Facts about Diagnosing, Managing, and Preventing Cardiovascular Disease, a Glossary of Related Medical Terms, and a Directory of Resources for Additional Information

Edited by Amy L. Sutton. 600 pages. 2010. 978-0-7808-1080-8.

Caregiving Sourcebook

Basic Consumer Health Information for Caregivers, Including a Profile of Caregivers, Caregiving Responsibilities and Concerns, Tips for Specific Conditions, Care Environments, and the Effects of Caregiving

Along with Facts about Legal Issues, Financial Information, and Future Planning, a Glossary, and a Listing of Additional Resources

Edited by Joyce Brennfleck Shannon. 583 pages. 2001. 978-0-7808-0331-2.

"Essential for most collections."
—*Library Journal, Apr 1 '02*

"An ideal addition to the reference collection of any public library. Health sciences information professionals may also want to acquire the Caregiving Sourcebook for their hospital or academic library for use as a ready reference tool by health care workers interested in aging and caregiving."
—*E-Streams, Jan '02*

Child Abuse Sourcebook, 2nd Edition

Basic Consumer Health Information about the Physical, Sexual, and Emotional Abuse of Children, Neglect, Münchhausen Syndrome by Proxy (MSBP), and Shaken Baby Syndrome, and Featuring Facts about Withholding Medical Care, Corporal Punishment, Child Maltreatment in Youth Sports, and Parental Substance Abuse

Along with Information about Child Protective Services, Foster Care, Adoption, Parenting Challenges, Abuse Prevention Programs, and Intervention, Treatment, and Recovery Guidelines, a Glossary of Related Terms, and Resources for Additional Help and Information

Edited by Joyce Brennfleck Shannon. 600 pages. 2009. 978-0-7808-1037-2.

SEE ALSO *Domestic Violence Sourcebook, 3rd Edition*

Childhood Diseases and Disorders Sourcebook, 2nd Edition

Basic Consumer Health Information about the Physical, Mental, and Developmental Health of Pre-Adolescent Children, Including Facts about Infectious Diseases, Asthma, Allergies, Diabetes, and Other Acute and Chronic Conditions Affecting the Gastrointestinal Tract, Ears, Nose, Throat, Liver, Kidneys, Heart, Blood, Brain, Muscles, Bones, and Skin

Along with Reports on Recommended Childhood Vaccinations, Wellness Guidelines, a Glossary of Related Medical Terms, and a List of Resources for Parents

Edited by Sandra J. Judd. 694 pages. 2009. 978-0-7808-1031-0.

"The strength of this source is the wide range of information given about childhood health issues... It is most appropriate for public libraries and academic libraries that field medical questions."
— *American Reference Books Annual, 2009*

SEE ALSO *Healthy Children Sourcebook*

Colds, Flu and Other Common Ailments Sourcebook

Basic Consumer Health Information about Common Ailments and Injuries, Including Colds, Coughs, the Flu, Sinus Problems, Headaches, Fever, Nausea and Vomiting, Menstrual Cramps, Diarrhea, Constipation, Hemorrhoids, Back Pain, Dandruff, Dry and Itchy Skin, Cuts, Scrapes, Sprains, Bruises, and More

Along with Information about Prevention, Self-Care, Choosing a Doctor, Over-the-Counter Medications, Folk Remedies, and Alternative Therapies, and Including a Glossary of Important Terms and a Directory of Resources for Further Help and Information

Edited by Chad T. Kimball. 622 pages. 2001. 978-0-7808-0435-7.

"A good starting point for research on common illnesses. It will be a useful addition to public and consumer health library collections."
— *American Reference Books Annual, 2002*

"Will prove valuable to any library seeking to maintain a current, comprehensive reference collection of health resources... Excellent reference."
— *The Bookwatch, Aug '01*

SEE ALSO *Contagious Diseases Sourcebook, 2nd Edition*

Communication Disorders Sourcebook

Basic Information about Deafness and Hearing Loss, Speech and Language Disorders, Voice Disorders, Balance and Vestibular Disorders, and Disorders of Smell, Taste, and Touch

Edited by Linda M. Ross. 533 pages. 1996. 978-0-7808-0077-9.

"This is skillfully edited and is a welcome resource for the layperson. It should be found in every public and medical library."
— *Booklist Health Sciences Supplement, Oct '97*

Complementary & Alternative Medicine Sourcebook, 4th Edition

Basic Consumer Health Information about Ayurveda, Acupuncture, Aromatherapy, Chiropractic Care, Diet-Based Therapies, Guided Imagery, Herbal and Vitamin Supplements, Homeopathy, Hypnosis, Massage, Meditation, Naturopathy, Pilates, Reflexology, Reiki, Shiatsu, Tai Chi, Traditional Chinese Medicine, Yoga, and Other Complementary and Alternative Medical Therapies

Along with Statistics, Tips for Selecting a Practitioner, Treatments for Specific Health Conditions, a Glossary of Related Terms, and a Directory of Resources for Additional Help and Information

Edited by Amy L. Sutton. 600 pages. 2010. 978-0-7808-1082-2.

Congenital Disorders Sourcebook, 2nd Edition

Basic Consumer Health Information about Nonhereditary Birth Defects and Disorders

590

Related to Prematurity, Gestational Injuries, Congenital Infections, and Birth Complications, Including Heart Defects, Hydrocephalus, Spina Bifida, Cleft Lip and Palate, Cerebral Palsy, and More

Along with Facts about the Prevention of Birth Defects, Fetal Surgery and Other Treatment Options, Research Initiatives, a Glossary of Related Terms, and Resources for Additional Information and Support

Edited by Sandra J. Judd. 619 pages. 2007. 978-0-7808-0945-1.

"Congenital Disorders Sourcebook provides an excellent, non-technical overview of many aspects of pregnancy with the focus on congenital disorders."
—American Reference Books Annual, 2008

"An excellent readable reference aimed at the lay public for difficult to understand medical problems. An excellent starting point for the interested parent or family member who may then be motivated to seek more information."
—Doody's Review Service, 2007

SEE ALSO Pregnancy and Birth Sourcebook, 3rd Edition

Contagious Diseases Sourcebook, 2nd Edition

Basic Consumer Health Information about Diseases Spread from Person to Person through Direct Physical Contact, Airborne Transmissions, Sexual Contact, or Contact with Blood or Other Body Fluids, Including Pneumococcal, Staphylococcal, and Streptococcal Diseases, Colds, Influenza, Lice, Measles, Mumps, Tuberculosis, and Others

Along with Facts about Self-Care and Over-the-Counter Medications, Antibiotics and Drug Resistance, Disease Prevention, Vaccines, and Bioterrorism, a Glossary, and a Directory of Resources for More Information

Edited by Joyce Brennfleck Shannon. 600 pages. 2010. 978-0-7808-1075-4.

SEE ALSO AIDS Sourcebook, 4th Edition, Hepatitis Sourcebook

Cosmetic and Reconstructive Surgery Sourcebook, 2nd Edition

Basic Consumer Information about Plastic Surgery and Non-Surgical Appearance-Enhancing Procedures, Including Facts about Botulinum Toxin, Collagen Replacement, Dermabrasion, Chemical Peels, Eyelid Surgery, Nose Reshaping, Lip Augmentation, Liposuction, Breast Enlargement and Reduction, Tummy Tucking, and Other Skin, Hair, Facial, and Body Shaping Procedures

Along with Information about Reconstructive Procedures for Congenital Disorders, Disfiguring Diseases, Burns, and Traumatic Injuries, a Glossary of Related Terms, and a Directory of Additional Resources

Edited by Karen Bellenir. 483 pages. 2007. 978-0-7808-0951-2.

"A comprehensive source for people considering cosmetic surgery... also recommended for medical students who will perform these procedures later in their careers; and public librarians and academic medical librarians who may assist patrons interested in this information."
—Medical Reference Services Quarterly, Fall '08

"A practical guide for health care consumers and health care workers... This easy-to-read reference guide would be useful for novice and veteran health care consumers, surgical technology students, nursing students, and perioperative nurses new to plastic and reconstructive surgery. It also may be helpful for medical-surgical nurses as a guide for patient teaching in their practices."
—AORN Journal, Aug '08

SEE ALSO Surgery Sourcebook, 2nd Edition

Death and Dying Sourcebook, 2nd Edition

Basic Consumer Health Information about End-of-Life Care and Related Perspectives and Ethical Issues, Including End-of-Life Symptoms and Treatments, Pain Management, Quality-of-Life Concerns, the Use of Life Support, Patients' Rights and Privacy Issues, Advance Directives, Physician-Assisted Suicide, Caregiving, Organ and Tissue Donation, Autopsies, Funeral Arrangements, and Grief

Along with Statistical Data, Information about the Leading Causes of Death, a Glossary, and Directories of Support Groups and Other Resources

Edited by Joyce Brennfleck Shannon. 626 pages. 2006. 978-0-7808-0871-3.

Dental Care and Oral Health Sourcebook, 3rd Edition

Basic Consumer Health Information about Dental Care and Oral Health Throughout the Lifespan, Including Facts about Cavities, Bad Breath, Cold and Canker Sores, Dry Mouth, Toothaches, Gum Disease, Malocclusion, Temporomandibular Joint and Muscle Disorders, Oral Cancers, and Dental Emergencies

Along with Information about Mouth Hygiene, Crowns, Bridges, Implants, and Fillings, Surgical, Orthodontic, and Cosmetic Dental Procedures, Pain Management, Health Conditions that Impact Oral Care, a Glossary of Related Terms, and a Directory of Additional Resources

Edited by Amy L. Sutton. 619 pages. 2008. 978-0-7808-1032-7.

"Could serve as turning point in the battle to educate consumers in issues concerning oral health. Tightly written in terms the average person can understand, yet comprehensive in scope and authoritative in tone, it is another excellent sourcebook in the Health Reference Series... Should be in the reference department of all public libraries, and in academic libraries that have a public constituency."
—American Reference Books Annual, 2009

Depression Sourcebook, 2nd Edition

Basic Consumer Health Information about Unipolar Depression, Bipolar Disorder, Dysthymia, Seasonal Affective Disorder, Postpartum Depression, and Other Depressive Disorders, Including Facts about Populations at Special Risk, Coexisting Medical Conditions, Symptoms, Treatment Options, and Suicide Prevention

Along with Statistical Data, a Glossary of Related Terms, and a Directory of Resources for Additional Help and Information

Edited by Sandra J. Judd. 646 pages. 2008. 978-0-7808-1003-7.

"Recommended for public libraries."
—American Reference Books Annual, 2009

SEE ALSO *Mental Health Disorders Sourcebook, 4th Edition*

Dermatological Disorders Sourcebook, 2nd Edition

Basic Consumer Health Information about Conditions and Disorders Affecting the Skin, Hair, and Nails, Such as Acne, Rosacea, Rashes, Dermatitis, Pigmentation Disorders, Birthmarks, Skin Cancer, Skin Injuries, Psoriasis, Scleroderma, and Hair Loss, Including Facts about Medications and Treatments for Dermatological Disorders and Tips for Maintaining Healthy Skin, Hair, and Nails

Along with Information about How Aging Affects the Skin, a Glossary of Related Terms, and a Directory of Resources for Additional Help and Information

Edited by Amy L. Sutton. 617 pages. 2006. 978-0-7808-0795-2.

"Well organized... presents a plethora of information in a manner that is appropriate in style and readability for the intended audience."
—Physical Therapy, Nov '06

"Helpfully brings together... sources in one convenient place, saving the user hours of research time."
—American Reference Books Annual, 2006

SEE ALSO *Burns Sourcebook*

Diabetes Sourcebook, 4th Edition

Basic Consumer Health Information about Type 1 and Type 2 Diabetes Mellitus, Gestational Diabetes, Monogenic Forms of Diabetes, and Insulin Resistance, with Guidelines for Lifestyle Modifications and the Medical Management of Diabetes, Including Facts about Insulin, Insulin Delivery Devices, Oral Diabetes Medications, Self-Monitoring of Blood Glucose, Meal Planning, Physical Activity Recommendations, Foot Care, and Treatment Options for People with Kidney Failure

Along with a Section about Diabetes Complications and Co-Occurring Conditions, a Glossary of Related Terms, and Directories of Resources for Additional Help and Information

Edited by Karen Bellenir. 627 pages. 2008. 978-0-7808-1005-1.

"Completely and comprehensively covering almost everything a student or physician would need to know... well worth the investment."
—*Internet Bookwatch, Dec '08*

SEE ALSO *Endocrine and Metabolic Disorders Sourcebook, 2nd Edition*

Diet and Nutrition Sourcebook, 3rd Edition

Basic Consumer Health Information about Dietary Guidelines and the Food Guidance System, Recommended Daily Nutrient Intakes, Serving Proportions, Weight Control, Vitamins and Supplements, Nutrition Issues for Different Life Stages and Lifestyles, and the Needs of People with Specific Medical Concerns, Including Cancer, Celiac Disease, Diabetes, Eating Disorders, Food Allergies, and Cardiovascular Disease

Along with Facts about Federal Nutrition Support Programs, a Glossary of Nutrition and Dietary Terms, and Directories of Additional Resources for More Information about Nutrition

Edited by Joyce Brennfleck Shannon. 605 pages. 2006. 978-0-7808-0800-3.

"A valuable resource tool for any individual."
—*Journal of Dental Hygiene, Apr '07*

"From different recommended eating habits to reduce disease and common ailments to nutrition advice for those with specific conditions, Diet and Nutrition Sourcebook is especially important because so much is changing in this area, and so rapidly."
—*California Bookwatch, Jun '06*

SEE ALSO *Eating Disorders Sourcebook, 2nd Edition, Vegetarian Sourcebook*

Digestive Diseases and Disorders Sourcebook

Basic Consumer Health Information about Diseases and Disorders that Impact the Upper and Lower Digestive System, Including Celiac Disease, Constipation, Crohn's Disease, Cyclic Vomiting Syndrome, Diarrhea, Diverticulosis and Diverticulitis, Gallstones, Heartburn, Hemorrhoids, Hernias, Indigestion (Dyspepsia), Irritable Bowel Syndrome, Lactose Intolerance, Ulcers, and More

Along with Information about Medications and Other Treatments, Tips for Maintaining a Healthy Digestive Tract, a Glossary, and Directory of Digestive Diseases Organizations

Edited by Karen Bellenir. 323 pages. 2000. 978-0-7808-0327-5.

"An excellent addition to all public or patient-research libraries."
—*American Reference Books Annual, 2001*

"Recommended reference source."
—*Booklist, May '00*

SEE ALSO *Gastrointestinal Diseases and Disorders Sourcebook, 2nd Edition*

Disabilities Sourcebook

Basic Consumer Health Information about Physical and Psychiatric Disabilities, Including Descriptions of Major Causes of Disability, Assistive and Adaptive Aids, Workplace Issues, and Accessibility Concerns

Along with Information about the Americans with Disabilities Act, a Glossary, and Resources for Additional Help and Information

Edited by Dawn D. Matthews. 602 pages. 2000. 978-0-7808-0389-3.

"A must for libraries with a consumer health section."
—*American Reference Books Annual, 2002*

"A much needed addition to the Omnigraphics Health Reference Series. A current reference work to provide people with disabilities, their families, caregivers or those who work with them, a broad range of information in one volume, has not been available until now... It is recommended for all public and academic library reference collections."
—*E-Streams, May '01*

"An excellent source book in easy-to-read format covering many current topics; highly recommended for all libraries."
—*CHOICE, Jan '01*

Disease Management Sourcebook

Basic Consumer Health Information about Coping with Chronic and Serious Illnesses, Navigating the Health Care System, Communicating with Health Care Providers, Assessing Health Care Quality, and Making Informed Health Care Decisions, Including Facts about Second Opinions, Hospitalization, Surgery, and Medications

Along with a Section about Children with Chronic Conditions, Information about Legal, Financial, and Insurance Issues, a Glossary of Related Terms, and Directories of Additional Resources

Edited by Joyce Brennfleck Shannon. 621 pages. 2008. 978-0-7808-1002-0.

"Consumers need to know how to manage their health care the same way they manage anything else in their lives. The text is very readable and is written for the layperson and consumer. The cost is not prohibitive. This book should be in all collections of health care libraries and public libraries."
— *American Reference Books Annual, 2009*

"The information is very current, and the selection of font and layout make the book easy to read. A hardback that will stand up to much usage, this is an excellent resource for consumers... Recommended. General readers."
—*CHOICE, Nov '08*

"Intended for lay readers, this resource clarifies the many confusing and overwhelming details associated with chronic disease care. Meticulous and clearly explained, the book even includes diagrams intended to ease comprehension of over-the-counter medication labels. An essential guide to navigating the health-care rapids."
—*Library Journal, Aug '08*

Domestic Violence Sourcebook, 3rd Edition

Basic Consumer Health Information about Warning Signs, Risk Factors, and Health Consequences of Intimate Partner Violence, Sexual Violence and Rape, Stalking, Human Trafficking, Child Maltreatment, Teen Dating Violence, and Elder Abuse

Along with Facts about Victims and Perpetrators, Strategies for Violence Prevention, and Emergency Interventions, Safety Plans, and Financial and Legal Tips for Victims, a Glossary of Related Terms, and Directories of Resources for Additional Information and Support

Edited by Joyce Brennfleck Shannon. 634 pages. 2009. 978-0-7808-1038-9.

"A recommended pick for any library interested in consumer health and social issues... A 'must' for any serious health collection."
—*California Bookwatch, Jul '09*

SEE ALSO *Child Abuse Sourcebook, 2nd Edition*

Drug Abuse Sourcebook, 3rd Edition

Basic Consumer Health Information about the Abuse of Cocaine, Club Drugs, Hallucinogens, Heroin, Inhalants, Marijuana, and Other Illicit Substances, Prescription Medications, and Over-the-Counter Medicines

Along with Facts about Addiction and Related Health Effects, Drug Abuse Treatment and Recovery, Drug Testing, Prevention Programs, Glossaries of Drug-Related Terms, and Directories of Resources for More Information

Edited by Joyce Brennfleck Shannon. 600 pages. 2010. 978-0-7808-1079-2.

SEE ALSO *Alcoholism Sourcebook, 3rd Edition*

Ear, Nose, and Throat Disorders Sourcebook, 2nd Edition

Basic Consumer Health Information about Disorders of the Ears, Hearing Loss, Vestibular Disorders, Nasal and Sinus Problems, Throat and Vocal Cord Disorders, and Otolaryngologic Cancers, Including Facts about Ear Infections and Injuries, Genetic and Congenital Deafness, Sensorineural Hearing Disorders, Tinnitus, Vertigo, Ménière Disease, Rhinitis, Sinusitis, Snoring, Sore Throats, Hoarseness, and More

Along with Reports on Current Research Initiatives, a Glossary of Related Medical Terms, and a Directory of Sources for Further Help and Information

Edited by Sandra J. Judd. 631 pages. 2007. 978-0-7808-0872-0.

"A resource book for the general public that provides comprehensive coverage of basic up-to-date medical information about the causes, symptoms, diagnosis, and treatment of diseases and disorders that affect the ears, nose, sinuses, throat, and voice... The majority of information is presented in question and answer format, much like questions a patient might ask of a health care provider. An extensive index facilitates the reader's ability to easily access information on any specific topic."
—*Journal of Dental Hygiene, Oct '07*

"A handy compilation of information on common and some not so common ailments of the ears, nose, and throat."
—*Doody's Review Service, 2007*

■

Eating Disorders Sourcebook, 2nd Edition

Basic Consumer Health Information about Anorexia Nervosa, Bulimia, Binge Eating, Compulsive Exercise, Female Athlete Triad, and Other Eating Disorders, Including Facts about Body Image and Other Cultural and Age-Related Risk Factors, Prevention Efforts, Adverse Health Effects, Treatment Options, and the Recovery Process

Along with Guidelines for Healthy Weight Control, a Glossary, and Directories of Additional Resources

Edited by Joyce Brennfleck Shannon. 557 pages. 2007. 978-0-7808-0948-2.

"Recommended for the reference collection of large public libraries."
—*American Reference Books Annual, 2008*

"A basic health reference any health or general library needs."
—*Internet Bookwatch, Jun '07*

SEE ALSO Diet and Nutrition Sourcebook, 3rd Edition, Mental Health Disorders Sourcebook, 4th Edition

■

Emergency Medical Services Sourcebook

Basic Consumer Health Information about Preventing, Preparing for, and Managing Emergency Situations, When and Who to Call for Help, What to Expect in the Emergency Room, the Emergency Medical Team,

Patient Issues, and Current Topics in Emergency Medicine

Along with Statistical Data, a Glossary, and Sources of Additional Help and Information

Edited by Jenni Lynn Colson. 472 pages. 2002. 978-0-7808-0420-3.

"Handy and convenient for home, public, school, and college libraries. Recommended."
—*CHOICE, Apr '03*

"This reference can provide the consumer with answers to most questions about emergency care in the United States, or it will direct them to a resource where the answer can be found."
—*American Reference Books Annual, 2003*

SEE ALSO Injury and Trauma Sourcebook

■

Endocrine and Metabolic Disorders Sourcebook, 2nd Edition

Basic Consumer Health Information about Hormonal and Metabolic Disorders that Affect the Body's Growth, Development, and Functioning, Including Disorders of the Pancreas, Ovaries and Testes, and Pituitary, Thyroid, Parathyroid, and Adrenal Glands, with Facts about Growth Disorders, Addison Disease, Cushing Syndrome, Conn Syndrome, Diabetic Disorders, Multiple Endocrine Neoplasia, Inborn Errors of Metabolism, and More

Along with Information about Endocrine Functioning, Diagnostic and Screening Tests, a Glossary of Related Terms, and Directories of Additional Resources

Edited by Joyce Brennfleck Shannon. 597 pages. 2007. 978-0-7808-0952-9.

SEE ALSO Diabetes Sourcebook, 4th Edition

■

Environmental Health Sourcebook, 3rd Edition

Basic Consumer Health Information about the Environment and Its Effects on Human Health, Including Facts about Air, Water, and Soil Contamination, Hazardous Chemicals, Foodborne Hazards and Illnesses, Household Hazards Such as Radon, Mold, and Carbon Monoxide, Consumer Hazards from Toxic Products and Imported Goods, and Disorders

Linked to Environmental Causes, Including Chemical Sensitivity, Cancer, Allergies, and Asthma

Along with Information about the Impact of Environmental Hazards on Specific Populations, a Glossary of Related Terms, and Resources for Additional Help and Information.

Edited by Laura Larsen. 600 pages. 2010. 978-0-7808-1078-5

Ethnic Diseases Sourcebook

Basic Consumer Health Information for Ethnic and Racial Minority Groups in the United States, Including General Health Indicators and Behaviors, Ethnic Diseases, Genetic Testing, the Impact of Chronic Diseases, Women's Health, Mental Health Issues, and Preventive Health Care Services

Along with a Glossary and a Listing of Additional Resources

Edited by Joyce Brennfleck Shannon. 648 pages. 2001. 978-0-7808-0336-7.

"Not many books have been written on this topic to date, and the Ethnic Diseases Sourcebook is a strong addition to the list. It will be an important introductory resource for health consumers, students, health care personnel, and social scientists. It is recommended for public, academic, and large hospital libraries."
— *American Reference Books Annual, 2002*

"Will prove valuable to any library seeking to maintain a current, comprehensive reference collection of health resources... An excellent source of health information about genetic disorders which affect particular ethnic and racial minorities in the U.S."
—*The Bookwatch, Aug '01*

Eye Care Sourcebook, 3rd Edition

Basic Consumer Health Information about Eye Care and Eye Disorders, Including Facts about the Diagnosis, Prevention, and Treatment of Refractive Disorders, Cataracts, Glaucoma, Macular Degeneration, and Problems Affecting the Cornea, Retina, and Lacrimal Glands

Along with Advice about Preventing Eye Injuries and Tips for Living with Low Vision or

Blindness, a Glossary of Related Terms, and Directories of Resources for More Help and Information

Edited by Amy L. Sutton. 646 pages. 2008. 978-0-7808-1000-6.

"A solid reference tool for eye care and a valuable addition to a collection."
—*American Reference Books Annual, 2009*

Family Planning Sourcebook

Basic Consumer Health Information about Planning for Pregnancy and Contraception, Including Traditional Methods, Barrier Methods, Hormonal Methods, Permanent Methods, Future Methods, Emergency Contraception, and Birth Control Choices for Women at Each Stage of Life

Along with Statistics, a Glossary, and Sources of Additional Information

Edited by Amy Marcaccio Keyzer. 503 pages. 2001. 978-0-7808-0379-4.

"Recommended for public, health, and undergraduate libraries as part of the circulating collection."
—*E-Streams, Mar '02*

"Will prove valuable to any library seeking to maintain a current, comprehensive reference collection of health resources... Excellent reference."
—*The Bookwatch, Aug '01*

SEE ALSO Pregnancy and Birth Sourcebook, 3rd Edition

Fitness and Exercise Sourcebook, 3rd Edition

Basic Consumer Health Information about the Physical and Mental Benefits of Fitness, Including Cardiorespiratory Endurance, Muscular Strength, Muscular Endurance, and Flexibility, with Facts about Sports Nutrition and Exercise-Related Injuries and Tips about Physical Activity and Exercises for People of All Ages and for People with Health Concerns

Along with Advice on Selecting and Using Exercise Equipment, Maintaining Exercise Motivation, a Glossary of Related Terms, and a Directory of Resources for More Help and Information

Edited by Amy L. Sutton. 635 pages. 2007. 978-0-7808-0946-8.

"Updates the consumer information on the physical and mental benefits of physical activity throughout the lifespan offered in earlier editions... Recommended. All readers; all levels."
—CHOICE, Oct '07

"An exceptionally well-rounded coverage perfect for any concerned about developing and understanding a fitness program."
—California Bookwatch, Jun '07

SEE ALSO Sports Injuries Sourcebook, 3rd Edition

Food Safety Sourcebook

Basic Consumer Health Information about the Safe Handling of Meat, Poultry, Seafood, Eggs, Fruit Juices, and Other Food Items, and Facts about Pesticides, Drinking Water, Food Safety Overseas, and the Onset, Duration, and Symptoms of Foodborne Illnesses, Including Types of Pathogenic Bacteria, Parasitic Protozoa, Worms, Viruses, and Natural Toxins

Along with the Role of the Consumer, the Food Handler, and the Government in Food Safety, a Glossary, and Resources for Additional Help and Information

Edited by Dawn D. Matthews. 327 pages. 1999. 978-0-7808-0326-8.

"Recommended reference source."
—Booklist, May '00

"This book takes the complex issues of food safety and foodborne pathogens and presents them in an easily understood manner. [It does] an excellent job of covering a large and often confusing topic."
— American Reference Books Annual, 2000

Forensic Medicine Sourcebook

Basic Consumer Information for the Layperson about Forensic Medicine, Including Crime Scene Investigation, Evidence Collection and Analysis, Expert Testimony, Computer-Aided Criminal Identification, Digital Imaging in the Courtroom, DNA Profiling, Accident Reconstruction, Autopsies, Ballistics, Drugs and Explosives Detection, Latent Fingerprints, Product Tampering, and Questioned Document Examination

Along with Statistical Data, a Glossary of Forensics Terminology, and Listings of Sources for Further Help and Information

Edited by Annemarie S. Muth. 574 pages. 1999. 978-0-7808-0232-2.

"Given the expected widespread interest in its content and its easy to read style, this book is recommended for most public and all college and university libraries."
—E-Streams, Feb '01

"A wealth of information, useful statistics, references are up-to-date and extremely complete. This wonderful collection of data will help students who are interested in a career in any type of forensic field. It is a great resource for attorneys who need information about types of expert witnesses needed in a particular case. It also offers useful information for fiction and nonfiction writers whose work involves a crime. A fascinating compilation. All levels."
—CHOICE, Jan '00

"There are several items that make this book attractive to consumers who are seeking certain forensic data... This is a useful current source for those seeking general forensic medical answers."
—American Reference Books Annual, 2000

Gastrointestinal Diseases and Disorders Sourcebook, 2nd Edition

Basic Consumer Health Information about the Upper and Lower Gastrointestinal (GI) Tract, Including the Esophagus, Stomach, Intestines, Rectum, Liver, and Pancreas, with Facts about Gastroesophageal Reflux Disease, Gastritis, Hernias, Ulcers, Celiac Disease, Diverticulitis, Irritable Bowel Syndrome, Hemorrhoids, Gastrointestinal Cancers, and Other Diseases and Disorders Related to the Digestive Process

Along with Information about Commonly Used Diagnostic and Surgical Procedures, Statistics, Reports on Current Research Initiatives and Clinical Trials, a Glossary, and Resources for Additional Help and Information

Edited by Sandra J. Judd. 654 pages. 2006. 978-0-7808-0798-3.

"The text is designed for the general reader seeking information on prevention, disease warning signs, diagnostic and therapeutic questions... It is an excellent resource for the general reader to conveniently locate credible, coordinated and indexed information... The sourcebook will prove very helpful for patients, caregivers and should be available in every physician waiting room."

—*Doody's Review Service, 2006*

SEE ALSO *Diet and Nutrition Sourcebook, 3rd Edition, Digestive Diseases and Disorders Sourcebook*

Genetic Disorders Sourcebook, 4th Edition

Basic Consumer Health Information about Hereditary Diseases and Disorders, Including Facts about the Human Genome, Genetic Inheritance Patterns, Disorders Associated with Specific Genes, Such as Sickle Cell Disease, Hemophilia, and Cystic Fibrosis, Chromosome Disorders, Such as Down Syndrome, Fragile X Syndrome, and Turner Syndrome, and Complex Diseases and Disorders Resulting from the Interaction of Environmental and Genetic Factors, Such as Allergies, Cancer, and Obesity

Along with Facts about Genetic Testing, Suggestions for Parents of Children with Special Needs, Reports on Current Research Initiatives, a Glossary of Genetic Terminology, and Resources for Additional Help and Information

Edited by Sandra J. Judd. 600 pages. 2010. 978-0-7808-1076-1.

Head Trauma Sourcebook

Basic Information for the Layperson about Open-Head and Closed-Head Injuries, Treatment Advances, Recovery, and Rehabilitation

Along with Reports on Current Research Initiatives

Edited by Karen Bellenir. 414 pages. 1997. 978-0-7808-0208-7.

Headache Sourcebook

Basic Consumer Health Information about Migraine, Tension, Cluster, Rebound and Other Types of Headaches, with Facts about the Cause and Prevention of Headaches, the Effects of Stress and the Environment, Headaches during Pregnancy and Menopause, and Childhood Headaches

Along with a Glossary and Other Resources for Additional Help and Information

Edited by Dawn D. Matthews. 342 pages. 2002. 978-0-7808-0337-4.

"Highly recommended for academic and medical reference collections."

—*Library Bookwatch, Sep '02*

SEE ALSO *Pain Sourcebook, 3rd Edition*

Healthy Aging Sourcebook

Basic Consumer Health Information about Maintaining Health through the Aging Process, Including Advice on Nutrition, Exercise, and Sleep, Help in Making Decisions about Midlife Issues and Retirement, and Guidance Concerning Practical and Informed Choices in Health Consumerism

Along with Data Concerning the Theories of Aging, Different Experiences in Aging by Minority Groups, and Facts about Aging Now and Aging in the Future; and Featuring a Glossary, a Guide to Consumer Help, Additional Suggested Reading, and Practical Resource Directory

Edited by Jenifer Swanson. 537 pages. 1999. 978-0-7808-0390-9.

"Recommended reference source."

—*Booklist, Feb '00*

SEE ALSO *Adult Health Sourcebook, Physical and Mental Issues in Aging Sourcebook*

Healthy Children Sourcebook

Basic Consumer Health Information about the Physical and Mental Development of Children between the Ages of 3 and 12, Including Routine Health Care, Preventative Health Services, Safety and First Aid, Healthy Sleep, Dental Care, Nutrition, and Fitness, and Featuring Parenting Tips on Such Topics as Bedwetting, Choosing Day Care, Monitoring TV and Other Media, and Establishing a Foundation for Substance Abuse Prevention

Along with a Glossary of Commonly Used Pediatric Terms and Resources for Additional Help and Information.

Edited by Chad T. Kimball. 624 pages. 2003. 978-0-7808-0247-6.

"Should be required reading for parents and teachers."
—*E-Streams, Jun '04*

"It is hard to imagine that any other single resource exists that would provide such a comprehensive guide of timely information on health promotion and disease prevention for children aged 3 to 12."
—*American Reference Books Annual, 2004*

"This easy-to-read volume is a tremendous resource."
—*AORN Journal, May '05*

SEE ALSO *Childhood Diseases and Disorders Sourcebook, 2nd Edition*

Healthy Heart Sourcebook for Women

Basic Consumer Health Information about Cardiac Issues Specific to Women, Including Facts about Major Risk Factors and Prevention, Treatment and Control Strategies, and Important Dietary Issues

Along with a Special Section Regarding the Pros and Cons of Hormone Replacement Therapy and Its Impact on Heart Health, and Additional Help, Including Recipes, a Glossary, and a Directory of Resources

Edited by Dawn D. Matthews. 321 pages. 2000. 978-0-7808-0329-9.

"A good reference source and recommended for all public, academic, medical, and hospital libraries."
—*Medical Reference Services Quarterly, Summer '01*

"Contains very important information about coronary artery disease that all women should know. The information is current and presented in an easy-to-read format. The book will make a good addition to any library."
—*American Medical Writers Association Journal, Summer '00*

SEE ALSO *Cardiovascular Diseases and Disorders Sourcebook, 4th Edition, Women's Health Concerns Sourcebook, 3rd Edition*

Hepatitis Sourcebook

Basic Consumer Health Information about Hepatitis A, Hepatitis B, Hepatitis C, and Other Forms of Hepatitis, Including Autoimmune Hepatitis, Alcoholic Hepatitis, Nonalcoholic Steatohepatitis, and Toxic Hepatitis, with Facts about Risk Factors, Screening Methods, Diagnostic Tests, and Treatment Options

Along with Information on Liver Health, Tips for People Living with Chronic Hepatitis, Reports on Current Research Initiatives, a Glossary of Terms Related to Hepatitis, and a Directory of Sources for Further Help and Information

Edited by Sandra J. Judd. 570 pages. 2006. 978-0-7808-0749-5.

"The breadth of information found in this one book would not be readily found in another source. Highly recommended."
—*American Reference Books Annual, 2006*

SEE ALSO *Contagious Diseases Sourcebook, 2nd Edition*

Household Safety Sourcebook

Basic Consumer Health Information about Household Safety, Including Information about Poisons, Chemicals, Fire, and Water Hazards in the Home

Along with Advice about the Safe Use of Home Maintenance Equipment, Choosing Toys and Nursery Furniture, Holiday and Recreation Safety, a Glossary, and Resources for Further Help and Information

Edited by Dawn D. Matthews. 587 pages. 2002. 978-0-7808-0338-1.

"As a sourcebook on household safety this book meets its mark. It is encyclopedic in scope and covers a wide range of safety issues that are commonly seen in the home."
—*E-Streams, Jul '02*

Hypertension Sourcebook

Basic Consumer Health Information about the Causes, Diagnosis, and Treatment of High Blood Pressure, with Facts about Consequences, Complications, and Co-Occurring Disorders, Such as Coronary Heart Disease, Diabetes, Stroke, Kidney Disease, and Hypertensive Retinopathy, and Issues in Blood Pressure

Control, Including Dietary Choices, Stress Management, and Medications

Along with Reports on Current Research Initiatives and Clinical Trials, a Glossary, and Resources for Additional Help and Information

Edited by Dawn D. Matthews and Karen Bellenir. 588 pages. 2004. 978-0-7808-0674-0.

"Academic, public, and medical libraries will want to add the Hypertension Sourcebook to their collections."
—E-Streams, Aug '05

"The strength of this source is the wide range of information given about hypertension."
—American Reference Books Annual, 2005

SEE ALSO Stroke Sourcebook, 2nd Edition

Immune System Disorders Sourcebook, 2nd Edition

Basic Consumer Health Information about Disorders of the Immune System, Including Immune System Function and Response, Diagnosis of Immune Disorders, Information about Inherited Immune Disease, Acquired Immune Disease, and Autoimmune Diseases, Including Primary Immune Deficiency, Acquired Immunodeficiency Syndrome (AIDS), Lupus, Multiple Sclerosis, Type 1 Diabetes, Rheumatoid Arthritis, and Graves' Disease

Along with Treatments, Tips for Coping with Immune Disorders, a Glossary, and a Directory of Additional Resources

Edited by Joyce Brennfleck Shannon. 643 pages. 2005. 978-0-7808-0748-8.

"Highly recommended for academic and public libraries."
—American Reference Books Annual, 2006

"The updated second edition is a 'must' for any consumer health library seeking a solid resource covering the treatments, symptoms, and options for immune disorder sufferers... An excellent guide."
—MBR Bookwatch, Jan '06

SEE ALSO AIDS Sourcebook, 4th Edition, Arthritis Sourcebook, 3rd Edition

Infant and Toddler Health Sourcebook

Basic Consumer Health Information about the Physical and Mental Development of Newborns, Infants, and Toddlers, Including Neonatal Concerns, Nutrition Recommendations, Immunization Schedules, Common Pediatric Disorders, Assessments and Milestones, Safety Tips, and Advice for Parents and Other Caregivers

Along with a Glossary of Terms and Resource Listings for Additional Help

Edited by Jenifer Swanson. 570 pages. 2000. 978-0-7808-0246-9.

"As a reference for the general public, this would be useful in any library."
—E-Streams, May '01

"Recommended reference source."
—Booklist, Feb '01

Infectious Diseases Sourcebook

Basic Consumer Health Information about Non-Contagious Bacterial, Viral, Prion, Fungal, and Parasitic Diseases Spread by Food and Water, Insects and Animals, or Environmental Contact, Including Botulism, E. Coli, Encephalitis, Legionnaires' Disease, Lyme Disease, Malaria, Plague, Rabies, Salmonella, Tetanus, and Others, and Facts about Newly Emerging Diseases, Such as Hantavirus, Mad Cow Disease, Monkeypox, and West Nile Virus

Along with Information about Preventing Disease Transmission, the Threat of Bioterrorism, and Current Research Initiatives, with a Glossary and Directory of Resources for More Information

Edited by Karen Bellenir. 610 pages. 2004. 978-0-7808-0675-7.

"This reference continues the excellent tradition of the Health Reference Series in consolidating a wealth of information on a selected topic into a format that is easy to use and accessible to the general public."
—American Reference Books Annual, 2005

"Recommended for public and academic libraries."
—E-Streams, Jan '05

SEE ALSO Environmental Health Sourcebook, 3rd Edition

Injury and Trauma Sourcebook

Basic Consumer Health Information about the Impact of Injury, the Diagnosis and Treatment of Common and Traumatic Injuries, Emergency Care, and Specific Injuries Related to Home, Community, Workplace, Transportation, and Recreation

Along with Guidelines for Injury Prevention, a Glossary, and a Directory of Additional Resources

Edited by Joyce Brennfleck Shannon. 675 pages. 2002. 978-0-7808-0421-0.

"Practitioners should be aware of guides such as this in order to facilitate their use by patients and their families."
—*Doody's Health Sciences Book Review Journal, Sep-Oct '02*

"Recommended reference source."
—*Booklist, Sep '02*

"Highly recommended for academic and medical reference collections."
—*Library Bookwatch, Sep '02*

SEE ALSO Emergency Medical Services Sourcebook, Sports Injuries Sourcebook, 3rd Edition

Learning Disabilities Sourcebook, 3rd Edition

Basic Consumer Health Information about Dyslexia, Auditory and Visual Processing Disorders, Communication Disorders, Dyscalculia, Dysgraphia, and Other Conditions That Impede Learning, Including Attention Deficit/Hyperactivity Disorder, Autism Spectrum Disorders, Hearing and Visual Impairments, Chromosome-Based Disorders, and Brain Injury

Along with Facts about Brain Function, Assessment, Therapy and Remediation, Accommodations, Assistive Technology, Legal Protections, and Tips about Family Life, School Transitions, and Employment Strategies, a Glossary of Related Terms, and Directories of Additional Resources

Edited by Joyce Brennfleck Shannon. 613 pages. 2009. 978-0-7808-1039-6.

"Intended to be a starting point for people who need to know about learning disabilities. Each chapter on a specific disability includes readable,

well-organized descriptions... The book is well indexed and a glossary is included. Chapters on organizations and helpful websites will aid the reader who needs more information."
—*American Reference Books Annual, 2009*

"This book provides the necessary information to better understand learning disabilities and work with children who have them... It would be difficult to find another book that so comprehensively explains learning disabilities without becoming incomprehensible to the average parent who needs this information."
—*Doody's Review Service, 2009*

SEE ALSO Attention Deficit Disorder Sourcebook, Autism and Pervasive Developmental Disorders Sourcebook

Leukemia Sourcebook

Basic Consumer Health Information about Adult and Childhood Leukemias, Including Acute Lymphocytic Leukemia (ALL), Chronic Lymphocytic Leukemia (CLL), Acute Myelogenous Leukemia (AML), Chronic Myelogenous Leukemia (CML), and Hairy Cell Leukemia, and Treatments Such as Chemotherapy, Radiation Therapy, Peripheral Blood Stem Cell and Marrow Transplantation, and Immunotherapy

Along with Tips for Life During and After Treatment, a Glossary, and Directories of Additional Resources

Edited by Joyce Brennfleck Shannon. 564 pages. 2003. 978-0-7808-0627-6.

"Unlike other medical books for the layperson... the language does not talk down to the reader... This volume is highly recommended for all libraries."
—*American Reference Books Annual, 2004*

"A fine title which ranges from diagnosis to alternative treatments, staging, and tips for life during and after diagnosis."
—*The Bookwatch, Dec '03*

SEE ALSO Blood & Circulatory Disorders Sourcebook, 3rd Edition, Cancer Sourcebook, 5th Edition

Liver Disorders Sourcebook

Basic Consumer Health Information about the Liver and How It Works; Liver Diseases, Including Cancer, Cirrhosis, Hepatitis, and

Toxic and Drug Related Diseases; Tips for Maintaining a Healthy Liver; Laboratory Tests, Radiology Tests, and Facts about Liver Transplantation

Along with a Section on Support Groups, a Glossary, and Resource Listings

Edited by Joyce Brennfleck Shannon. 580 pages. 2000. 978-0-7808-0383-1.

"This title is recommended for health sciences and public libraries with consumer health collections."
— E-Streams, Oct '00

"Recommended reference source."
— Booklist, Jun '00

SEE ALSO Gastrointestinal Diseases and Disorders Sourcebook, 2nd Edition, Hepatitis Sourcebook

Lung Disorders Sourcebook

Basic Consumer Health Information about Emphysema, Pneumonia, Tuberculosis, Asthma, Cystic Fibrosis, and Other Lung Disorders, Including Facts about Diagnostic Procedures, Treatment Strategies, Disease Prevention Efforts, and Such Risk Factors as Smoking, Air Pollution, and Exposure to Asbestos, Radon, and Other Agents

Along with a Glossary and Resources for Additional Help and Information

Edited by Dawn D. Matthews. 657 pages. 2002. 978-0-7808-0339-8.

"Highly recommended for academic and medical reference collections."
— Library Bookwatch, Sep '02

SEE ALSO Asthma Sourcebook, 2nd Edition, Respiratory Disorders Sourcebook, 2nd Edition

Medical Tests Sourcebook, 3rd Edition

Basic Consumer Health Information about X-Rays, Blood Tests, Stool and Urine Tests, Biopsies, Mammography, Endoscopic Procedures, Ultrasound Exams, Computed Tomography, Magnetic Resonance Imaging (MRI), Nuclear Medicine, Genetic Testing, Home-Use Tests, and More

Along with Facts about Preventive Care and Screening Test Guidelines, Screening and

Assessment Tests Associated with Such Specific Concerns as Cancer, Heart Disease, Allergies, Diabetes, Thyroid Disfunction, and Infertility, a Glossary of Related Terms, and a Directory of Resources for Additional Help and Information

Edited by Karen Bellenir. 627 pages. 2008. 978-0-7808-1040-2

"This volume has a wide scope that makes it useful... Can be a valuable reference guide."
— American Reference Books Annual, 2009

"Would be a valuable contribution to any consumer health or public library."
— Doody's Book Review Service, 2009

Men's Health Concerns Sourcebook, 3rd Edition

Basic Consumer Health Information about Wellness in Men and Gender-Related Differences in Health, With Facts about Heart Disease, Cancer, Traumatic Injury, and Other Leading Causes of Death in Men, Reproductive Concerns, Sexual Dysfunction, Disorders of the Prostate, Penis, and Testes, Sex-Linked Genetic Disorders, and Other Medical and Mental Concerns of Men

Along with Statistical Data, a Glossary of Related Terms, and a Directory of Resources for Additional Information

Edited by Sandra J. Judd. 632 pages. 2009. 978-0-7808-1033-4.

"A good addition to any reference shelf in academic, consumer health, or hospital libraries."
— ARBAOnline, Oct '09

SEE ALSO Prostate and Urological Disorders Sourcebook

Mental Health Disorders Sourcebook, 4th Edition

Basic Consumer Health Information about the Causes and Symptoms of Mental Health Problems, Including Depression, Bipolar Disorder, Anxiety Disorders, Posttraumatic Stress Disorder, Obsessive-Compulsive Disorder, Eating Disorders, Addictions, and Personality and Psychotic Disorders

Along with Information about Medications and Treatments, Mental Health Concerns in

Children, Adolescents, and Adults, Tips on Living with Mental Health Disorders, a Glossary of Related Terms, and a Directory of Resources for Additional Help and Information

Edited by Amy L. Sutton. 680 pages. 2009. 978-0-7808-1041-9.

"Mental health concerns are presented in everyday language and intended for patients and their families as well as the general public... This resource is comprehensive and up to date... The easy-to-understand writing style helps to facilitate assimilation of needed facts and specifics on often challenging topics."
—*ARBAOnline, Oct '09*

"No health collection should be without this resource, which will reach into many a general lending library as well."
—*Internet Bookwatch, Oct '09*

SEE ALSO Depression Sourcebook, 2nd Edition, Stress-Related Disorders Sourcebook, 2nd Edition

Mental Retardation Sourcebook

Basic Consumer Health Information about Mental Retardation and Its Causes, Including Down Syndrome, Fetal Alcohol Syndrome, Fragile X Syndrome, Genetic Conditions, Injury, and Environmental Sources

Along with Preventive Strategies, Parenting Issues, Educational Implications, Health Care Needs, Employment and Economic Matters, Legal Issues, a Glossary, and a Resource Listing for Additional Help and Information

Edited by Joyce Brennfleck Shannon. 627 pages. 2000. 978-0-7808-0377-0.

"Public libraries will find the book useful for reference and as a beginning research point for students, parents, and caregivers."
—*American Reference Books Annual, 2001*

"The strength of this work is that it compiles many basic fact sheets and addresses for further information in one volume. It is intended and suitable for the general public."
—*E-Streams, Nov '00*

"An invaluable overview."
—*Reviewer's Bookwatch, Jul '00*

Movement Disorders Sourcebook, 2nd Edition

Basic Consumer Health Information about the Symptoms and Causes of Movement Disorders, Including Parkinson Disease, Amyotrophic Lateral Sclerosis, Cerebral Palsy, Muscular Dystrophy, Multiple Sclerosis, Myasthenia, Myoclonus, Spina Bifida, Dystonia, Essential Tremor, Choreatic Disorders, Huntington Disease, Tourette Syndrome, and Other Disorders That Cause Slowed, Absent, or Excessive Movements

Along with Information about Surgical and Nonsurgical Interventions, Physical Therapies, Strategies for Independent Living, a Glossary of Related Terms, and a Directory of Resources for Additional Help and Information

Edited by Amy L. Sutton. 618 pages. 2009. 978-0-7808-1034-1.

"The second updated edition of Movement Disorders Sourcebook is a winner, providing the latest research and health findings on all kinds of movement disorders in children and adults... a top pick for any health or general lending library's health reference collection."
—*California Bookwatch, Aug '09*

SEE ALSO Muscular Dystrophy Sourcebook

Multiple Sclerosis Sourcebook

Basic Consumer Health Information about Multiple Sclerosis (MS) and Its Effects on Mobility, Vision, Bladder Function, Speech, Swallowing, and Cognition, Including Facts about Risk Factors, Causes, Diagnostic Procedures, Pain Management, Drug Treatments, and Physical and Occupational Therapies

Along with Guidelines for Nutrition and Exercise, Tips on Choosing Assistive Equipment, Information about Disability, Work, Financial, and Legal Issues, a Glossary of Related Terms, and a Directory of Additional Resources

Edited by Joyce Brennfleck Shannon. 553 pages. 2007. 978-0-7808-0998-7.

Muscular Dystrophy Sourcebook

Basic Consumer Health Information about Congenital, Childhood-Onset, and Adult-Onset

603

Forms of Muscular Dystrophy, Such as Duchenne, Becker, Emery-Dreifuss, Distal, Limb-Girdle, Facioscapulohumeral (FSHD), Myotonic, and Ophthalmoplegic Muscular Dystrophies, Including Facts about Diagnostic Tests, Medical and Physical Therapies, Management of Co-Occurring Conditions, and Parenting Guidelines

Along with Practical Tips for Home Care, a Glossary, and Directories of Additional Resources

Edited by Joyce Brennfleck Shannon. 552 pages. 2004. 978-0-7808-0676-4.

"This book is highly recommended for public and academic libraries as well as health care offices that support the information needs of patients and their families."
—E-Streams, Apr '05

"Excellent reference."
—The Bookwatch, Jan '05

SEE ALSO Movement Disorders Sourcebook, 2nd Edition

Obesity Sourcebook
Basic Consumer Health Information about Diseases and Other Problems Associated with Obesity, and Including Facts about Risk Factors, Prevention Issues, and Management Approaches

Along with Statistical and Demographic Data, Information about Special Populations, Research Updates, a Glossary, and Source Listings for Further Help and Information

Edited by Wilma Caldwell and Chad T. Kimball. 360 pages. 2001. 978-0-7808-0333-6.

"The book synthesizes the reliable medical literature on obesity into one easy-to-read and useful resource for the general public."
—American Reference Books Annual, 2002

"Well suited for the health reference collection of a public library or an academic health science library that serves the general population."
—E-Streams, Sep '01

Osteoporosis Sourcebook
Basic Consumer Health Information about Primary and Secondary Osteoporosis and Juvenile Osteoporosis and Related Conditions, Including Fibrous Dysplasia, Gaucher Disease, Hyperthyroidism, Hypophosphatasia,

Myeloma, Osteopetrosis, Osteogenesis Imperfecta, and Paget's Disease

Along with Information about Risk Factors, Treatments, Traditional and Non-Traditional Pain Management, a Glossary of Related Terms, and a Directory of Resources

Edited by Allan R. Cook. 568 pages. 2001. 978-0-7808-0239-1.

"This resource is recommended as a great reference source for public, health, and academic libraries, and is another triumph for the editors of Omnigraphics."
—American Reference Books Annual, 2002

"Will prove valuable to any library seeking to maintain a current, comprehensive reference collection of health resources... From prevention to treatment and associated conditions, this provides an excellent survey."
—The Bookwatch, Aug '01

SEE ALSO Healthy Aging Sourcebook, Women's Health Concerns Sourcebook, 3rd Edition

---

Pain Sourcebook, 3rd Edition
Basic Consumer Health Information about Acute and Chronic Pain, Including Nerve Pain, Bone Pain, Muscle Pain, Cancer Pain, and Disorders Characterized by Pain, Such as Arthritis, Temporomandibular Muscle and Joint (TMJ) Disorder, Carpal Tunnel Syndrome, Headaches, Heartburn, Sciatica, and Shingles, and Facts about Diagnostic Tests and Treatment Options for Pain, Including Over-the-Counter and Prescription Drugs, Physical Rehabilitation, Injection and Infusion Therapies, Implantable Technologies, and Complementary Medicine

Along with Tips for Living with Pain, a Glossary of Related Terms, and a Directory of Additional Resources

Edited by Joyce Brennfleck Shannon. 644 pages. 2008. 978-0-7808-1006-8.

"Excellent for ready-reference users and can be used for beginning students in health fields... appropriate for the consumer health collection in both public and academic libraries."
—American Reference Books Annual, 2009

SEE ALSO Arthritis Sourcebook, 3rd Edition; Back and Neck Sourcebook, 2nd Edition;

Headache Sourcebook; Sports Injuries Sourcebook, 3rd Edition

Pediatric Cancer Sourcebook

Basic Consumer Health Information about Leukemias, Brain Tumors, Sarcomas, Lymphomas, and Other Cancers in Infants, Children, and Adolescents, Including Descriptions of Cancers, Treatments, and Coping Strategies

Along with Suggestions for Parents, Caregivers, and Concerned Relatives, a Glossary of Cancer Terms, and Resource Listings

Edited by Edward J. Prucha. 575 pages. 1999. 978-0-7808-0245-2.

"An excellent source of information. Recommended for public, hospital, and health science libraries with consumer health collections."
—E-Streams, Jun '00

"A valuable addition to all libraries specializing in health services and many public libraries."
—American Reference Books Annual, 2000

SEE ALSO *Childhood Diseases and Disorders Sourcebook, 2nd Edition, Healthy Children Sourcebook*

Physical and Mental Issues in Aging Sourcebook

Basic Consumer Health Information on Physical and Mental Disorders Associated with the Aging Process, Including Concerns about Cardiovascular Disease, Pulmonary Disease, Oral Health, Digestive Disorders, Musculoskeletal and Skin Disorders, Metabolic Changes, Sexual and Reproductive Issues, and Changes in Vision, Hearing, and Other Senses

Along with Data about Longevity and Causes of Death, Information on Acute and Chronic Pain, Descriptions of Mental Concerns, a Glossary of Terms, and Resource Listings for Additional Help

Edited by Jenifer Swanson. 660 pages. 1999. 978-0-7808-0233-9.

"This is a treasure of health information for the layperson."
—CHOICE Health Sciences Supplement, May '00

"Recommended for public libraries."
—American Reference Books Annual, 2000

SEE ALSO *Healthy Aging Sourcebook*

Podiatry Sourcebook, 2nd Edition

Basic Consumer Health Information about Disorders, Diseases, and Deformities that Affect the Foot and Ankle, Including Sprains, Corns, Calluses, Bunions, Plantar Warts, Plantar Fasciitis, Neuromas, Clubfoot, Flat Feet, Achilles Tendonitis, and Much More

Along with Information about Selecting a Foot Care Specialist, Foot Fitness, Shoes and Socks, Diagnostic Tests and Corrective Procedures, Financial Assistance for Corrective Devices, a Glossary of Related Terms, and a Directory of Resources for Additional Help and Information

Edited by Ivy L. Alexander. 516 pages. 2007. 978-0-7808-0944-4.

"An excellent resource... Although there have been various types of 'foot books' published in the past, none are as comprehensive as this one. 5 Stars (out of 5)!"
—Doody's Review Service, 2007

"Perfect for both health libraries and general-interest lending collections."
—Internet Bookwatch, Jul '07

Pregnancy and Birth Sourcebook, 3rd Edition

Basic Consumer Health Information about Pregnancy and Fetal Development, Including Facts about Fertility and Conception, Physical and Emotional Changes during Pregnancy, Prenatal Care and Diagnostic Tests, High-Risk Pregnancies and Complications, Labor, Delivery, and the Postpartum Period

Along with Tips on Maintaining Health and Wellness during Pregnancy and Caring for Newborn Infants, a Glossary of Related Terms, and Directories of Resources for Additional Help and Information

Edited by Amy L. Sutton. 645 pages. 2009. 978-0-7808-1074-7.

SEE ALSO *Breastfeeding Sourcebook, Congenital Disorders Sourcebook, 2nd Edition, Family Planning Sourcebook, Women's Health Concerns Sourcebook, 3rd Edition*

Prostate and Urological Disorders Sourcebook

Basic Consumer Health Information about Urogenital and Sexual Disorders in Men, Including Prostate and Other Andrological Cancers, Prostatitis, Benign Prostatic Hyperplasia, Testicular and Penile Trauma, Cryptorchidism, Peyronie Disease, Erectile Dysfunction, and Male Factor Infertility, and Facts about Commonly Used Tests and Procedures, Such as Prostatectomy, Vasectomy, Vasectomy Reversal, Penile Implants, and Semen Analysis

Along with a Glossary of Andrological Terms and a Directory of Resources for Additional Information

Edited by Karen Bellenir. 604 pages. 2006. 978-0-7808-0797-6.

"Certain to be a popular pick among library reference holdings... No prior knowledge is assumed for any of the conditions or terms herein, making it a most accessible general-interest reference."
—California Bookwatch, Apr '06

SEE ALSO *Men's Health Concerns Sourcebook, 3rd Edition, Urinary Tract and Kidney Diseases and Disorders Sourcebook, 2nd Edition*

Prostate Cancer Sourcebook

Basic Consumer Health Information about Prostate Cancer, Including Information about the Associated Risk Factors, Detection, Diagnosis, and Treatment of Prostate Cancer

Along with Information on Non-Malignant Prostate Conditions, and Featuring a Section Listing Support and Treatment Centers and a Glossary of Related Terms

Edited by Dawn D. Matthews. 340 pages. 2001. 978-0-7808-0324-4.

"Recommended reference source."
—Booklist, Jan '02

"A valuable resource for health care consumers seeking information on the subject... All text is written in a clear, easy-to-understand language that avoids technical jargon. Any library that collects consumer health resources would strengthen their collection with the addition of the Prostate Cancer Sourcebook."
—American Reference Books Annual, 2002

SEE ALSO *Cancer Sourcebook, 5th Edition, Men's Health Concerns Sourcebook, 3rd Edition*

Rehabilitation Sourcebook

Basic Consumer Health Information about Rehabilitation for People Recovering from Heart Surgery, Spinal Cord Injury, Stroke, Orthopedic Impairments, Amputation, Pulmonary Impairments, Traumatic Injury, and More, Including Physical Therapy, Occupational Therapy, Speech/Language Therapy, Massage Therapy, Dance Therapy, Art Therapy, and Recreational Therapy

Along with Information on Assistive and Adaptive Devices, a Glossary, and Resources for Additional Help and Information

Edited by Dawn D. Matthews. 519 pages. 2000. 978-0-7808-0236-0.

"This is an excellent resource for public library reference and health collections."
—American Reference Books Annual, 2001

"Recommended reference source."
—Booklist, May '00

Respiratory Disorders Sourcebook, 2nd Edition

Basic Consumer Health Information about Infectious, Inflammatory, and Chronic Conditions Affecting the Lungs and Respiratory System, Including Pneumonia, Bronchitis, Influenza, Tuberculosis, Sarcoidosis, Asthma, Cystic Fibrosis, Chronic Obstructive Pulmonary Disease, Lung Abscesses, Pulmonary Embolism, Occupational Lung Diseases, and Other Bacterial, Viral, and Fungal Infections

Along with Facts about the Structure and Function of the Lungs and Airways, Methods of Diagnosing Respiratory Disorders, and Treatment and Rehabilitation Options, a Glossary of Related Terms, and a Directory of Resources for Additional Help and Information

Edited by Sandra L. Judd. 638 pages. 2008. 978-0-7808-1007-5.

"An excellent book for patients, their families, or for those who are just curious about respiratory disease. Public libraries and physician offices would find this a valuable resource as well. 4 Stars! (out of 5)"
—Doody's Review Service, 2009

"A great addition for public and school libraries because it provides concise health information... readers can start with this reference source and get satisfactory answers before proceeding to other medical reference tools for

more in depth information... A good guide for health education on lung disorders."
—*American Reference Books Annual, 2009*

SEE ALSO *Asthma Sourcebook, 2nd Edition, Lung Disorders Sourcebook*

Sexually Transmitted Diseases Sourcebook, 4th Edition

Basic Consumer Health Information about Chlamydial Infections, Gonorrhea, Hepatitis, Herpes, HIV/AIDS, Human Papillomavirus, Pubic Lice, Scabies, Syphilis, Trichomoniasis, Vaginal Infections, and Other Sexually Transmitted Diseases, Including Facts about Risk Factors, Symptoms, Diagnosis, Treatment, and the Prevention of Sexually Transmitted Infections

Along with Updates on Current Research Initiatives, a Glossary of Related Terms, and Resources for Additional Help and Information

Edited by Laura Larsen. 623 pages. 2009. 978-0-7808-1073-0.

"Extremely beneficial... The question-and-answer format along with the index and table of contents make this well-organized resource extremely easy to reference, read, and comprehend... an invaluable medical reference source for lay readers, and a highly appropriate addition for public library collections, health clinics, and any library with a consumer health collection"
—*ARBAOnline, Oct '09*

SEE ALSO *AIDS Sourcebook, 4th Edition, Contagious Diseases Sourcebook, 2nd Edition, Men's Health Concerns Sourcebook, 3rd Edition, Women's Health Concerns Sourcebook, 3rd Edition*

Sleep Disorders Sourcebook, 3rd Edition

Basic Consumer Health Information about Sleep Disorders, Including Insomnia, Sleep Apnea and Snoring, Jet Lag and Other Circadian Rhythm Disorders, Narcolepsy, and Parasomnias, Such as Sleep Walking and Sleep Talking, and Featuring Facts about Other Health Problems that Affect Sleep, Why Sleep Is Necessary, How Much Sleep Is Needed, the Physical and Mental Effects of Sleep Deprivation, and Pediatric Sleep Issues

Along with Tips for Diagnosing and Treating Sleep Disorders, a Glossary of Related Terms, and a List of Resources for Additional Help and Information

Edited by Sandra J. Judd. 600 pages. 2010. 978-0-7808-1084-6.

Smoking Concerns Sourcebook

Basic Consumer Health Information about Nicotine Addiction and Smoking Cessation, Featuring Facts about the Health Effects of Tobacco Use, Including Lung and Other Cancers, Heart Disease, Stroke, and Respiratory Disorders, Such as Emphysema and Chronic Bronchitis

Along with Information about Smoking Prevention Programs, Suggestions for Achieving and Maintaining a Smoke-Free Lifestyle, Statistics about Tobacco Use, Reports on Current Research Initiatives, a Glossary of Related Terms, and Directories of Resources for Additional Help and Information

Edited by Karen Bellenir. 595 pages. 2004. 978-0-7808-0323-7.

"Provides everything needed for the student or general reader seeking practical details on the effects of tobacco use."
—*The Bookwatch, Mar '05*

"Public libraries and consumer health care libraries will find this work useful."
—*American Reference Books Annual, 2005*

SEE ALSO *Respiratory Disorders Sourcebook, 2nd Edition*

Sports Injuries Sourcebook, 3rd Edition

Basic Consumer Health Information about Sprains and Strains, Fractures, Growth Plate Injuries, Overtraining Injuries, and Injuries to the Head, Face, Shoulders, Elbows, Hands, Spinal Column, Knees, Ankles, and Feet, and with Facts about Heat-Related Illness, Steroids and Sport Supplements, Protective Equipment, Diagnostic Procedures, Treatment Options, and Rehabilitation

Along with a Glossary of Related Terms and a Directory of Resources for Additional Help and Information

Edited by Sandra J. Judd. 623 pages. 2007. 978-0-7808-0949-9.

SEE ALSO *Fitness and Exercise Sourcebook, 3rd Edition, Podiatry Sourcebook, 2nd Edition*

Stress-Related Disorders Sourcebook, 2nd Edition

Basic Consumer Health Information about Stress and Stress-Related Disorders, Including Types of Stress, Sources of Acute and Chronic Stress, the Impact of Stress on the Body's Systems, and Mental and Emotional Health Problems Associated with Stress, Such as Depression, Anxiety Disorders, Substance Abuse, Posttraumatic Stress Disorder, and Suicide

Along with Advice about Getting Help for Stress-Related Disorders, Information about Stress Management Techniques, a Glossary of Stress-Related Terms, and a Directory of Resources for Additional Help and Information

Edited by Amy L. Sutton. 608 pages. 2007. 978-0-7808-0996-3.

"Accessible to the lay reader. Highly recommended for medical and psychiatric collections."
—*Library Journal, Mar '08*

"Well-written for a general readership, the 2nd Edition of Stress-Related Disorders Sourcebook is a useful addition to the health reference literature."
—*American Reference Books Annual, 2008*

SEE ALSO *Mental Health Disorders Sourcebook, 4th Edition*

Stroke Sourcebook, 2nd Edition

Basic Consumer Health Information about Stroke, Including Ischemic, Hemorrhagic, and Mini Strokes, as Well as Risk Factors, Prevention Guidelines, Diagnostic Tests, Medications and Surgical Treatments, and Complications of Stroke

Along with Rehabilitation Techniques and Innovations, Tips on Staying Healthy and Maintaining Independence after Stroke, a Glossary of Related Terms, and a Directory of Resources for Stroke Survivors and Their Families

Edited by Amy L. Sutton. 626 pages. 2008. 978-0-7808-1035-8.

"An encyclopedic handbook on stroke that is written in a language the layperson can understand... This is one of the most helpful, readable books on stroke. This volume is highly recommended and should be in every medical, hospital and public library; in addition, every family practitioner should have a copy in his or her office."
—*American Reference Books Annual, 2009*

SEE ALSO *Brain Disorders Sourcebook, 3rd Edition, Hypertension Sourcebook*

Surgery Sourcebook, 2nd Edition

Basic Consumer Health Information about Common Inpatient and Outpatient Surgeries, Including Critical Care and Trauma, Gastrointestinal, Gynecologic and Obstetric, Cardiac and Vascular, Neurologic, Ophthalmologic, Orthopedic, Reconstructive and Cosmetic, and Other Major and Minor Surgeries

Along with Information about Anesthesia and Pain Relief Options, Risks and Complications, Postoperative Recovery Concerns, and Innovative Surgical Techniques and Tools, a Glossary of Related Terms, and a Directory of Additional Resources

Edited by Amy L. Sutton. 645 pages. 2008. 978-0-7808-1004-4.

"Large public libraries and medical libraries would benefit from this material in their reference collections."
—*American Reference Books Annual, 2009*

SEE ALSO *Cosmetic and Reconstructive Surgery Sourcebook, 2nd Edition*

Thyroid Disorders Sourcebook

Basic Consumer Health Information about Disorders of the Thyroid and Parathyroid Glands, Including Hypothyroidism, Hyperthyroidism, Graves Disease, Hashimoto Thyroiditis, Thyroid Cancer, and Parathyroid Disorders, Featuring Facts about Symptoms, Risk Factors, Tests, and Treatments

Along with Information about the Effects of Thyroid Imbalance on Other Body Systems, Environmental Factors That Affect the Thyroid Gland, a Glossary, and a Directory of Additional Resources

Edited by Joyce Brennfleck Shannon. 573 pages. 2005. 978-0-7808-0745-7.

"Recommended for consumer health collections."
—*American Reference Books Annual, 2006*

"Highly recommended pick for Basic Consumer health reference holdings at all levels."
—*The Bookwatch, Aug '05*

SEE ALSO *Endocrine and Metabolic Disorders Sourcebook, 2nd Edition*

Transplantation Sourcebook

Basic Consumer Health Information about Organ and Tissue Transplantation, Including Physical and Financial Preparations, Procedures and Issues Relating to Specific Solid Organ and Tissue Transplants, Rehabilitation, Pediatric Transplant Information, the Future of Transplantation, and Organ and Tissue Donation

Along with a Glossary and Listings of Additional Resources

Edited by Joyce Brennfleck Shannon. 610 pages. 2002. 978-0-7808-0322-0.

"Recommended for libraries with an interest in offering consumer health information."
—*E-Streams, Jul '02*

"This is a unique and valuable resource for patients facing transplantation and their families."
—*Doody's Review Service, Jun '02*

Traveler's Health Sourcebook

Basic Consumer Health Information for Travelers, Including Physical and Medical Preparations, Transportation Health and Safety, Essential Information about Food and Water, Sun Exposure, Insect and Snake Bites, Camping and Wilderness Medicine, and Travel with Physical or Medical Disabilities

Along with International Travel Tips, Vaccination Recommendations, Geographical Health Issues, Disease Risks, a Glossary, and a Listing of Additional Resources

Edited by Joyce Brennfleck Shannon. 619 pages. 2000. 978-0-7808-0384-8.

"Recommended reference source."
—*Booklist, Feb '01*

"This book is recommended for any public library, any travel collection, and especially any collection for the physically disabled."
—*American Reference Books Annual, 2001*

SEE ALSO *Worldwide Health Sourcebook*

Urinary Tract and Kidney Diseases and Disorders Sourcebook, 2nd Edition

Basic Consumer Health Information about the Urinary System, Including the Bladder, Urethra, Ureters, and Kidneys, with Facts about Urinary Tract Infections, Incontinence, Congenital Disorders, Kidney Stones, Cancers of the Urinary Tract and Kidneys, Kidney Failure, Dialysis, and Kidney Transplantation

Along with Statistical and Demographic Information, Reports on Current Research in Kidney and Urologic Health, a Summary of Commonly Used Diagnostic Tests, a Glossary of Related Terms, and a Directory of Resources for Additional Help and Information

Edited by Ivy L. Alexander. 621 pages. 2005. 978-0-7808-0750-1.

"A good choice for a consumer health information library or for a medical library needing information to refer to their patients."
—*American Reference Books Annual, 2006*

SEE ALSO *Prostate and Urological Disorders Sourcebook*

Vegetarian Sourcebook

Basic Consumer Health Information about Vegetarian Diets, Lifestyle, and Philosophy, Including Definitions of Vegetarianism and Veganism, Tips about Adopting Vegetarianism, Creating a Vegetarian Pantry, and Meeting Nutritional Needs of Vegetarians, with Facts Regarding Vegetarianism's Effect on Pregnant and Lactating Women, Children, Athletes, and Senior Citizens

Along with a Glossary of Commonly Used Vegetarian Terms and Resources for Additional Help and Information

Edited by Chad T. Kimball. 337 pages. 2002. 978-0-7808-0439-5.

"Organizes into one concise volume the answers to the most common questions concerning vegetarian diets and lifestyles. This title is

609

recommended for public and secondary school libraries."

—*E-Streams, Apr '03*

"Invaluable reference for public and school library collections alike."
—*Library Bookwatch, Apr '03*

"The articles in this volume are easy to read and come from authoritative sources. The book does not necessarily support the vegetarian diet but instead provides the pros and cons of this important decision... Recommended for public libraries and consumer health libraries."
—*American Reference Books Annual, 2003*

SEE ALSO *Diet and Nutrition Sourcebook, 3rd Edition*

Women's Health Concerns Sourcebook, 3rd Edition

Basic Consumer Health Information about Issues and Trends in Women's Health and Health Conditions of Special Concern to Women, Including Endometriosis, Uterine Fibroids, Menstrual Irregularities, Menopause, Sexual Dysfunction, Infertility, Cancer in Women, and Other Such Chronic Disorders as Lupus, Fibromyalgia, and Thyroid Disease

Along with Statistical Data, Tips for Maintaining Wellness, a Glossary, and a Directory of Resources for Further Help and Information

Edited by Sandra J. Judd. 679 pages. 2009. 978-0-7808-1036-5.

"This useful resource provides information about a wide range of topics that will help women understand their bodies, prevent or treat disease, and maintain health... A detailed index helps readers locate information. This is a useful addition to public and consumer health library collections"
—*ARBAOnline, Jun '09*

SEE ALSO *Breast Cancer Sourcebook, 3rd Edition, Cancer Sourcebook for Women, 4th Edition, Healthy Heart Sourcebook for Women*

Workplace Health and Safety Sourcebook

Basic Consumer Health Information about Workplace Health and Safety, Including the Effect of Workplace Hazards on the Lungs,

Skin, Heart, Ears, Eyes, Brain, Reproductive Organs, Musculoskeletal System, and Other Organs and Body Parts

Along with Information about Occupational Cancer, Personal Protective Equipment, Toxic and Hazardous Chemicals, Child Labor, Stress, and Workplace Violence

Edited by Chad T. Kimball. 610 pages. 2000. 978-0-7808-0231-5.

"As a reference for the general public, this would be useful in any library."
—*E-Streams, Jun '01*

"Provides helpful information for primary care physicians and other caregivers interested in occupational medicine... General readers; professionals."
—*CHOICE, May '01*

Worldwide Health Sourcebook

Basic Information about Global Health Issues, Including Malnutrition, Reproductive Health, Disease Dispersion and Prevention, Emerging Diseases, Risky Health Behaviors, and the Leading Causes of Death

Along with Global Health Concerns for Children, Women, and the Elderly, Mental Health Issues, Research and Technology Advancements, and Economic, Environmental, and Political Health Implications, a Glossary, and a Resource Listing for Additional Help and Information

Edited by Joyce Brennfleck Shannon. 597 pages. 2001. 978-0-7808-0330-5.

"Named an Outstanding Academic Title."
—*CHOICE, Jan '02*

"Yet another handy but also unique compilation in the extensive Health Reference Series, this is a useful work because many of the international publications reprinted or excerpted are not readily available. Highly recommended."
—*CHOICE, Nov '01*

SEE ALSO *Traveler's Health Sourcebook*

Teen Health Series
Complete Catalog
List price $69 per volume. School and library price $62 per volume.

Abuse and Violence Information for Teens
Health Tips about the Causes and Consequences of Abusive and Violent Behavior
Including Facts about the Types of Abuse and Violence, the Warning Signs of Abusive and Violent Behavior, Health Concerns of Victims, and Getting Help and Staying Safe

Edited by Sandra Augustyn Lawton. 411 pages. 2008. 978-0-7808-1008-2.

"A useful resource for schools and organizations providing services to teens and may also be a starting point in research projects."
—*Reference and Research Book News, Aug '08*

"Violence is a serious problem for teens... This resource gives teens the information they need to face potential threats and get help—either for themselves or for their friends."
—*American Reference Books Annual, 2009*

Accident and Safety Information for Teens
Health Tips about Medical Emergencies, Traumatic Injuries, and Disaster Preparedness
Including Facts about Motor Vehicle Accidents, Burns, Poisoning, Firearms, Natural Disasters, National Security Threats, and More

Edited by Karen Bellenir. 420 pages. 2008. 978-0-7808-1046-4.

"Aimed at teenage audiences, this guide provides practical information for handling a comprehensive list of emergencies, from sport injuries and auto accidents to alcohol poisoning and natural disasters."
—*Library Journal, Apr 1, '09*

"Useful in the young adult collections of public libraries as well as high school libraries."
—*American Reference Books Annual, 2009*

SEE ALSO *Sports Injuries Information for Teens, 2nd Edition*

Alcohol Information for Teens, 2nd Edition
Health Tips about Alcohol and Alcoholism
Including Facts about Alcohol's Effects on the Body, Brain, and Behavior, the Consequences of Underage Drinking, Alcohol Abuse Prevention and Treatment, and Coping with Alcoholic Parents

Edited by Lisa Bakewell. 410 pages. 2009. 978-0-7808-1043-3.

"This handbook, written for a teenage audience, provides information on the causes, effects, and preventive measures related to alcohol abuse among teens... The chapters are quick to make a connection to their teenage reading audience. The prose is straightforward and the book lends itself to spot reading. It should be useful both for practical information and for research, and it is suitable for public and school libraries."
—*ARBAOnline, Jun '09*

SEE ALSO *Drug Information for Teens, 2nd Edition*

Allergy Information for Teens
Health Tips about Allergic Reactions Such as Anaphylaxis, Respiratory Problems, and Rashes
Including Facts about Identifying and Managing Allergies to Food, Pollen, Mold, Animals, Chemicals, Drugs, and Other Substances

Edited by Karen Bellenir. 410 pages. 2006. 978-0-7808-0799-0.

"This is a comprehensive, readable text on the subject of allergic diseases in teenagers. 5 Stars (out of 5)!"
—*Doody's Review Service, Jun '06*

"This authoritative and useful self-help title is a solid addition to YA collections, whether for personal interest or reports."
—*School Library Journal, Jul '06*

Asthma Information for Teens, 2nd Ed.
Health Tips about Managing Asthma and Related Concerns

Including Facts about Asthma Causes, Triggers and Symptoms, Diagnosis, and Treatment

Edited by Kim Wohlenhaus. 400 pages. 2010. 978-0-7808-1086-0.

Body Information for Teens
Health Tips about Maintaining Well-Being for a Lifetime
Including Facts about the Development and Functioning of the Body's Systems, Organs, and Structures and the Health Impact of Lifestyle Choices

Edited by Sandra Augustyn Lawton. 458 pages. 2007. 978-0-7808-0443-2.

Cancer Information for Teens, 2nd Edition
Health Tips about Cancer Awareness, Symptoms, Prevention, Diagnosis, and Treatment
Including Facts about Common Cancers Affecting Teens, Causes, Detection, Coping Strategies, Clinical Trials, Nutrition and Exercise, Cancer in Friends or Family, and More

Edited by Karen Bellenir and Lisa Bakewell. 445 pages. 2010. 978-0-7808-1085-3.

Complementary and Alternative Medicine Information for Teens
Health Tips about Non-Traditional and Non-Western Medical Practices
Including Information about Acupuncture, Chiropractic Medicine, Dietary and Herbal Supplements, Hypnosis, Massage Therapy, Prayer and Spirituality, Reflexology, Yoga, and More

Edited by Sandra Augustyn Lawton. 407 pages. 2007. 978-0-7808-0966-6.

"This volume covers CAM specifically for teenagers but of general use also. It should be a welcome addition to both public and academic libraries."
—*American Reference Books Annual, 2008*

"This volume provides a solid foundation for further investigation of the subject, making it useful for both public and high school libraries."
—*VOYA: Voice of Youth Advocates, Jun '07*

Diabetes Information for Teens
Health Tips about Managing Diabetes and Preventing Related Complications
Including Information about Insulin, Glucose Control, Healthy Eating, Physical Activity, and Learning to Live with Diabetes

Edited by Sandra Augustyn Lawton. 410 pages. 2006. 978-0-7808-0811-9.

"A comprehensive instructional guide for teens... some of the material may also be directed towards parents or teachers. 5 stars (out of 5)!"
—*Doody's Review Service, 2006*

"Students dealing with their own diabetes or that of a friend or family member or those writing reports on the topic will find this a valuable resource."
—*School Library Journal, Aug '06*

"This text is directed to the teen population and would be an excellent library resource for a health class or for the teacher as a reference for class preparation. It can, however, serve a much wider audience. The clinical educator on diabetes may find it valuable to educate the newly diagnosed client regardless of age. It also would be an excellent reference and education tool for a preventive medicine seminar on diabetes."
—*Physical Therapy, Mar '07*

Diet Information for Teens, 2nd Edition
Health Tips about Diet and Nutrition
Including Facts about Dietary Guidelines, Food Groups, Nutrients, Healthy Meals, Snacks, Weight Control, Medical Concerns Related to Diet, and More

Edited by Karen Bellenir. 432 pages. 2006. 978-0-7808-0820-1.

"A very quick and pleasant read in spite of the fact that it is very detailed in the information it gives... A book for anyone concerned about diet and nutrition."
—*American Reference Books Annual, 2007*

SEE ALSO *Eating Disorders Information for Teens, 2nd Edition*

Drug Information for Teens, 2nd Edition

Health Tips about the Physical and Mental Effects of Substance Abuse

Including Information about Marijuana, Inhalants, Club Drugs, Stimulants, Hallucinogens, Opiates, Prescription and Over-the-Counter Drugs, Herbal Products, Tobacco, Alcohol, and More

Edited by Sandra Augustyn Lawton. 468 pages. 2006. 978-0-7808-0862-1.

"As with earlier installments in Omnigraphics' Teen Health Series, Drug Information for Teens is designed specifically to meet the needs and interests of middle and high school students... Strongly recommended for both academic and public libraries."
—*American Reference Books Annual, 2007*

"Solid thoughtful advice is given about how to handle peer pressure, drug-related health concerns, and treatment strategies."
—*School Library Journal, Dec '06*

SEE ALSO *Alcohol Information for Teens, 2nd Edition, Tobacco Information for Teens, 2nd Edition*

Eating Disorders Information for Teens, 2nd Edition

Health Tips about Anorexia, Bulimia, Binge Eating, And Other Eating Disorders

Including Information about Risk Factors, Diagnosis and Treatment, Prevention, Related Health Concerns, and Other Issues

Edited by Sandra Augustyn Lawton. 377 pages. 2009. 978-0-7808-1044-0.

"This handy reference offers basic information and addresses specific disorders, consequences, prevention, diagnosis and treatment, healthy eating, and more. It is written in a conversational style that is easy to understand... Will provide plenty of facts for reports as well as browsing potential for students with an interest in the topic."
—*School Library Journal, Jun '09*

"Written in a straightforward style that will appeal to its teenage audience. The author does not play down the danger of living with an eating disorder and urges those struggling with this problem to seek professional help.

This work, as well as others in this series, will be a welcome addition to high school and undergraduate libraries."
—*American Reference Books Annual, 2009*

SEE ALSO *Diet Information for Teens, 2nd Edition*

Fitness Information for Teens, 2nd Edition

Health Tips about Exercise, Physical Well-Being, and Health Maintenance

Including Facts about Conditioning, Stretching, Strength Training, Body Shape and Body Image, Sports Nutrition, and Specific Activities for Athletes and Non-Athletes

Edited by Lisa Bakewell. 432 pages. 2009. 978-0-7808-1045-7.

"This no-nonsense guide packs a great deal into its pages... This is a helpful reference for basic diet and exercise information for health reports or personal use."
—*School Library Journal, April 2009*

"An excellent source for general information on why teens should be active, making time to exercise, the equipment people might need, various types of activities to try, how to maintain health and wellness, and how to avoid barriers to becoming healthier... This would still be an excellent addition to a public library ready-reference collection or a high school health library collection."
—*American Reference Books Annual, 2009*

"This easy to read, well-written, up-to-date overview of fitness for teenagers provides excellent wellness and exercise tips, information, and directions... It is a useful tool for them to obtain a base knowledge in fitness topics and different sports."
—*Doody's Review Service, 2009*

SEE ALSO *Diet Information for Teens, 2nd Edition, Sports Injuries Information for Teens, 2nd Edition*

Learning Disabilities Information for Teens

Health Tips about Academic Skills Disorders and Other Disabilities That Affect Learning

Including Information about Common Signs of Learning Disabilities, School Issues, Learning to Live with a Learning Disability, and Other Related Issues

Edited by Sandra Augustyn Lawton. 400 pages. 2006. 978-0-7808-0796-9.

"This book provides a wealth of information for any reader interested in the signs, causes, and consequences of learning disabilities, as well as related legal rights and educational interventions... Public and academic libraries should want this title for both students and general readers."
—*American Reference Books Annual, 2006*

Mental Health Information for Teens, 3rd Edition
Health Tips about Mental Wellness and Mental Illness
Including Facts about Mental and Emotional Health, Depression and Other Mood Disorders, Anxiety Disorders, Behavior Disorders, Self-Injury, Psychosis, Schizophrenia, and More

Edited by Karen Bellenir. 400 pages. 2010. 978-0-7808-1087-7.

SEE ALSO *Stress Information for Teens, Suicide Information for Teens, 2nd Edition*

Pregnancy Information for Teens
Health Tips about Teen Pregnancy and Teen Parenting
Including Facts about Prenatal Care, Pregnancy Complications, Labor and Delivery, Postpartum Care, Pregnancy-Related Lifestyle Concerns, and More

Edited by Sandra Augustyn Lawton. 434 pages. 2007. 978-0-7808-0984-0.

Sexual Health Information for Teens, 2nd Edition
Health Tips about Sexual Development, Reproduction, Contraception, and Sexually Transmitted Infections
Including Facts about Puberty, Sexuality, Birth Control, Chlamydia, Gonorrhea, Herpes, Human Papillomavirus, Syphilis, and More

Edited by Sandra Augustyn Lawton. 430 pages. 2008. 978-0-7808-1010-5.

"This offering represents the most up-to-date information available on an array of topics including abstinence-only sexual education and pregnancy-prevention methods... The range of coverage—from puberty and anatomy to sexually transmitted diseases—is thorough and extensive. Each chapter includes a bibliographic citation, and the three back sections containing additional resources, further reading, and the index are all first-rate... This volume will be well used by students in need of the facts, whether for educational or personal reasons."
—*School Library Journal, Nov '08*

"Presents information related to the emotional, physical, and biological development of both males and females that occurs during puberty. It also strives to address some of the issues and questions that may arise... The text is easy to read and understand for young readers, with satisfactory definitions within the text to explain new terms."
—*American Reference Books Annual, 2009*

Skin Health Information for Teens, 2nd Edition
Health Tips about Dermatological Concerns and Skin Cancer Risks
Including Facts about Acne, Warts, Hives, and Other Conditions and Lifestyle Choices, Such as Tanning, Tattooing, and Piercing, That Affect the Skin, Nails, Scalp, and Hair

Edited by Edited by Kim Wohlenhaus. 418 pages. 2009. 978-0-7808-1042-6.

"The material in this work will be easily understood by teenagers and young adults. The publisher has liberally used bulleted lists and sidebars to keep the reader's attention... A useful addition to school and public library collections."
—*ARBAOnline, Oct '09*

Sleep Information for Teens
Health Tips about Adolescent Sleep Requirements, Sleep Disorders, and the Effects of Sleep Deprivation
Including Facts about Why People Need Sleep, Sleep Patterns, Circadian Rhythms, Dreaming, Insomnia, Sleep Apnea, Narcolepsy, and More

Edited by Karen Bellenir. 355 pages. 2008. 978-0-7808-1009-9.

"Clear, concise, and very readable and would be a good source of sleep information for anyone—not just teenagers. This work is highly recommended for medical libraries, public school libraries, and public libraries."
—*American Reference Books Annual, 2009*

SEE ALSO *Body Information for Teens*

Sports Injuries Information for Teens, 2nd Edition
Health Tips about Acute, Traumatic, and Chronic Injuries in Adolescent Athletes
Including Facts about Sprains, Fractures, and Overuse Injuries, Treatment, Rehabilitation, Sport-Specific Safety Guidelines, Fitness Suggestions, and More

Edited by Karen Bellenir. 429 pages. 2008. 978-0-7808-1011-2.

"An engaging selection of informative articles about the prevention and treatment of sports injuries... The value of this book is that the articles have been vetted and are often augmented with inserts of useful facts, definitions of technical terms, and quick tips. Sensitive topics like injuries to genitalia are discussed openly and responsibly. This revised edition contains updated articles and defines sport more broadly than the first edition."
—*School Library Journal, Nov '08*

"This work will be useful in the young adult collections of public libraries as well as high school libraries... A useful resource for student research."
—*American Reference Books Annual, 2009*

SEE ALSO *Accident and Safety Information for Teens*

Stress Information for Teens
Health Tips about the Mental and Physical Consequences of Stress
Including Information about the Different Kinds of Stress, Symptoms of Stress, Frequent Causes of Stress, Stress Management Techniques, and More

Edited by Sandra Augustyn Lawton. 392 pages. 2008. 978-0-7808-1012-9.

"Understanding what stress is, what causes it, how the body and the mind are impacted by it, and what teens can do are the general categories addressed here... The chapters are brief but informative, and the list of community-help organizations is exhaustive. Report writers will find information quickly and easily, as will those who have personal concerns. The print is clear and the format is readable, making this an accessible resource for struggling readers and researchers."
—*School Library Journal, Dec '08*

"The articles selected will specifically appeal to young adults and are designed to answer their most common questions."
— *American Reference Books Annual, 2009*

SEE ALSO *Mental Health Information for Teens, 3rd Edition*

Suicide Information for Teens, 2nd Edition
Health Tips about Suicide Causes and Prevention
Including Facts about Depression, Risk Factors, Getting Help, Survivor Support, and More

Edited by Kim Wohlenhaus. 400 pages. 2010. 978-0-7808-1088-4.

SEE ALSO *Mental Health Information for Teens, 3rd Edition*

Tobacco Information for Teens, 2nd Edition
Health Tips about the Hazards of Using Cigarettes, Smokeless Tobacco, and Other Nicotine Products
Including Facts about Nicotine Addiction, Nicotine Delivery Systems, Secondhand Smoke, Health Consequences of Tobacco Use, Related Cancers, Smoking Cessation, and Tobacco Use Statistics

Edited by Karen Bellenir. 400 pages. 2010. 978-0-7808-1153-9.

SEE ALSO *Drug Information for Teens, 2nd Edition*